BODY MECHANICS
in
HEALTH and DISEASE

Joel E. Goldthwait M.D., F.A.C.S., LL.D., SC.D.
Lloyd T. Brown M.D., F.A.C.S.
Loring T. Swaim M.D.
John G. Kuhns M.D., F.A.C.S., SC.D.

Pioneers of Manual Therapy Volume III

MWI Publishing

Published in the USA and UK
by
MASTERWORKS INTERNATIONAL
27 Old Gloucester Street
London
WC1N 3XX

Email: admin@mwipublishing.com
Web: http://www.mwipublishing.com

ISBN: 978-0-9933465-1-4

Copyright © 1934, 1937, 1941, 1945, 1952 & 2016 Masterworks International Publishing

This edition is a composite of the 1945 and 1952 editions.

All rights reserved.

No part of this book or other material may be reproduced in any form without written permission of the publishers.

Cover by MWI Design
Front Cover Graphics: Human Bones Radiography Scans Images©Videodoctor - Dreamstime.com

This book is an historic document and is intended for use by health care professionals and should not be regarded as a guide to self-diagnosis or treatment.

Contents

PREFACE TO THE FIFTH AND FIRST EDITION

1.THE PROBLEM OF CHRONIC ILLNESS	12
Relation of Recovery to Treatment	12
2 .BODY TYPES	16
The Intermediate Type.	16
Slender and Stocky Types.	18
The Slender Type	19
The Stocky Type	24
Differentiation of Types	26
Postural Differences	27
Differences in Physiologic Processes	28
Susceptibility to Disease	30
Anatomic and Functional Features	30
3.BODY MECHANICS	32
General Considerations	32
The Bones	35
The Spine	39
The Chest	46
The Diaphragm	49
The Abdominal Viscera	53
4.DEVELOPMENTAL DEFORMITIES.	58
The Head	58
The Thorax	60
The Spine	62
The Extremities	66

5.BACKACHE AND OTHER SPINAL SPRAINS.   68

Backache   68
Other Spinal Sprains   74
Operative Treatment of Backache   79
Lesions of the Intervertebral Disks   82

6.THE CIRCULATORY SYSTEM   84

The Heart and the Diaphragm   85
The Vascular System   91

7. ANGINA PECTORIS and POSTURAL EMPHYSEMA RELATED TO OBESITY   98

Causative Factors   98
Kerr-Lagen Belt   103
Angina Pectoris   104

8.DISEASES OF THE ABDOMINAL VISCERA   106

Position of the Organs and the Vessels   106
The Diaphragm   108
The Liver   109
The Pancreas   110
Case Reports   111
The Spleen   115
The Stomach   115
The Duodenum   123
The Small Intestine   123
The Cecum   125
The Kidneys   126
The Pelvis   126
Conclusions   128

9.DISEASES OF THE NERVOUS SYSTEM   130

Changes in Structure   130
Circulatory Disturbance   131
Venous Drainage   132
Divisions of the Nervous System   134
Vegetative Nervous System   134
Sympathetic Nervous System   135
Illustrative Cases   142

10. CHRONIC ARTHRITIS — 148
Causes — 148
The Adrenal Cortex and Arthritis — 150
Treatment — 150
Atrophic (Rheumatoid, Proliferative) Arthritis — 150
Hypertrophic Arthritis — 158
Illustrative Cases — 159

11. TREATMENT — 172
General Considerations — 172
Supports and Braces — 178
Muscle Re-education — 181
Exercises — 188
Lying on the Back — 188
Arm, Neck and Shoulder — 191
Sitting — 192
Standing — 192

12. THE FOOT AND BODY MECHANICS — 196
Introduction — 196
Development and Anatomy — 196
Types of Disabilities — 199
Symptoms and Signs of Disability — 202
Treatment — 204
Exercises — 205
Supports and Operative Treatment — 207

13. PUBLIC HEALTH ASPECTS OF BODY MECHANICS — 210

14. GERIATRICS AND BODY MECHANICS — 220
Introduction — 220
Changes in the Aging Body — 220
General Management — 221
Circulatory Disturbances — 221
Tumors — 222
Gastro-intestinal Disturbances — 222
Diabetes — 222
Lung Diseases — 223

Nervous Diseases	224
Mental Disease	226
Arthritis	226
Myositis (Fibrositis)	227
Bursitis	227
Skeletal Disturbances	227
Summary	229
INDEX	

The Authors

Joel E. Goldthwait, M.D., F.A.C.S., LL.D.

member, Board of Consultants, Massachusetts General Hospital; Ex-President, American Orthopedic Association; Organizer and First Chief, Orthopedic Service, Massachusetts General Hospital; Member, American Academy of Orthopedic Surgery; Member, British Orthopedic Association.

Lloyd T.Brown, M.D. F.A.C.S.

President, Robert B. Brigham Hospital; Member, American Orthopedic Association, Member, American Academy of Orthopedic Surgery, Member, Board of Orthopedic Surgery; Instructor in Orthopedics, Harvard Medical School.

Loring T. Swaim M.D.

Secretary, American Rheumatism Association; Member, American Orthopedic Association; Member American Academy of Orthopedic Surgery; Instructor, Orthopedic Surgery, Harvard Medical School; Chief Orthopedic Consultant, Robert B. Brigham Hospital.

John G. Kuhns, M.D., F.A.C.S.

Member, American Orthopedic Association; Member Academy of orthopedic Surgery,; Assistant in Orthopedic Surgery, Harvard Medical School; Chief of Orthopedic Staff, Robert B. Brigham Hospital.

William J. Kerr, M.D., F.A.C.P.

Professor of Medicine, University of California Medical School; Physician in Chief, University of California Hospital; Member, American Board of Internal medicine; formerly President, American Heart Association, American Rheumatism Association, and American College of Physicians.

Preface to the Fifth Edition

Since the publication of the latest edition of this book, World War II with its aftermath of crippling injuries and consequent disability has given impetus to the study and the application of mechanical principles in medical treatment. Great advances have been made in physiotherapeutic technics and in plans for the improvement of those with severe disability. While these procedures have proved to be useful and worthwhile, for the most part they have failed to improve or correct the alignment and the proper working of the whole body. A number of new antibiotics have been found, and new and more potent hormones have been synthesized or discovered. Some of these agents have prevented disease or have made easier the treatment of certain acute or chronic diseases. However, they have not added to the endurance or stamina of the individual whose resistance would be puny indeed without their constant availability. The widespread use of these medicinal substances has served to bring into greater prominence the need for the understanding and the treatment which will lead to lasting improvement of the health of the individual and a better response to the demands of the environment. A steadily increasing segment of older individuals in our population presents to the medical profession a great challenge to maintain the physical fitness and the usefulness of these persons who are more advanced in years. While the problems which command our attention in medicine vary in each decade, the mechanical principles which govern the well-being of the body remain unchanged. We have endeavoured to present these mechanical principles as simply and lucidly as possible in this edition. These principles of body mechanics have proved to be of value in the treatment of many varied conditions. Wee encouraged by the continued demand for this book which has required this revision.

The Authors

Preface to the First Edition

With the increasing number of persons afflicted with the chronic diseases, the problem of treatment is becoming more and more difficult for the medical profession, and the results of the diseases causing such conditions are presenting an ever increasing economic problem both to the patient and the community. For the understanding and relief of these conditions, it is hoped that this publication may suggest new lines of study and treatment, which will prove as helpful to the general practitioner as they have to the authors.

Acute medicine in the past generation has made great advances, but with chronic medicine relatively little actual advance has been made as far as the general understanding of the disease is concerned. It is perfectly true that with many of the chronic disease today some of the symptoms, such as the control of the results of imperfect sugar metabolism of the body by the use of insulin or diet, have been relieved, but the actual disease behind the difficulty is little better understood than it was a generation ago. The same thing is true with reference to the so-called pernicious anemia; in which condition, with special diets, varying degrees of relief are brought about but actually the knowledge of the disease itself has changed but little.

In the latter part of the Nineteenth Century, typhoid fever, diphtheria, and scarlet fever were the most common of the so called acute diseases, and they required much time for their treatment and for their convalescence. Practically all wounds were infected, and long treatment was necessary to bring about healing from operations or injuries. Obviously, the treatment that was required for such "acute" cases trained the physician to think in terms of long-time healing, with long-time recovery, and prepared him to handle the problems of the chronic patient. Today it is expected that rapid relief of the medical symptoms will occur, as well as rapid healing of the wounds. There has developed a distinct rivalry in the hospitals looking toward the shortest possible number of days for a patient to recover from acute disease or from operation. The result is that physicians are interested almost entirely in the acute part of both disease and healing, and have very little understanding of the basic principles of health upon which recovery in long-time disease is to be brought about.

No one who has studied the work of the various hospital clinics can fail to be impressed with the relatively small number of patients suffering from chronic disease who are accepted for treatment or are receiving benefit from the treatment given. When one realizes that the majority of such patients are seeking treatment for what, basically, are chronic conditions for which little interest or knowledge is held by the average practitioner, it is not surprising that so many seek relief at the hands of irregular practitioners.

That the profession has too little real interest in chronic medicine is obvious not only from the present-day organization at our hospitals, but in the study of the textbooks of medicine or surgery as they exist today. The small amount of space allotted to this branch of our work means lack of interest, or lack of knowledge of the diseases, or -of the lines of investigation to obtain such knowledge.

In the studies that are made of the chronic patient in the majority of our clinics today, we should consider most seriously that unless something is done other than to report the negative findings, the patients are harmed rather than helped by the usual hopeless or indifferent prognoses given. No one can have had much to do with chronic patients without being conscious of this fact. Such patients commonly have had the most elaborate tests for chemical or bacterial disturbances, with the result that most of the tests have been practically negative and the condition is, therefore, considered functional. The many sheets of the most carefully prepared papers showing the latest kidney or heart tests, the various blood tests, the basal metabolism, the intestinal contents, the visceral roentgenology, etc., etc., which the patients so frequently thrust into our presence as a challenge, must either go further in the interpretation of the findings, or most of the work must be considered purposeless. In studying many such records, that which has led to the greatest surprise is the lack of consideration of the anatomic structure or the general appearance of the patient. One of the basic principles in the study or teaching of medicine, theoretically, has always been proper foundation in anatomy, but with very few exceptions, this is still being taught on the basis of one human type to which all must conform. It should cause little surprise that the advance has been so slight in the knowledge or treatment of chronic disease when the great variations from this textbook normal are appreciated, and when, in so far as our experience is concerned, practically none of the cases of chronic disease are of this so-called normal structure. Sufficient studies have been made to take this variation in type out of the position of speculation, but in no textbook, in so far as we know, is it mentioned, nor is anatomy taught with reference to it.

Still further, the function or physiology of the body is also supposed to be of basic importance; nevertheless, rarely is any attention given to the probable difference in the physiology of the widely different anatomic structures. An intestine, for instance, of ten feet in length should hardly be expected to function similarly to one of thirty-five feet. Similar questions should occur with the differences in the other organs. Not only is little attention paid to such differences in structure but practically no consideration is given to what should happen to the function of the various organs when the easily demonstrable malposition of them is considered. With an automobile the proper running of the engine depends upon the right mixture. Too rich a mixture, the engine stalls; too thin a mixture, it stalls. Is it not possible that much of that which concerns chronic medicine has to do with the imperfect functioning of sagged or misplaced organs? Is it not possible that such sagging results in imperfect general secretions, or mixtures which at first are purely functional but which, long continued, may produce actual pathology?

It seems to us that in a better understanding of the special structure and the special physiology of the individual, and in a broader knowledge of the changing physiology that should be part of the varying mechanics of the body, the solution of the problem of chronic disease is largely to be found.

The Authors
Boston, Massachusetts

1

The Problem of Chronic Illness

An individual is in the best health only when the body is so used that there is no strain on any of its parts. This means that, when standing, the body is held fully erect, with no strain on the joints, the bones, the ligaments, the muscles or any other structures. There should be adequate room for all the viscera, so that their function can be performed normally unless there be some congenital defect.

In the beginning our study was carried on chiefly to improve the mechanics of the body so that health might be restored and so that the diseases which had resulted from the wrong use of the parts might be arrested. As the work continued it became obvious that the prevention of such conditions before disease has become evident is of the utmost importance. Therefore, emphasis must be put upon the proper training of the body so that the best possible state of health may be obtained.

Since it has become clear that there are many variations from the so-called textbook normal, or better, intermediate, body type, and since very few chronically ill patients conform to this standard, it is necessary to study each individual with reference to his special type of anatomy and then to interpret the function or the physiology to be expected under those conditions. Such an approach should be of great value in preventing the deformities commonly developed during childhood and early adult life, as well as all that concerns the development of the best general health of the individual.

RELATION OF RECOVERY TO TREATMENT

It has been shown with chronic arthritis, for example, that wherever groups of such cases were treated, a large proportion recovered irrespective of the form of treatment, but also that there was always a certain proportion of patients who were not controlled and went on to greater and greater helplessness. This was irrespective of the country or of the method of treatment. The percentage of hopeless cases was about the same, so that it very soon became obvious that with reasonably good care a generous majority recovered entirely. However, there was always that group of discouraging cases which grew worse in spite of the special methods of treatment. These represented the failures.

In the early days of our work the results of the various methods of treatment tried were no different from those obtained elsewhere. Nature, practically unaided, was able to cure the majority of the cases. However, there were a considerable number which represented failures, not only of the physician but also of Nature.

In the belief that there must be some solution to the problem, all that medical science had to offer in those days was tried, still with disappointment. Careful pathologic study of the special manifestations of the disease showed clearly the nature of the bone, the joint and the muscular condition but gave no clue to the real cause of the disease or its control. Bacteriologic study also was disappointing except that it seemed to show that only in rare cases was the disease primarily due to bacterial life. Biochemical study was also most carefully carried out for several years, with disappointing results. The findings checked with the pathologic picture, but what was behind each was still a mystery.

Varying Anatomic Features. After following the accepted lines of study of such cases without results, and with the appeal of these seemingly hopeless cases as a constant incentive, we turned to anatomy in the hope of finding something not previously recognized that would be of help. It had been noted previously that the types of disease as they were recognized commonly occurred in individuals of physical structure different from the so-called normal. Those of slender or stocky build were most common among the arthritics, and the type of build was associated so commonly with the special type of disease that it was hoped that a better knowledge of the anatomy might throw some valuable light on the subject. In this study Dr. Thomas Dwight, then Professor of Anatomy at the Harvard Medical School, was of the greatest assistance, and as the work progressed it became apparent that very few of those afflicted with these chronic diseases were of the structure described in the textbooks on anatomy.

Body Mechanics. Once the varying anatomic features were recognized, it became apparent that the position of the organs in the body was of importance for their function. This led to that which is now called body mechanics, or the mechanics of the function of all the parts of the human body: bones, joints, muscles, viscera and nerves. This naturally deals largely with the general physiology of the body. This study has shown that many of the other chronic diseases are probably part of the disturbances which at times result in arthritis or the progressive paralyses but at other times may result in diabetes, the chronic blood diseases, various skin lesions or cardiorenal diseases. With the general increase in the common chronic diseases, such as diabetes and chronic blood and cardiorenal diseases, it would seem possible that a similar study of anatomy, body mechanics and physiology in these cases might be of help.

Since this line of study has been followed the results of treatment in the arthritics and the paralytics usually have been so much better as to make it probable that the real control of these and many of the other chronic, as well as acute, diseases is to be found along -these lines. It would seem to be a matter of simple common sense to expect better health with the body so poised or balanced that all the organs are in their proper positions, and the muscles are in proper balance; whereas, with the poise such that the viscera of both the abdomen and the thorax are thrown out of place, as can be demonstrated easily with the roentgenogram, the best health hardly could be expected.

Body Sag. In the incidental study of diabetes or the cardiorenal disturbances that has been carried on by us, all cases have shown the sagged, commonly considered heavy, abdomen. With these, as well as with the arthritic cases, a large, prominent abdomen does not represent great actual increase in bulk. It represents sag, for if the patient is made to draw the chin in and the chest up and forward, the abdomen is drawn up into place, and the girth is reduced by several inches. In other words, in these cases body sag instead of overweight is commonly the chief difficulty. From the common improvement of such cases, once the faulty mechanics are corrected, it is apparent that in the beginning at least, the pathologic symptoms are not the result of actual disease or damage of the organ but are due to malposition of the organ, with resulting disturbance of its function.

Visceral Damage. It is recognized, of course, with visceral conditions, as with articular or spinal-cord conditions, that if the malposition with the malfunction be kept up long enough, permanent damage of the organ will result. Therefore, it does not seem unreasonable to expect that, if the faulty mechanics be corrected early, the visceral damage will be prevented. However, in the cases in which undoubted damage of the viscera has occurred, the correction of the faulty mechanics many times leads to compensatory adjustments that make possible fairly satisfactory health, as an arthritic becomes well for practical purposes even though a joint may be damaged.

The purpose of this book is to put before the profession those factors which have been of the greatest help to the writers in the treatment of the chronically ill patient and to indicate the lines along which a most promising study lies for the further increase of our knowledge.

Disturbances of the Special Systems. In the succeeding chapters the features indicated here are discussed in detail, and since such visceral malpositions must result in general disturbances, the effect of these is discussed, not as individual diseases, but as disturbances of the special systems: circulatory, cardiorenal, osseous, nervous, digestive, and so forth. Rarely is only one organ or tissue at fault in chronic disease. The joints may be most conspicuous, but the changes in the general skeleton, usually those of atrophy, are present also, as well as atrophy of the muscles, irregular temperature, irregularities of circulation, basal metabolic disturbances and digestive disturbances.

Once we hold this conception of the problem of chronic medicine, the study of our patient becomes interesting, with a definite line of study and treatment to carry out with the expectation of improvement and of a real cure if the treatment can be started early.

2

Body Types

As stated in the previous chapter, not all human beings are made alike, and a study of these anatomic and physiologic differences is helpful in the understanding and the treatment of disease. The recognition of structural differences is also of value in the maintenance of health and physical well-being, for differences in the organs within the body accompanying those changes in form seen externally. This leads to a somewhat different normal function and a different reaction to environment. Individuals of different body types show different susceptibility to various diseases. The pattern of the body is inherited and depends upon the body type of the ancestors. However, while the type of body cannot be changed, the manner in which it is used can be modified greatly. The health of the individual depends largely on this, as well as whether or not he will succumb to one of the diseases of which he is a potential victim. Good health is possible in all the variations from the so-called normal or intermediate body type.

THE INTERMEDIATE TYPE

In order to understand better the variations that are found among human beings, a description will be given of what is commonly called normal but is better termed intermediate. In textbooks of anatomy the torso is described as being of moderate length and breadth, with the proportion of the anteroposterior diameter to the lateral diameter at the ninth rib as The thorax is full and moderately rounded; the upper abdomen is rounded and of equal circumference with the thorax at the mammary line. The subcostal border usually forms an angle of from 70° to 90°. The diaphragm is high, and there is a generous space for the viscera below the lower ribs. All the abdominal viscera except the lower portion of the colon, the sigmoid and a small part of the small intestine are above the umbilicus. Around the viscera are well-defined masses of fat, provided for protection and support. The lower abdomen is flat, while the upper abdomen is firm and rounded, there being no marked depression below the lower border of the ribs. The ribs incline downward about 30° from the horizontal.

The spine shows a mild curve forward in the lumbar region, with the apex of the curve in the midlumbar region. This produces an inclination of the abdominal cavity downward and forward about 30° from the perpendicular. The sacrum is inclined downward and backward, also about 30° from the perpendicular. The diagonal conjugate (superior strait) of the pelvis is inclined forward and downward about 30° from the horizontal. The dorsal spine shows a slight backward curve, with the apex of the curve in the mid-dorsal region. The long axis of the thoracic cavity should be almost perpendicular, any deviation consisting of a slight forward inclination of a few degrees. There is a slight forward curve in the cervical spine.

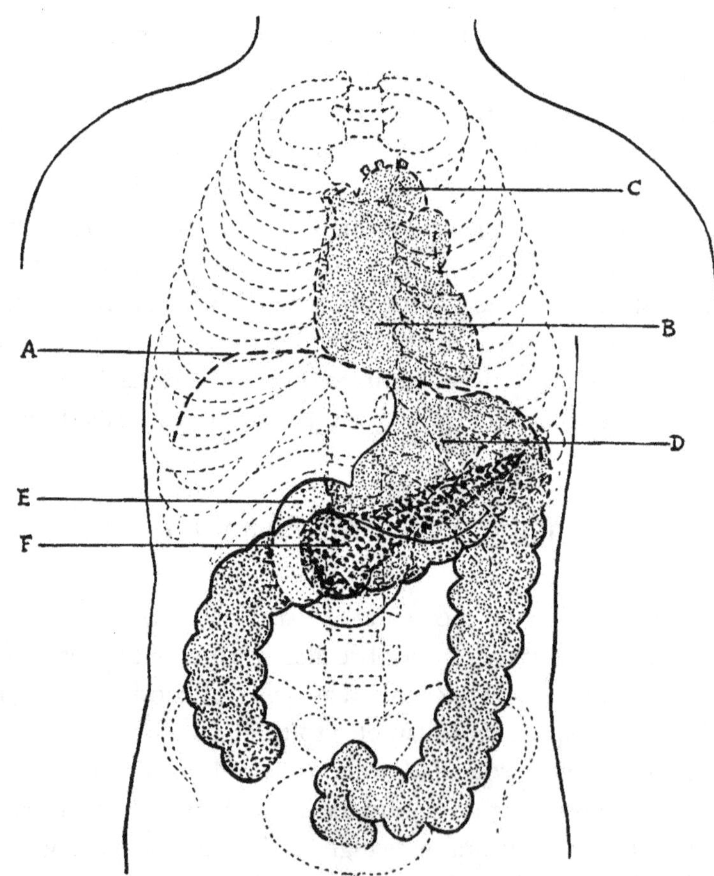

FIG. 1. Diagram of the normal type of anatomy. Note the position and the size of the various organs. The top of the diaphragm, **A**, is between the eighth and the ninth ribs posteriorly. The heart, **B**, is slightly to the left of the midportion of the chest, with the aortic arch, **C**, at the second rib. The stomach, **D**, is well up under the costal border. The duodenum, **E**, is at the level of the first lumbar vertebra where, in its second and third parts, it encircles the head of the pancreas. The pancreas, **F**, is retroperitoneal and crosses the spine at the level of the first lumbar vertebra.

The thoracic and the abdominal viscera are composed as follows: The stomach is pear-shaped and is placed under the lower ribs in such a position that little effort is required to empty its contents into the duodenum (Fig. 1). The small intestine is about 20 feet long. The large intestine, five or six feet in length, is adherent to the posterior abdominal wall on the right side until it reaches the region of the liver, where it crosses the abdomen with only a slight downward and forward sag to the splenic flexure; from this point it again is attached to the posterior abdominal wall until it reaches the sigmoid portion. The stomach and the liver are attached to the diaphragm; the latter is covered by the lower ribs and should not be felt below them. The kidneys are found in the posterior abdominal cavity, reaching at their lower margin to the upper edge of the third lumbar vertebra. They are surrounded by, and firmly embedded in, a mass of fat. The diaphragm is attached to the pericardium and the suspensory ligament on its upper surface. The suspensory ligament in turn is attached to the cervical fascia and the low-cervical spine. The heart lies in the middle mediastinum, resting on the diaphragm below; its long axis runs obliquely forward, downward and to the left. The arch of the aorta is posterior to the right margin of the sternum at the level of the second costal cartilage. While the heart changes its position and its shape with each breath, the general relationships mentioned should be maintained. Each lung lies freely in the pleural cavity. The apices lie above the level of the first costal arch and present a semi-lunar outline on the diaphragmatic surface. At expiration, the lungs reach the inferior border of the sixth rib anteriorly, the eighth rib in the axillary line and the tenth thoracic vertebra posteriorly.

SLENDER AND STOCKY TYPES

There are many individuals who differ in body type from the intermediate, but these variations are reducible to two distinct groups: slender and stocky. Such differences are seen not only in outward configuration but also in the heaviness or the lightness of the skeleton and in the shape, the position and the firmness of attachment of the internal organs. The amount of motion possible in the joints of the body, the nature of the muscular attachments and the relative size of the muscles differ greatly in slender and in stocky individuals; their temperaments and their degrees of susceptibility to various diseases are also unlike.

Various names have been given to these two types, depending on the point of view from which they are studied-phylogenetically, physiologically or psychologically. The slender type has been termed splanchnoptotic (by Glénard); congenital visceroptotic (by Goldthwait and Smith); carnivorous (by Treves, Werner and Bryant); hyperontomorph (by Bean); macroscelous (by Montessori); narrow-back (an industrial term) and linear (by Lucas). The heavy type has been called sthenic, herbivorous (by Goldthwait and Bryant); hypo-ontomorph (by Bean); brachyskelous (by Montessori); broad-backed (an industrial term) and lateral (by Lucas).

The Slender Type

The slender type differs from the intermediate in that the entire body is more slender and sparsely built (Fig.2). The individual is either small and delicate or tall and slender. The extremities, while they vary greatly in length, are usually long for the general proportions of the body. The muscles on the limbs are small in bulk, increasing the slenderness. The fingers and the toes are long and tapering; the hands are small; the feet are long and narrow and usually have a high arch. The joints of the body have loose ligamentous attachments, and their range of motion is from 15° to 30° more than is considered normal. In this type is found the scaphoid scapula described by Graves.

The skin is commonly soft and thin, with an abundant growth of hair. The head is large, and the face and the jaws are narrow. The arch of the palate is high. The torso is longer and

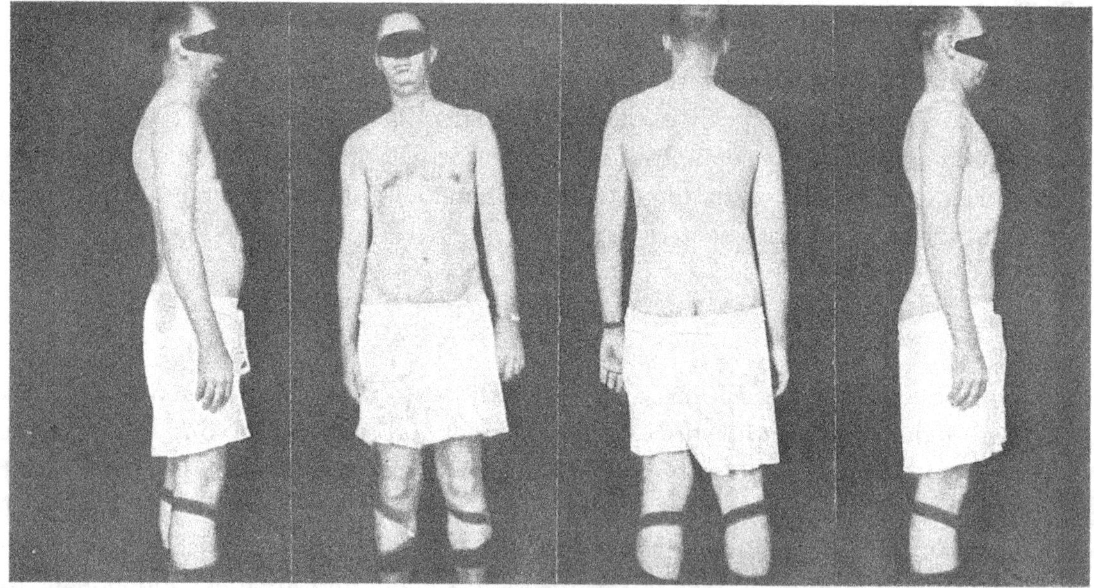

FIG. 2. The slender type. Compare with Figure 7. Note that the vertical length of the body is long in comparison with the anteroposterior depth. (Upper left) Lateral view of habitual relaxed faulty posture. (Upper right) Lateral view. Note the narrowing of the lower portion of the chest and the upper part of the abdominal cavity; the narrow subcostal angle. (Lower left) Posterior view, showing the folds in the skin in the region of the lower ribs, as well as the asymmetrical standing position which is due to faulty posture. (Lower right) The best corrected position possible for this patient. The hollow under the ribs shows that this position could have been habitual because, when the ribs are pulled up, the organs do not come with them.

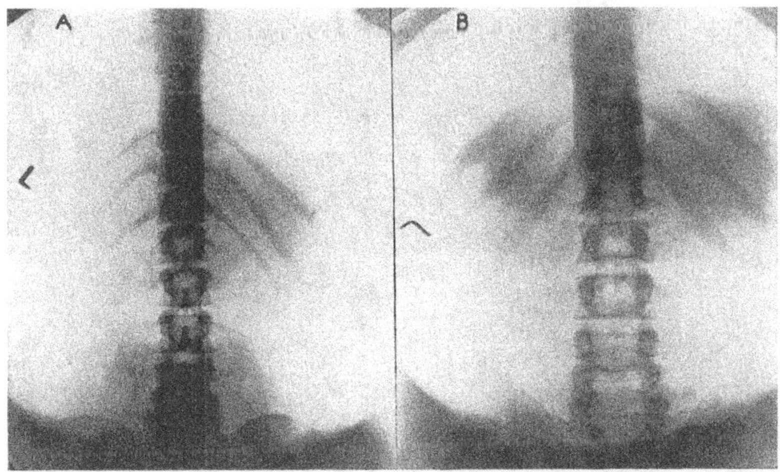

F1G. 3. Anatomic types of spine. (A) Slender type of spine. (B) Stocky type of spine. Note that the lumbar vertebrae in the slender type, A, are more nearly square, like the dorsal vertebrae; that in the stocky type, B, the width of the vertebral bodies is much greater than the height. Note the slender ribs of A as compared with the broader ones of B.

narrower than in the intermediate type. The ratio of the antero-posterior diameter of the chest to its lateral diameter is often 1:2. The subcostal angle of the chest is often less than 70°. The sternum and the costal cartilages form a flat surface instead of a convex arc anteriorly. The ribs are long and slender. The tenth rib is almost always free. The downward inclination of the ribs is greater than in the intermediate type. The articulations of the ribs with the spine commonly show a greater range of motion than is usually described.

The entire spine is lighter and more slender in form (Fig.3) The lumbar vertebrae resemble the dorsal vertebrae of the normal. The vertebral bodies in the lumbar region are of about equal depth and width. An increase in the number of vertebrae, particularly in the lumbar region, is not uncommon, with no decrease in the number of vertebrae in other parts of the spine. The transverse processes are small and slender, and the articular processes are usually flat. The anatomic modifications make for greater motion in the lumbar spine than that which is considered the normal range. It is from this type that the acrobat and the artistic dancer come.

While the thorax may be of fair size when well developed, the lungs are smaller than in the intermediate type. The heart is smaller and is in the midportion of the chest. Its long axis approaches the perpendicular when the patient is upright (Fig. 4). In the abdomen there are peculiarities in the shape and the attachment of the viscera. The stomach is long and tubular, and its attachments are longer than in the intermediate type, rendering possible its greater

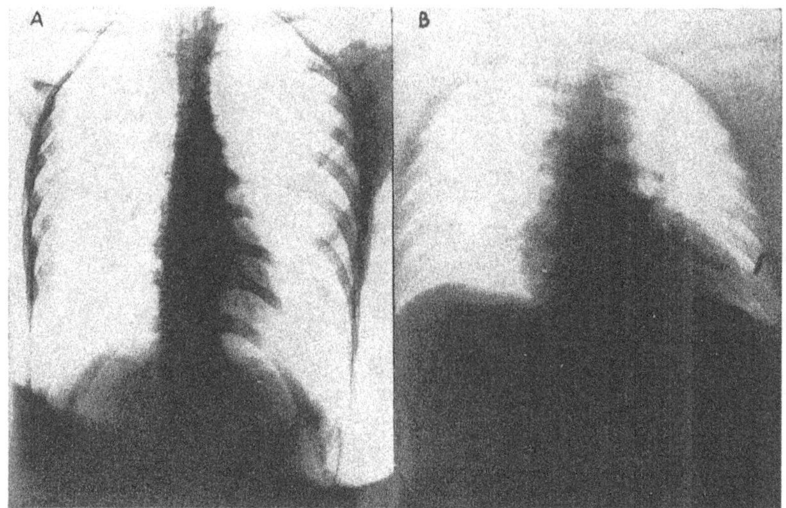

F1G. 4. Roentgenograms showing differences in size and shape of heart: (A) slender or vertical type, (B) heavy or horizontal type. Note in A, the slender type, the "droplet" or vertical type of heart associated with a very long chest cavity. The long chest cavity is always present with a low diaphragm. B shows the heavy or horizontal type of heart which is in a more nearly transverse position in the chest. In this type the chest is broader and less long, and the diaphragm is not nearly so low, and the vertical length of the chest cavity is relatively short.

downward displacement in the standing position (Fig. 5); the small intestine is shorter. According to Bean, its length varies from 12 to 15 feet; according to Bryant, from 10 to 15 feet; Swaim has found the shortest length to be 10 feet. The walls of the small intestine are thin, and its lumen is small; its mesentery is longer than in the intermediate type, permitting it to sag into the pelvic cavity on standing. The large intestine also is shorter than in the intermediate type, measuring from 3 to 5 feet. Its attachments of the large intestine are longer and permit greater mobility (Fig. 6). The entire colon may be below the iliac crests when the individual is standing. The transverse colon, while it usually is attached to the stomach, may have an entirely free mesentery. The vermiform appendix is long and well developed. Very little retroperitoneal fat is found. The kidneys often are mobile and at a lower level than in the intermediate type. The liver is small and frequently sags downward and to the right. In individuals who have poor body mechanics it is not uncommon to find in roentgenograms or at autopsy that the right lobe of the liver rests upon the right iliac crest. Differences from the so-called normal are found also in the pelvic organs of both sexes.

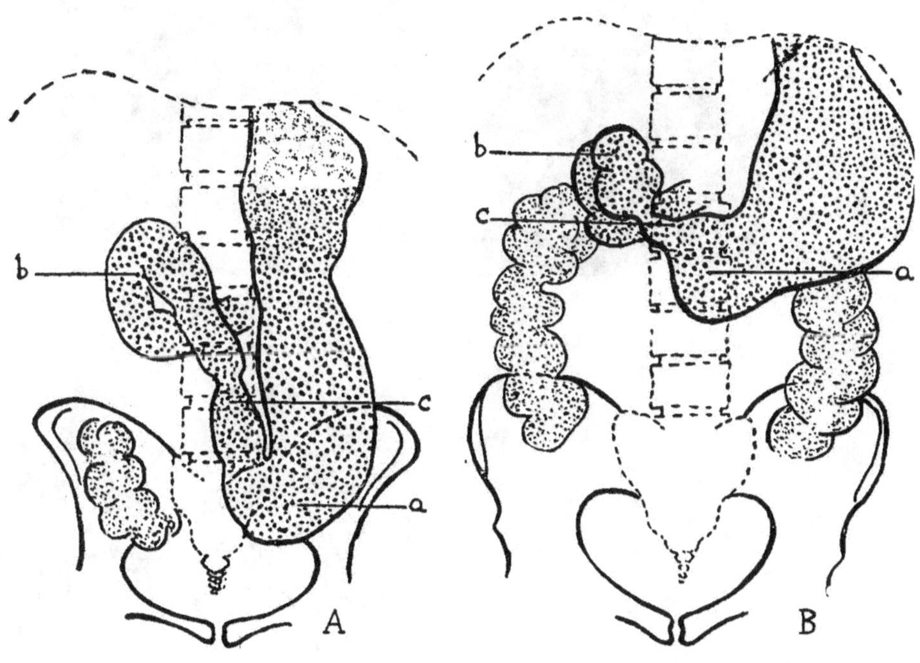

FIG. 5. (A) Diagrams of slender or fishhook type of stomach, taken in the standing position alter a barium meal. Note that the lower border of the stomach, a, is in the true pelvis; note the sharp angle between the first and the second portion of the duodenum; b, the second portion, is retroperitoneal and is adherent to the posterior abdominal wall and is at the level of the second lumbar vertebra. The first portion of the duodenum and the pyloric end of the stomach, c, are freely movable. (B) Heavy or transverse type of stomach. Compare the shape and the position with the slender type. Note that with the higher position of the stomach there may be less tendency for dragging on the second part of the duodenum. This position would suggest less mechanical difficulty in emptying the contents of the stomach.

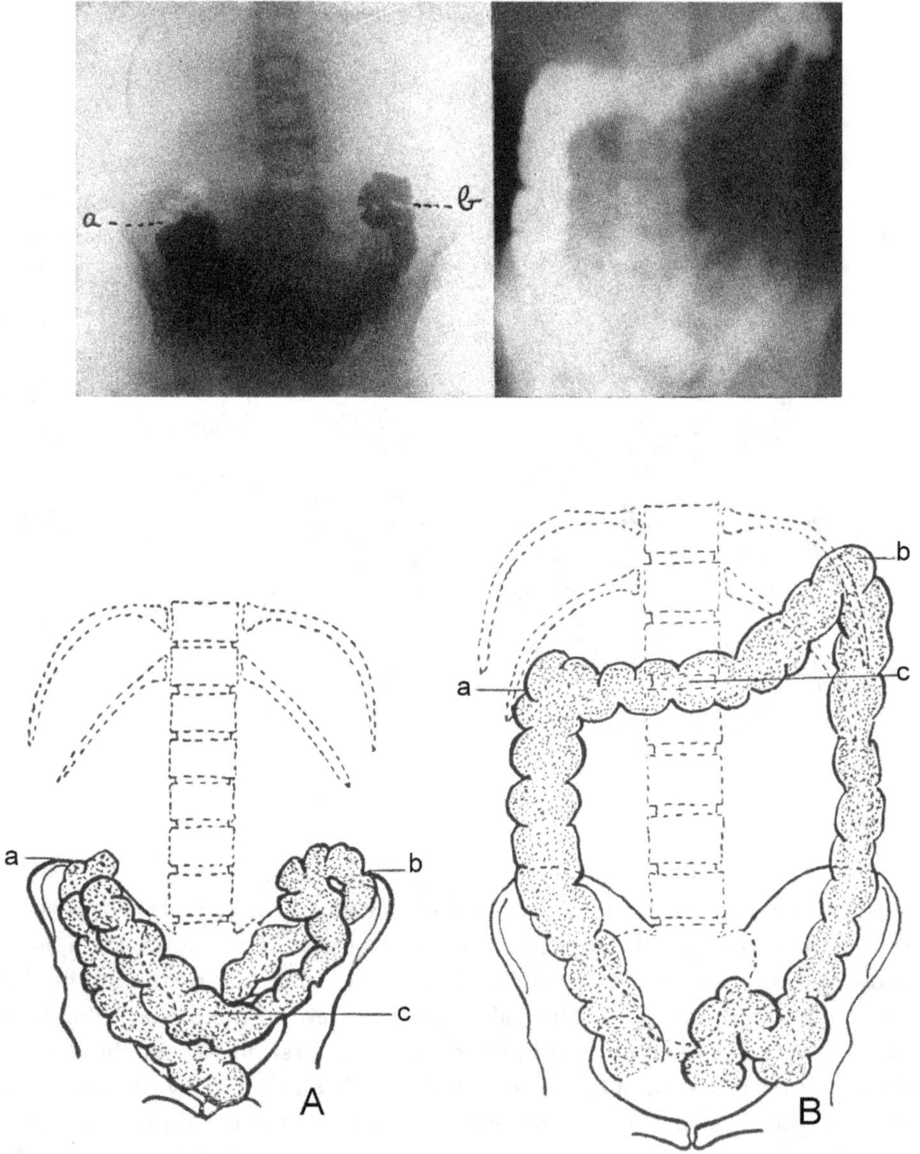

Fig.6 Roentgenograms and diagrams of the two types of large intestine after a barium enema: (A) slender, (B) stocky. Note that the hepatic flexure, a, and the splenic flexure, b, are practically in the pelvis in A. The transverse colon, c, which is in the omentum and is attached to the lower border of the stomach, also must be in the pelvis. (B) The heavy type of intestine, showing the hepatic flexor, a, and the splenic flexure, b, both under the ribs, and the transverse colon, c, as high as the lower border of the stomach.

The Stocky Type

The second deviation from the intermediate type is that represented by the stocky, heavily built individual. The general proportions show a much greater width in relation to the height. The limbs are large and heavy; the muscles are large, and their fibers are coarser (Fig. 7). The hands are broad, and the fingers are relatively short and thick. The feet are broad, and the long arch is usually low. The joints are deeply set, the articular ligaments are short, and the range of motion is often from 10° to 20° less than in the intermediate type.

As a rule, the skin is thicker, with the hair less abundant and more readily lost than in the slender type. Often there is an excess of fat throughout the body, but this is bound together with connective tissue, so that the flesh feels hard and firm. The head is usually rounded, with a broad face, a square jaw and small, closely set ears. The neck is short and thick in proportion to the body length. The ratio of the anteroposterior diameter of the chest to the transverse

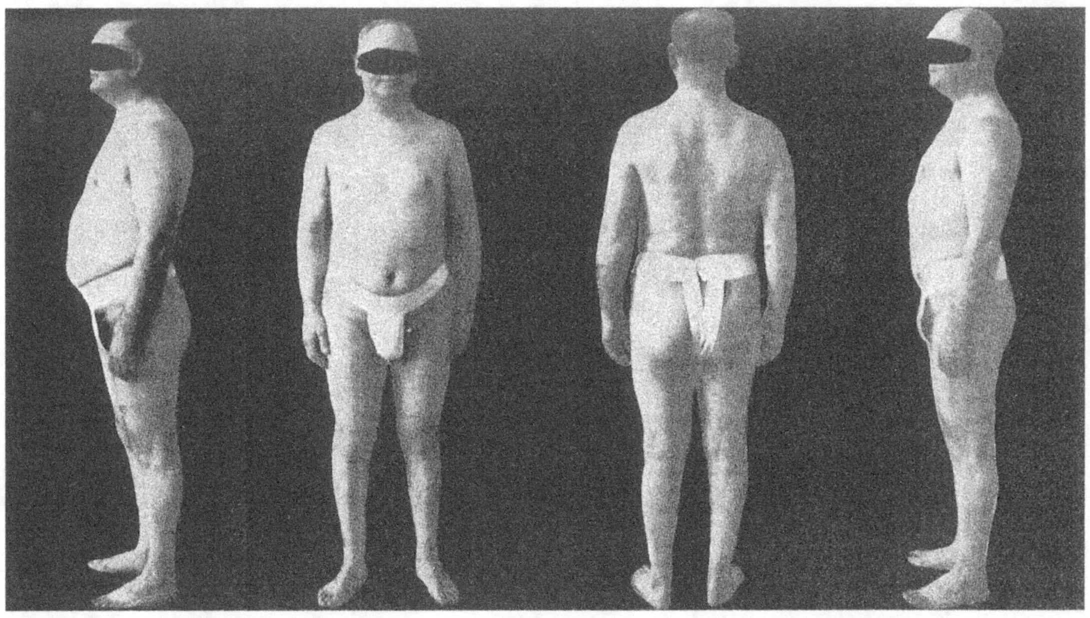

Fig.7. Stocky types of anatomy. Compare with FIG.2. Note the depth of the chest and the relatively short torso. (A) Lateral view showing the habitually relaxed faulty position. The apparent sag of the body is not so great as in the slender type, but, considering the anatomic structure, the potential of strain on the body and the viscera is equally as great. (B) Anterior view. The subcostal angle is not so narrow as in the slender type, nor is the lower chest so narrowed and small. (C) Posterior view. Note the folds in the skin of the back. these are due to the droop of the chest and the abdomen. (D) Best corrected posture. Note the lack of fullness in the epigastrium

diameter is usually less than that found in the intermediate type. The subcostal angle is frequently more than a right angle. The surface of the chest anteriorly is usually convex. The tenth rib is attached to the subjoined cartilage in front. The ribs are broad and heavy; their downward inclination from the vertebrae is often less than 30°. The costovertebral articulation is more frequently above than to the anterior side of the transverse process of the vertebra.

The vertebrae are large and heavy. The lumbar spine is relatively short and is set deeply between the ilia (Fig.3) There may be only four lumbar vertebrae.

There is usually very little lumbar lordosis, owing partly to the massiveness and the relative shortness of the lumbar spine and partly to the decreased motion possible in the articular facets. The transverse processes are large. The articular processes are large and crescentic (Fig. 8A).

The body cavities are larger and deeper than in the intermediate type, and the internal organs are larger. The stomach is roughly oval, and its greater diameter is transverse (Fig. 5). It is firmly attached, and little downward displacement can take place. The small intestine is longer than

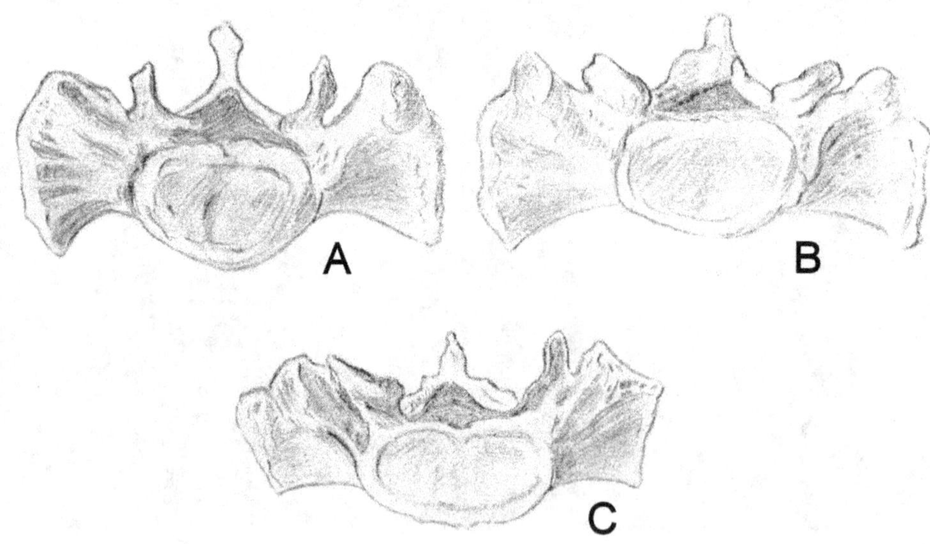

F1G. 8. The sacrum as seen from above, showing, A, the crescentic type of articular facets; B, the flat type of articular facets; C, the fiat type on the left, and the crescentic on the right. A, The deep, crescentic articulations permit less motion and usually are found in the stocky type. B, The shallow, flat articulations are more common in the slender type. Variations in the depth and the directional slant may occur in any type.

in the intermediate type, measuring from 25 to 35 feet; its walls are thick, and its lumen is relatively large. The large intestine also is longer, measuring from 5 to 8 1/2 feet in length. Here the retro-peritoneal attachments are short and firm, permitting very little sag (Fig. 6). The liver is large but is attached firmly beneath the diaphragm. There is much retro-peritoneal and abdominal fat. The diaphragm is usually high, with its dome at the eighth or the ninth thoracic vertebra. The heart and the lungs are large. The long axis of the heart often approaches the horizontal (FIG. 4B).

DIFFERENTIATION OF TYPES

There are a number of methods with which to determine the anatomic type. Draper has suggested a complex series of measurements to secure a satisfactory estimate of body build, whereas Naccaroti has attempted to classify the different types of individuals by obtaining the ratio of the length of the arm and the leg to the volume of the trunk. Simple measurements of height or of girth are inadequate, since they give information only as to the tallness or the nutritional status, and since either of the types may be thin or fat. Davenport believes that the relation of volume to stature is a satisfactory means of measuring body build and, on this basis, classifies individuals as very fleshy, medium, slender and very slender. Lucas simplifies the measurement still more by comparing the width of the body to its height, the former being measured by ascertaining the widest distance between the iliac crests. From such measurements he groups children into a linear (slender) type and a lateral (heavy) one. A fairly good estimate of the body type can be obtained from observation and from roentgenograms of the lumbar spine.

Because they are of different body types, many individuals show wide variations from the averages given in height-weight tables. In a study of the 11,585 officers in the United States Army, Dear found that most of them did not conform to the usual tables for their height and age and that it was necessary to consider build and musculature in those who were underweight or overweight. The slender and the stocky types could be recognized in all age periods but, in a pure form, were almost as rare as the intermediate type, although the proportion of individuals of slender type was increasing. Mixtures and gradations of types were common. The roentgenographic studies of Goldthwait and Brown have shown that skeletal differences among the various body types occur frequently, and Stockard has observed many such variations in the animal world. At times, this mixture of types makes the problem of differentiation somewhat difficult.

POSTURAL DIFFERENCES

The habits of posture are different in the three classes of anatomic build—-intermediate, slender and stocky. (Figs. 8 and 9.) A proper adjustment and relationship of the various parts of the body probably are most easily maintained in the intermediate type. In the slender type while the ideal standing position is the same as for the intermediate, the position commonly assumed is one in which the general relationship of the parts is much disturbed. The body inclines backward from the low lumbar region, increasing the lumbar lordosis and the forward inclination of the pelvis, with an increased rounding of the mid-dorsal or the upper dorsal region and a forward projection of the neck; the chest is flattened, and the subcostal angle is narrowed. The vital capacity is decreased more than in the stocky and the intermediate types. With the droop of the ribs and the clavicles, there is inadequate support of the shoulders, so that they sink forward and downward, and the scapulae rotate outward. In the lower extremities the knees are often hyperextended, and the feet are pronated and strained. Developmental deformities are seen most commonly in this type. There is also more extensive downward displacement of the viscera. With the sagging of the chest and the forward droop of the head, the diaphragm assumes a lower position in the thorax, and its excursions are decreased. The heart and the aortic arch are lowered. The abdomen shows a depression just below the costal border anteriorly, with a prominence below the umbilicus. The liver often is rotated forward and downward to the right. The kidneys are frequently immobile—the so-called floating kidneys. Displacements of the pelvic viscera are common.

In the stocky type of individual with heavy bones, thick muscles, shorter ligamentous attachments and decreased motion in the joints, one would expect a lessened tendency to the assumption of faulty carriage and to displacement of the viscera. In posture clinics the children who come for treatment are rarely of this type. Deformity and disturbances from faulty carriage as a rule develop much later in life than in the slender type, since the general structure of the body withstands strain much better. Occasionally in children but more commonly in adults, a backward inclination of the spine and the thorax on the pelvis is observed as the body weight increases; this takes place at the hip joints or at the dorsolumbar region as a compensation for the heavy abdominal viscera anteriorly. There never is any great increase in the forward inclination of the pelvis. The ribs do not change much in their inclination, and the vital capacity is decreased slightly. There may be a decrease in the anteroposterior diameter of the upper abdomen, which causes a crowding rather than a downward displacement of the heavy abdominal organs. The firm attachments and the short ligaments do not permit much sagging of the Organs Developmental are not common and appear late.

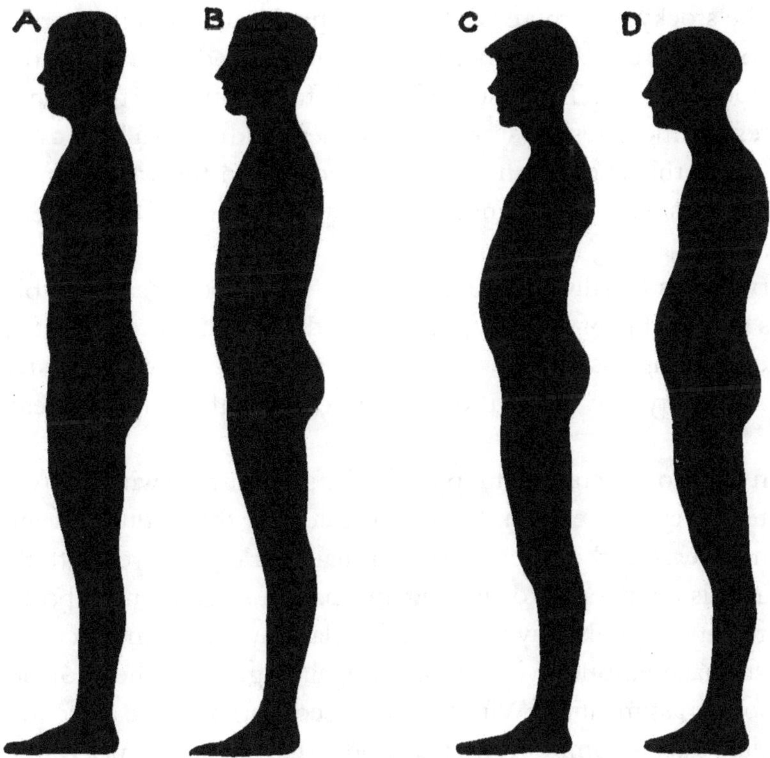

FIG. 9. The Harvard University chart for grading body mechanics. (A) Excellent mechanical use of the body: (l) head straight above chest, hips and feet; (2) chest up and forward; (3) abdomen in or fiat; (4) back, usual curves not exaggerated. (B) Good mechanical use of the body (compare with A): (l) head too far forward; (2) chest not so well up or forward; abdomen, very little change; (4) back, very little change. (C) Poor mechanical use of the body (compare with A): (1) head forward of chest; (2) chest flat; (3) abdomen relaxed and forward; (4) back curves exaggerated. (D) Very poor mechanical use of the body (compare with A): (1) head still farther forward; (2) chest still flatter and farther back; (3) abdomen completely relaxed, "slouchy;" (4) back, all curves exaggerated to the extreme.

DIFFERENCES IN PHYSIOLOGIC PROCESSES

Not only are-the mechanics of the body and the potentialities of strain different in the various types of body structure but the physiologic processes differ also.

Probably the greatest variation lies in the functioning of the gastro-intestinal tract. In the slender type it short, as in carnivorous animals; here a more concentrated kind of diet is indicated since the ingested fibre passes quickly through the tract, and therefore assimilation must be rapid. In the stocky type there is a long intestinal tract, as in the herbivore; here a less concentrated type of diet is indicated, since the passage of food is slower, and assimilation can be carried on for a longer time. The result of this differentiation in the length of the tract is shown by the protest of the digestive system of slender children to a high caloric, high fat diet in large amounts when this is given in an attempt to obtain the weight specified in height-weight tables. Other physiologic differences are shown in the circulatory, the nervous and the muscular systems.

The Circulatory rate is usually more rapid in the slender type and the blood pressure is lower; the muscles are capable of more rapid motion than are those of the stocky type but are not so well adapted to long-sustained action. Lucas and Pryor have suggested that some of our problems in immunity may lie in the recognition of differences in reaction in certain anatomic types.

Disturbances in function occur most rapidly in the slender type with faulty body mechanics there is a greater tendency to eyestrain. Howe has said that this is due to venous congestion, which produces an increase in the anteroposterior diameter of the eye. With the more marked sag in this type, there is a tendency to slowing and partial stagnation of both the pulmonary and the venous circulations. This may lead to cold, clammy hands and feet and to varicosities in the veins. The stomach empties with difficulty against gravity. The shortness of the small intestine leads to poorer assimilation. With the increased length of the mesenteric attachments, ptosis of the intestinal tract is common and may lead to constipation. As a rule, puberty appears early, and, in the female, dysmenorrhea is common. In the male, the voice is usually bass, and the change of voice comes early. Psychologically this type is quick to learn, and, with this, often comes impatience with the slower, heavy type. Such people are inclined to be dogmatic and fanatical; the leaders of movements usually come from among them. They become angry quickly and have a limited endurance but recover from fatigue rapidly. They adjust quickly to changes in environment.

In the stocky type the circulation is usually adequate, with a tendency to high blood pressure. The countenance is ruddy and plethoric. There is a greater development of the left side of the heart. The stomach generally has no difficulty in emptying. Because the small intestine is long, there is good nutrition, with a tendency to become fat. Puberty occurs at a later age. The basal metabolism is often less than the normal reading. Many males have tenor voices. People with this body type get along well socially; they are easy going and even-tempered, with a good sense of humor; they are tolerant and make poor reformers. They work more slowly but have greater endurance than those of the slender type. Their recovery from fatigue is usually less rapid. They are not self-conscious and tend to be extroverts and do not adjust easily to changes in environment.

SUSCEPTIBILITY TO DISEASE

There is a difference between the slender and the stocky types in susceptibility to disease. Those of the former type show a greater tendency to contract influenza, bronchitis and tuberculosis. They fall victims to acute infectious diseases more frequently, fevers are more common, and hypotension often occurs. In the intestinal tract such disorders as inadequate gastric secretions, gastric and duodenal ulcer, and spastic colitis are found frequently. Hyperglandular disturbances and atrophic rheumatoid) arthritis are frequent findings, It is in this type that melancholia depression and the nervous and mental disorders are prone to occur.

In the stocky type, on the other hand, there is less tendency to contract acute infectious diseases. Chronic bronchitis and emphysema are more common than in the slender type, as are hypertension with arteriosclerosis, myocardial degeneration chronic nephritis, gall stones and gallbladder disease. In the male, hypertrophy of the prostate is seen more often and also gout and hypertrophic arthritis (osteo-arthritis). Disturbances in the glands of internal secretion usually assume the nature of a hypofunction. Early loss of hair and baldness are common. Cerebral hemorrhage and the chronic degenerative nervous and mental disorders occur almost exclusively in this type.

ANATOMIC AND FUNCTIONAL FEATURES

From this discussion and these findings, which have been verified amply by numerous observers, it is readily apparent that a broader understanding of anatomic and functional features is necessary. The physician rarely is called on by patients having the anatomy of the intermediate type. The physiologic and the psychological peculiarities of each type and its tendency to disturbances in function must be kept in mind. For centuries a relationship has been sought between form and function. More recently the trend has been to disregard the individual and to focus the entire study on the micro-organism or other agent supposedly responsible for the disease. Both methods are necessary. A study of anatomic types will throw light on individual differences in susceptibility and resistance. These differences still await solution, since they are bound up in the physics and the chemistry of each type. The same diet has varying effects on individuals of different body build, as was found by Weir Mitchell and Salisbury in their attempts to help the chronically ill. The pharmacologic reaction to various therapeutic substances also is different.

The analysis of signs and symptoms will result in a more rational interpretation, particularly in circulatory disturbances, if the anatomic peculiarities of the individual are considered. In disturbances in the abdominal or the thoracic viscera, not only must the inadequacies of the organ be noted, but the conditions under which it works must be studied also. In different body types, marked variations in mental and nervous diseases will be found; these variations will require different therapeutic procedures. These differences are shown in the functioning of the endocrine glands and in their regulation by the sympathetic nervous system. In the preservation of health and in the treatment of disease, the study of anatomic types and their functional variations offers great help in the understanding of the basic problems which they present.

3

Body Mechanics

GENERAL CONSIDERATIONS

Every individual, be he layman or physician, knows instinctively that when a person breaks a leg or an arm the first and most important step is to reduce the fracture and to correct as well as possible any deformity that is present. He knows that this is necessary in order to obtain the maximum function.If this is true of the extremities, it is equally if not more true of the body as a whole. It is easy to recognize a deformity in the extremity. However, because of lack of knowledge, it is difficult to recognise as deformities the conditions that are found so commonly in the examination of the body as a whole. If the viscera are displaced, or if the pelvis is tipped forward markedly, so that the spinal nerves are compressed, and their function is disturbed, there is definitely a deformity as there is in a twisted foot. In the next few chapters we shall show how these deformities may be recognised and corrected.

The standard tables based on age, weight and height, although made up from the averages of many thousands of measurements, are not applicable to all types of the human body, even allowing a 10 per cent deviation from the scale either up or down. However, it is necessary to have some standard or basis to work from, and such a standard can be established easily when the individual is looked upon as a machine and is judged from the viewpoint of a mechanical engineer. A mechanical engineer, in testing a machine, first looks it over to see how it is made and then examines it to see how nearly perfect it is in alignment and function. from the point of view of the commercial value of the machine, he is less interested in its actual efficiency at the time of examination than he is in its mechanical alignment and in signs of wear in its vital parts. He knows very well that, although to all outward appearances it may be working to full capacity, there may be detectable signs of wear which must mean a breakdown in the near future. The less well aligned a machine, the more strain and wear there must be, and the greater the probability of trouble. The misalignment or faulty mechanics of the human machine is likewise a potential of trouble and it should be recognised as such by the physician.

Mechanical Correlation. Body mechanics, as defined by the White House Conference on Child Health and Protection, is "the mechanical correlation of the various systems of the body with special reference to the skeletal, muscular, and visceral systems and their neurological associations. Normal body mechanics may be said to obtain when this mechanical correlation is most favourable to the function of these systems."

It is necessary to explain what s meant by mechanical correlation. To understand this we must examine certain fundamental structures of the body: the bones, the muscles and the ligaments. Most of the bones in the body are separated from each other by joints and are held in contact by ligaments. The ligaments, being fibrous, non-elastic structures, must be protected by shock absorbers, that is the muscles. the amount of motion in a joint depends (1) on the shape of the joint surfaces, which vary in every type of individual; (2) on the laxity or the tightness of the ligaments; and (3) on the condition of the protective muscles.

. In every joint in the body there is a range of motion which, because of the three elements mentioned above, varies with every individual as shown in the wrist joints in Figure 10, whether the motion is as slight as that in the sacro-iliac joint or as great as that in the hip joint. Any joint, no matter how much or how little motion it may have, is in danger of being injured if

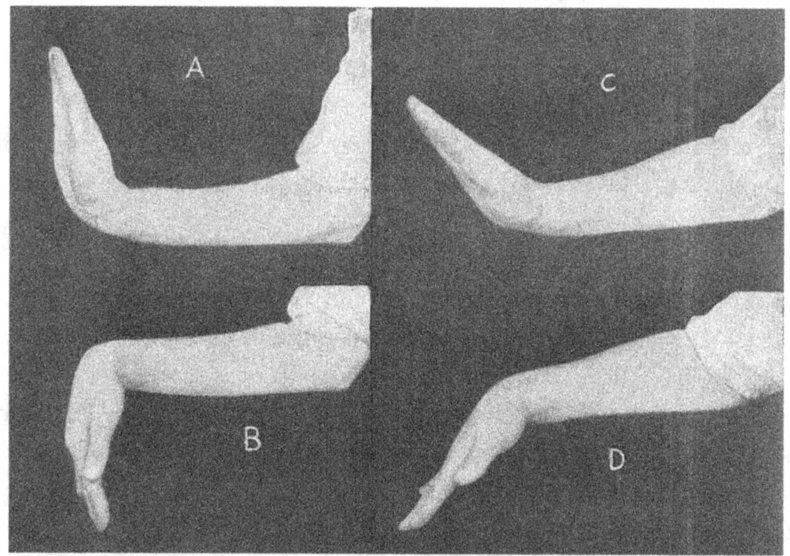

FIG. 10. Two normal wrists in the position of greatest extension, A and C, and of greatest flexion, B and D. Note the normal difference in the total possible amount of motion. This difference in motion occurs because of the difference in the type of bony structure. (A) Amount of extension possible in wrist No. 1. (B) Amount of flexion possible in wrist No. 1. (C) Amount of extension possible in wrist No. 2. Amount of flexion possible in wrist No. 2. Position A could not be assumed by wrist No. 2 without injury. Position C. Full extension for this wrist could be assumed by Wrist No. 1 with no injury, as there would still be a factor-of-safety motion.

for any reason its motion is forced beyond the normal range. For purposes of description we may compare a joint to the hinge on the door of an automobile. Automobile doors all have stops to prevent the door from swinging too far open; these stops are like the ligaments. Many of us have had the experience of seeing an automobile door left open, so that the stop strap. or ligament, is tight, and then pushed still farther open. The result is a broken strap, a broken hinge, or a broken door or all three. The potential reason for this accident is that the door was at one extreme of its motion, and since the stop strap, or ligament, was tight, there was no so-called factor-of-safety motion left. The actual reason was the blow on the door; the same blow, if the door had not been at one extreme of its range of motion and so had had a factor-of-safety motion, might not have caused any damage. Therefore, from the point of view of safety or health, the significant fact here is not the blow but the position of the door when it was struck in relation to the limits of the possible range of motion in its hinges (Fig. 11).

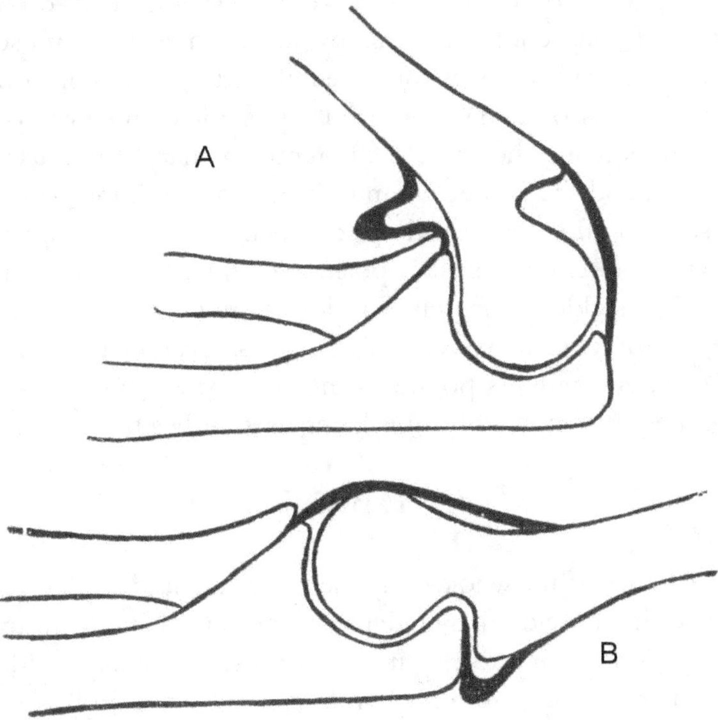

FIG. 11. Schematic diagram showing how motion in a joint is limited by the ligaments. (A) Elbow joint at the extreme of flexion, showing the tautness of the posterior ligaments and the laxness of the anterior ligaments. (B) Elbow joint in full extension, showing the opposite condition of the ligaments. There is no factor-of-safety motion, and attempts at further motion in flexion, in A, and in ex tension, in B, would tend to produce ligamentous injury.

Factor-of-safety Motion. Good body mechanics imply that all the joints of the body are used in such a position in relation to their total range of motion that the possibility of further motion in either direction — the factor-of-safety motion — is always present. Like the bones and the teeth, ligaments, although fibrous and nonelastic, are affected not only by the nutrition of the body but also by the position in which they are used habitually. They may become shortened on one side of a joint and lengthened on the other. In this way the range of motion may be diminished in one direction and increased in the other. This possible change, caused by habitual faulty use, always must be considered in the examination of any joint.

Muscle Functions. Muscles have two main functions: the mobilization and the protection of the joints. The physiology of muscular action is beyond the scope of this book, but some features influencing their action will be taken up. When a muscle contracts, it shortens, thus lessening the distance between its origin and its insertion.

If for any reason the origin and the insertion of a muscle were brought as close together as they could be, no contraction of these muscles would have any effect on the position of the bones and the joints. If long continued, this would mean that the muscle would become permanently shorter, and its usefulness would be nullified or at least impaired seriously. Such shortening, or contracture, associated with the faulty position of the joint, of necessity reduces its normal range of motion and therefore is a potential of danger because it has reduced the factor-of-safety motion and the protective muscle action to a minimum. The possibility of overstretching or straining the contracted or stretched muscles and ligaments is very great when, with such factors present, an extreme position of the joint, be it flexion or extension, is increased suddenly. This sudden change in position is undoubtedly the most common cause of acute back-ache and other acute strains (Fig. 11). Thus, it can be seen that in examining any joint one must observe not only its possible range of motion but also—and this is of the utmost importance the position in which it is being used or has been used habitually.

THE BONES

Bone Changes. The bones of the whole body-the spine, the head and the extremities—exactly like the ligaments and the muscles, may undergo changes in shape from their use in habitual faulty mechanical positions, owing to Nature's ever-present attempt to adapt the part to the function imposed on it, as has been shown by Wolff and subsequent observers. For this reason, the answer to the common question, "What is normal posture?" must be that there is not and cannot be one posture which is normal for all individuals and to which all individuals should conform. The reason for this can be understood readily when the anatomy of each section of the spine and its attachments is examined the two roentgenograms of so-called normal female pelves given in Fig.12 show the extreme differences which may occur, differences which may affect the entire spine. Note the relatively vertical iliac bones of the slender type as compared

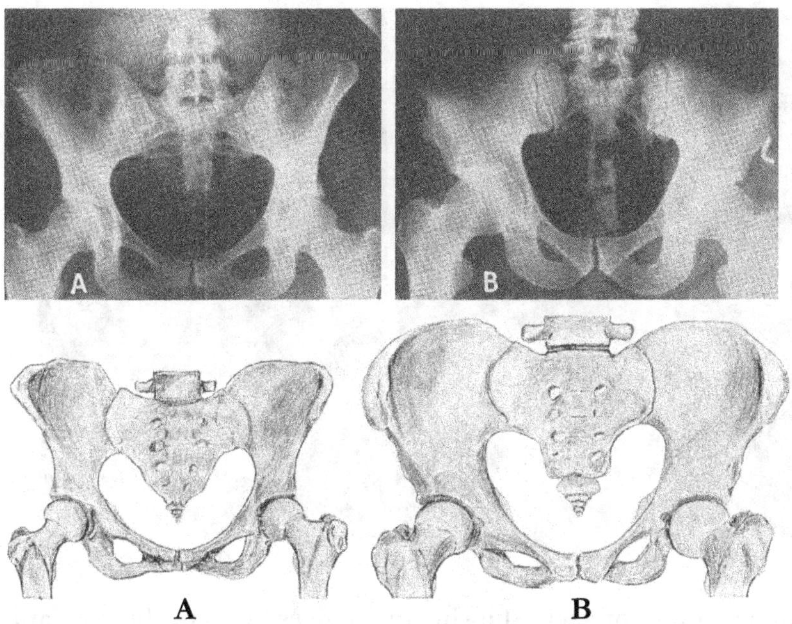

Fig. 12. Roentgenograms and diagrams of two normal female pelves (A) slender type, (B) heavy type, in A (slender type) the iliac bones are relatively vertical as compared with the flaring ilia in the heavy type, B. There is also a marked difference in the structure and the shape of the femora. The femoral neck in the slender type is longer and thinner.

with the wide, flaring ilia in the stocky type; in the former, the structure of the bones is distinctly lighter than in the latter; a similar difference is also present in the femora.

Differences in the Vertebrae. In the vertebrae themselves a similar difference is found in their shape and also in the shape, position and the inclination of the articular facets. These differences must cause a great variation in the actual curves that are present in the spine, and in the amount of motion that is possible in its various parts. If the element of faulty body mechanics of many years duration enters in, the changes in the shape of the bones may be even more marked, so that, in the adult at least, the complete correction of the faulty curves may be impossible. However, no matter how bad the curves, or how extensive the changes in shape, it is always possible to improve the body, mechanics and to prevent the further damage caused by it. These differences, due to Nature s adapting the shape of the bones to the function they have to perform, are shown in anatomic specimens of sacra. One sacrum may be concave anteriorly, and another, more nearly flat (Fig- 13), depending on the position in which the pelvis has been used. In some individuals with bad body mechanics, a much greater lumbar lordosis and a greater forward inclination of the pelvis are always present because of the shape of the articular facets of the sacrum and the vertebrae. This means that the lower end of the sacrum

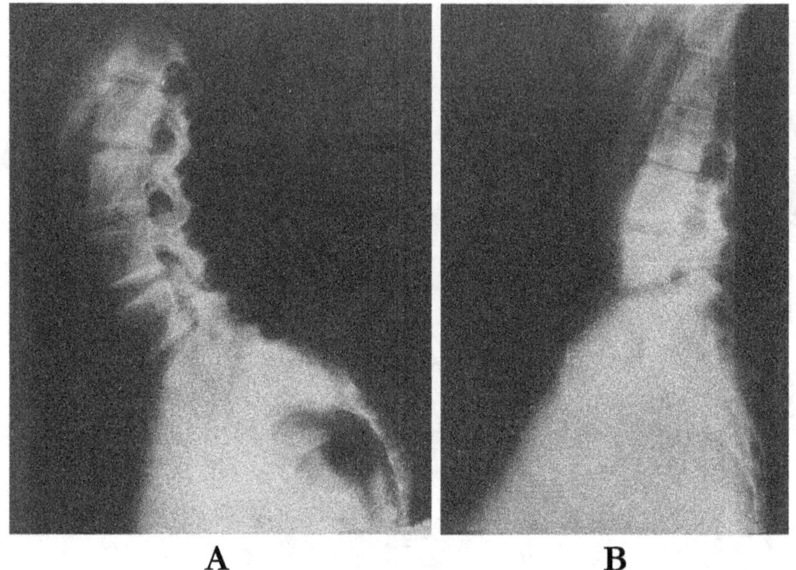

FIG. 13. Roentgenograms of sacra showing differences in shape due to Nature's adaptation to function. (Left) Markedly concave sacrum which is found in long-standing bad body mechanics where there is extreme lumbar lordosis. These are vertebrae of the slender type. The shallow articular facets permit this amount of lordosis. (Right) Almost flat sacrum found where marked lordosis is not possible.

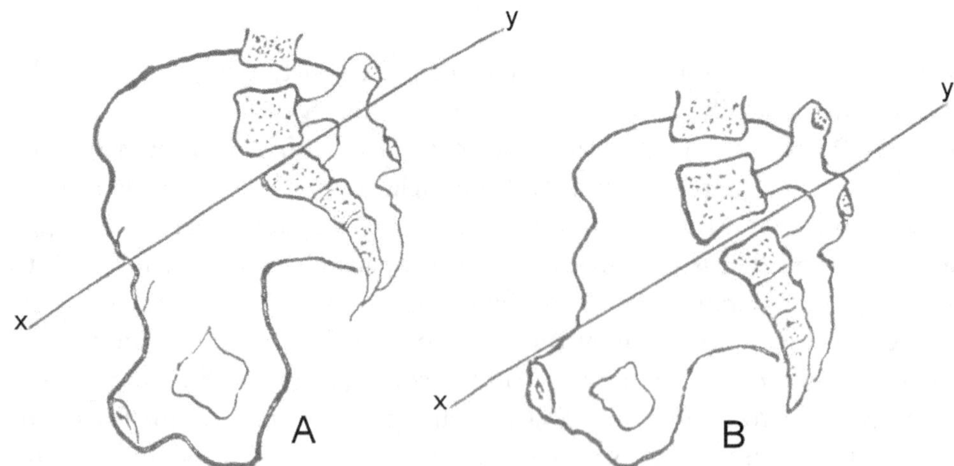

FIG 14. Diagrammatic drawings of pelves showing changes in relation of symphyses to the top of the sacrum. In A, the slender type, note that the symphysis pubis is considerably below the top surface of the first sacral body, X-Y. In B, the stocky type, the two are nearly on the same level. (See text.)

is pulled downward by muscular action, while the upper end is pushed downward by the weight of the lumbar spine and the body, thus causing a tendency to concavity. In other cases where, because of the size and the shape of the articular facets of the sacrum and the lumbar vertebrae, as well as the spinous processes, the marked lordosis is not possible, the mechanical forces which cause the concavity are not present.

The Sacrum. The upper surface of the sacrum, on which the fifth lumbar vertebra rests, varies greatly in relation to the symphysis pubis. In some pelves, as shown in Figure 14A, the symphysis pubis is on a plane considerably below that of the top of the sacrum. This occurs in the slender type because, in the lordotic position assumed in childhood, the forward inclination of the pelvis, caused by the pull of the Y ligaments and the anterior thigh muscles, holds the pubis down, while the weight of the body and the trunk, which is posterior to the pelvis because of the lordosis, tends to pull the sacrum upward. This constant strain during the growing period when the bones are soft makes possible the above relation of pubis and sacrum. In the stocky type of pelvis (Fig. 14 B), the pubis is practically on the same plane as the top of the sacrum because, during the growing period, there has not been that kind of strain which occurs in the slender type as the result of the extreme lordosis.

The position of the top of the sacrum in relation to the crests of the ilia is also subject to marked variation (Fig.15). If a line is drawn between the crests in some cases the sacrum will be found on the level of this line . In others, it will be the width of a vertebra below ff. The high position of the sacrum, as would be expected occurs more commonly in the slender type and thus makes possible the greater lordotic curves. The low- placed sacrum occurs more

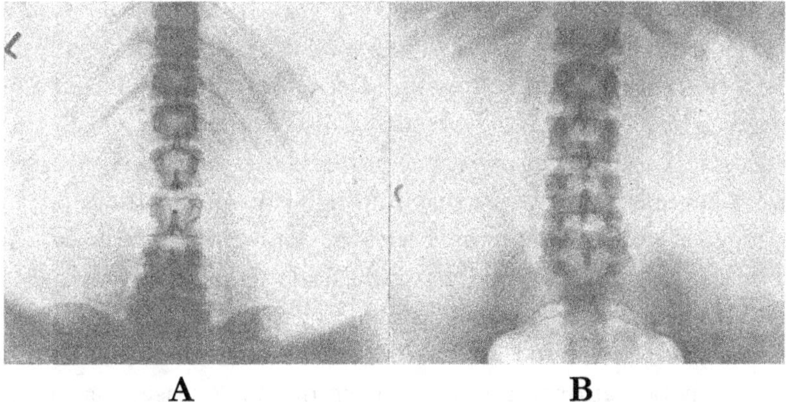

A   **B**

F1G. I5. Roentgenograms showing the relation of the fifth lumbar vertebra to the crests of the ilia; (A) The fifth lumbar vertebra is at the level of the crests; (B) the fifth lumbar vertebra is considerably below the level of the crests. Such normal structural differences must mean differences in the mechanics of this region. The ribs in A are slender and have a much greater downward inclination from the spine than is seen in B.

commonly in the stocky type, and this is one of the reasons why extreme lordotic curves are not found there. With these differences in mind, it appears that it is not the actual amount of lordosis present that must be considered but the amount in relation to the type of spine and sacrum.

THE SPINE

The spine offers much that is of interest from a mechanical point of view. In good body mechanics (Fig. 16), the weight of the trunk and the head rests mostly on the bodies of the vertebrae and the intervertebral disks (A). The articular facets normally act only as stabilizers. This is true in all parts of the spine. In the lumbar region the articular facets are perhaps the most important structures from a mechanical as well as a pathologic point of view. Their size, shape and obliquity may vary markedly. They are not designed to carry much of the body weight but, because of their shape, they have an extremely marked influence on the amount and the kind of motion of the spine.

Articular Processes. The articular processes of the adjoining lumbar vertebrae, with their facets, form the posterior wall of the intervertebral foramina. Where these two processes come together there is a true joint with a capsule and ligaments. The joints have a normal range of motion, its extent varying with the shape of the facets. In the lordotic position of the lumbar spine (Fig. 16 B), the weight of the body is thrown backward on the articular facets and the joint capsule instead of on the body of the vertebrae. If this strain is great enough to cause inflammatory reaction and swelling of these ligaments and joints, the possibility of narrowing the size of the intervertebral foramina will be very real. Inflammatory reaction from such a cause is undoubtedly a contributory factor in many cases of so-called sciatica and lumbago. In some forms of arthritis actual bony narrowing of the foramina can be seen.

Spinous Processes. These vary greatly in size and also in the angle which they form with the bodies of the vertebrae. In the lower lumbar region and the cervical region, where the lordotic curves are found, the spinous processes may impinge on one another and, in habitual faulty body mechanics, may act even as one of the points of support. The large bulbous and flattened ends of spinous processes seen in roentgenograms and in anatomic specimens may have been caused by this. The spinous processes may impinge not only at their tips but also throughout their length. It is conceivable that in extreme lumbar lordotic curves, where the weight of the upper spine is decidedly posterior to the hips, the spinous processes may act as a fulcrum and cause a stretching strain on the joints of the articular processes. If this backward strain were severe enough, these joints might be subluxed or even dislocated.

Transverse Processes. These also vary greatly in size, and in direction and shape (Fig. 17). It is not uncommon to find the transverse processes of the fifth lumbar vertebrae either symmetrically or asymmetrically enlarged, so much so that they impinge on the wings of the

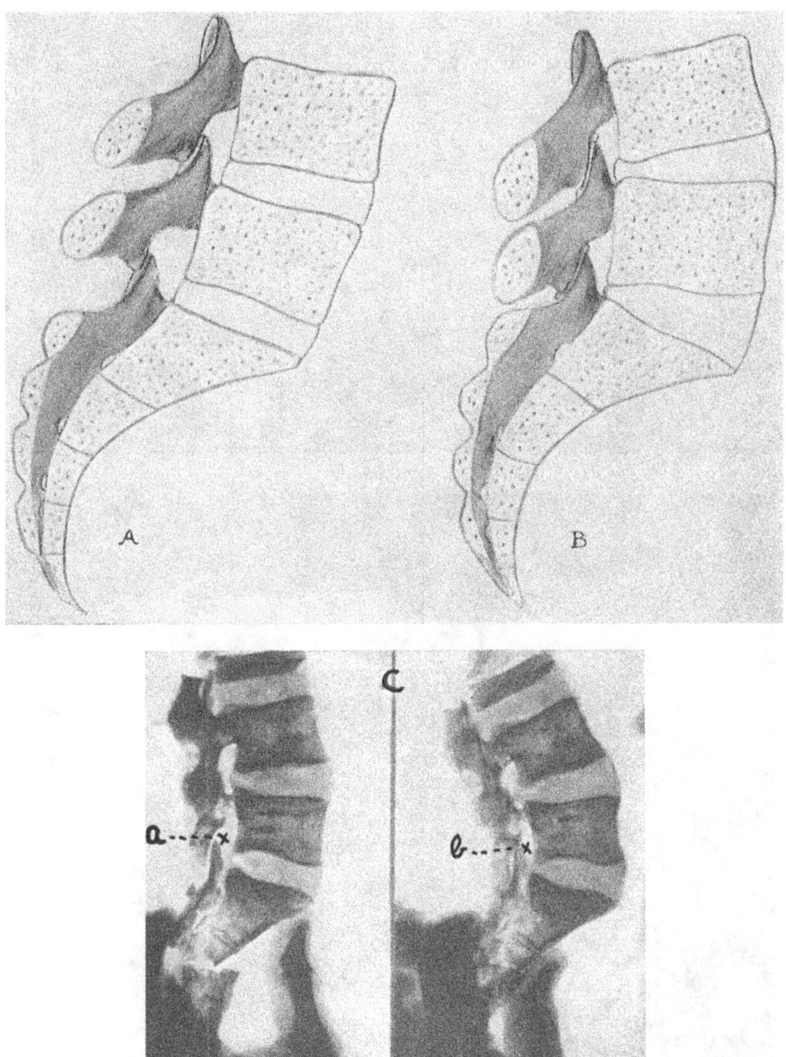

FIG. 16. Diagrammatic drawing of lumbosacral spine. (A) Good body mechanics. Note that the weight of the body is carried evenly on the intervertebral disks; that the articular processes and facets are not crowded together and that the intervertebral foramina are large. (B) Faulty body mechanics. Note that the weight is carried largely on the posterior part of the intervertebral disk, as shown by its wedge shape; that the articular processes and facets are crowded together, thereby decreasing the size of the intervertebral foramina. Note also that the spinous processes particularly rest upon each other. There is little or no factor-of-safety motion in extension in this position. (C) Anatomic specimen showing the same conditions as in diagrams. In B there is narrowing of the intervertebral space posteriorly. This is a common "trophostatic" cause of degeneration of the inter-vertebral disk.

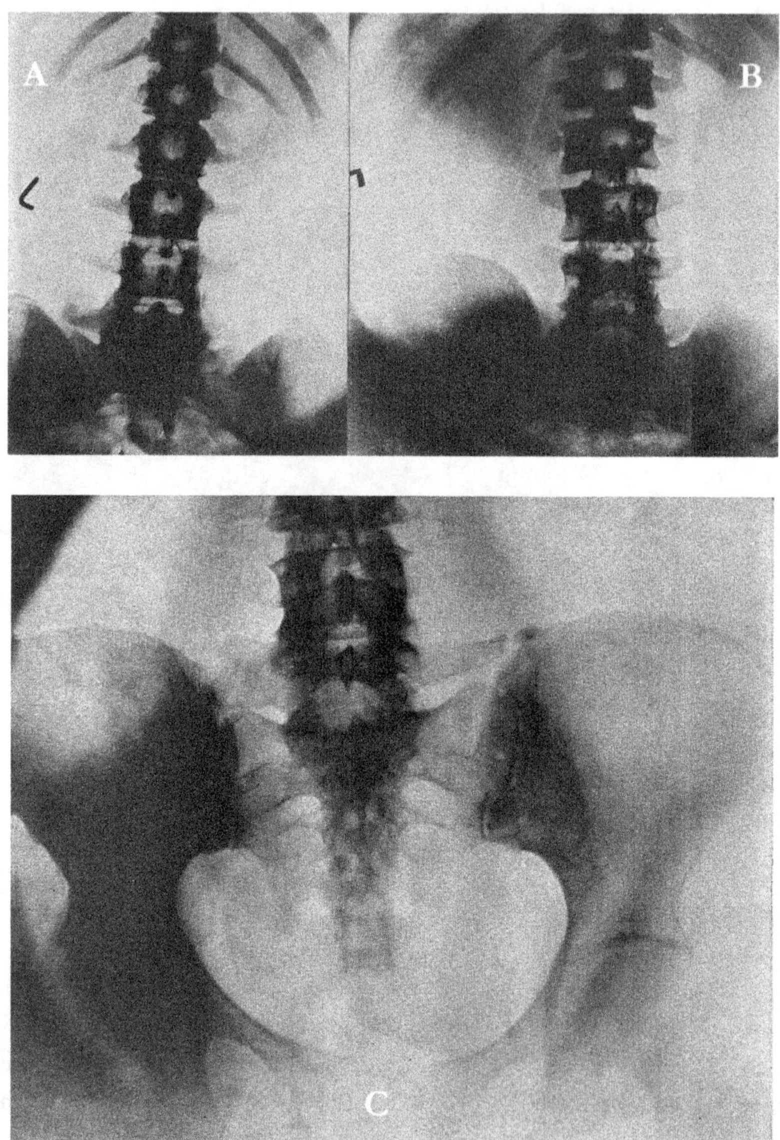

F1G. 17. Roentgenograms showing differences in the sizes and the shapes of the transverse processes in the lumbar region. (A) The wide transverse processes of the fifth lumbar vertebra. (B) The short, thick transverse processes. (C) The asymmetrical so-called sacralized transverse process on the right, with an articulation with the iliac crest on the left.

sacrum, forming a true joint; or they may be firmly fused or sacralized. Their importance is wholly potential. They limit the amount of possible motion in all directions at this region of the spine, and if, as so often occurs as one gets older, the curves of the spine become habitually increased, the abnormality, by limiting the amount of possible motion and thus lessening the factor of safety, may make strains or irritations in this region more probable. In treating backs with such an abnormality, it is well to remember that, since the abnormality has undoubtedly always been present, it is not the most potent factor, although it is easy to see it in roentgenograms. The governing factor from the point of view of treatment is likewise, not the acute strain, but the long standing and slowly increasing faulty body mechanics. When the body is used properly, the weight is carried on the bodies of the vertebrae. When it is used wrongly, the weight in the lumbar and the cervical regions is displaced backward, so that it comes to an increasing degree on the articular facets, forcing the joints more and more to the extreme position of their range of motion (Fig. 16 B).Whether this extreme position will be reached at the last lumbar vertebra and the sacrum or higher-up, or in the lower- or the upper-cervical region, depends entirely on the type of structure and the shape of the individual bones

Dorsal Spine. In the dorsal spine, the natural anterior curve increases, and the body weight comes on the front part of the vertebral bodies as the mechanics of the body becomes faulty. Therefore, instead of being crowded together, the articular facets are pulled apart- the reverse of what happens in the lumbar and the cervical regions. The possibility of strain in faulty body mechanics is equally great, for these joints are used also at one extreme of their possible range of motion. An examination of anatomic specimens shows evidence of strain in the region of the facets or the laminae, such as hypertrophic spurs, and the bodies themselves show changes in shape, such as narrowing of the anterior depth in comparison with the posterior, due to carrying the weight wrongly for a long time (Fig. 18).

The intervertebral disks are the most efficient shock absorbers, but when the weight rests on them at bad mechanical angles, their efficiency is lessened proportionately, and their work must be done by other parts of the body, thus causing unnecessary strain and fatigue.

The mechanics of the dorsal spine differ from those of the lumbar spine because of the ribs which are attached to it, and the irregular method of their articulation. The location of the articulation for the head of the rib is fairly constant, but that of the articulation for the transverse process varies. At times, it is on the anterior surface of the process. However, at other times it is on top of it, making a very different potential of joint strain at the head of the rib as the body is drooped or bent. The dorsal vertebrae differ in shape from the lumbar, since they do not have to carry so much weight and having to support the ribs do not need to exert so much motion. The vertebral bodies are smaller, the intervertebral foramina larger, and the laminae flatter; the articular facets face anteriorly and posteriorly and allow flexion and extension. The spinous processes may show interesting effects of long-standing faulty mechanics on the shape of bones; in such cases it will be found that, in the mid-dorsal region,

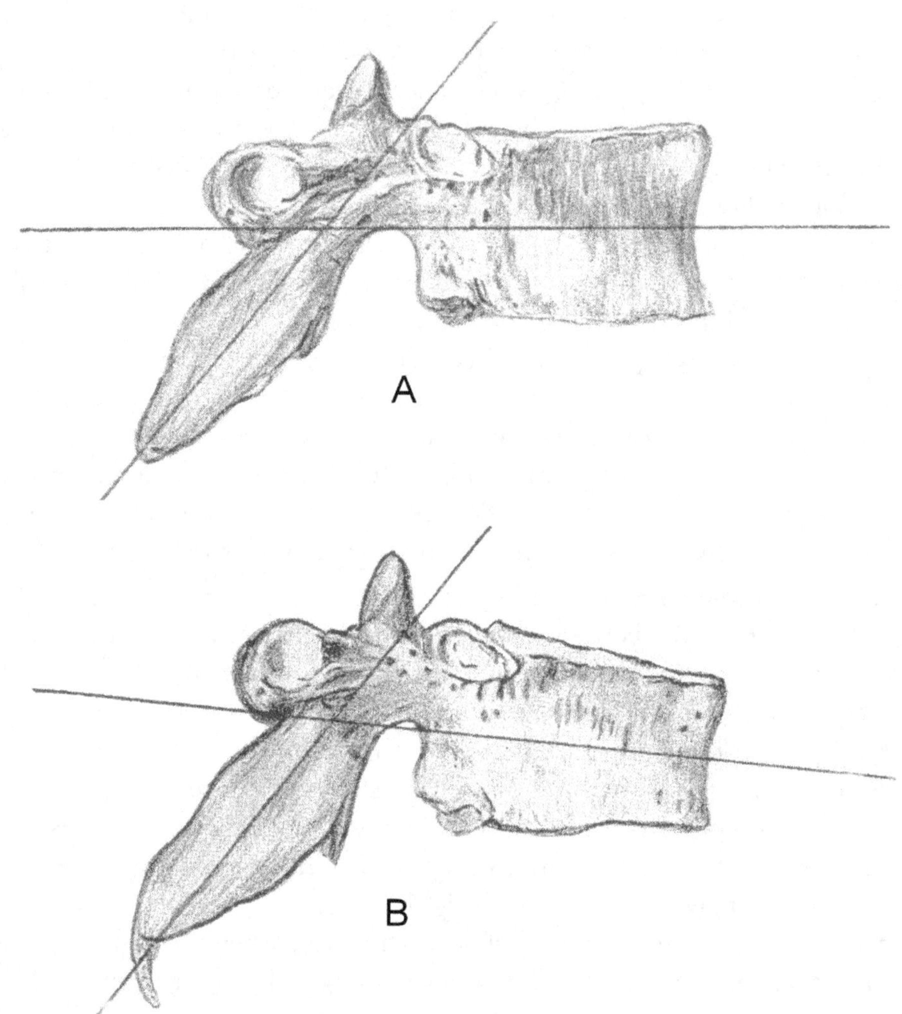

F1G. 18. Drawing of thoracic vertebra. (A) Normal vertebra. (B) Vertebra showing results of long-standing pressure and strain from faulty body mechanics. Note the narrowing of the anterior portion of the vertebra, that the spinous process of B comes away from the body at a more acute angle than in A and that the arch of the intervertebral foramen of B is narrower than that of A; that there are evidences of strain, such as hypertrophic spurs on the articular facets and the top of the spinous process in B. All of these changes can be caused by the long-standing strain of faulty body mechanics such as must occur in a rounded or drooped dorsal spine.

the angle at which the spinous processes leave the body of the vertebra (Fig. 18) varies. In cases of good body mechanics, with a nearly flat or straight dorsal spine, the angle is more obtuse, while in a spine with an habitual rounded curve, it is nearly 90°. The tips of the spinous processes may be elongated because of Nature's reaction to the long-continued pull of the faulty position of the spine.

Dorsolumbar Region. One of the most important parts of the spine from the mechanical point of view is the dorsolumbar region. Here comes the change from the dorsal to the lumbar type of vertebra. Here is the point of greatest mobility-that where the extremes of motion seen in contortionists and fancy dancers takes place. Because of this flexibility, there are great possibilities of strain in faulty body mechanics. Exactly where the greatest amount of motion will occur whether at the twelfth dorsal or the first lumbar vertebra in the intermediate type, the second and the third lumbar vertebrae in the slender, or the tenth and the eleventh dorsal vertebrae in the stocky—varies with the anatomic type. This region is the common site of fractures of the spine, and exactly which vertebra is to give way will depend on the point of greatest mobility. As the dorsolumbar region is the most mobile part of the spine, and as habitual faulty mechanics always tends sooner or later to cause strain, with its accompanying inflammatory processes around the articular facets and the joints of the spine, it is possible to have irritation at the spinal nerve roots in this region, with accompanying referred pain in the abdomen. It is beginning to be realized that many of the painful symptoms in the region of the appendix, the lower abdomen and the gall bladder may be due to this cause rather than to any pathology in the viscera themselves.

Cervical Spine. The cervical spine, like the lumbar spine, is one in which the habitual position tends to be in extension. The shape of the vertebrae varies markedly in the different types of anatomy, and their number may vary also, there being at times five or even eight, instead of the usual seven. Because of the differences in the anatomic structure, the point at which the greatest curve in extension may take place varies (Fig. 19). In some cases the apex of the curve is in the lower cervical spine and, in others, in the mid-cervical or the upper-cervical spine. Exactly where it occurs is a vital matter in the diagnosis of painful referred symptoms. As the greatest strain and its accompanying inflammatory processes usually occur at the apex of the curves, the referred symptoms will depend on whether the cervical or the brachial plexus is involved. In faulty body mechanics, as seen in the roentgenograms, the spinous processes are extremely close together or actually may impinge. Such impingement, of course, limits the amount of motion in extension and makes the possibility of strain much greater. This limited motion will be rotatory, if the point of greatest curve is in the upper-cervical spine, and lateral if in the lower- cervical spine. The amount of curve and the position in which it occurs depend primarily on the angle of inclination of the articular facets and of the spinous processes.

Cervical Vertebrae. The cervical vertebrae differ markedly in shape from the dorsal and the lumbar vertebrae, since their function requires greater ranges of motion. The vertebral artery

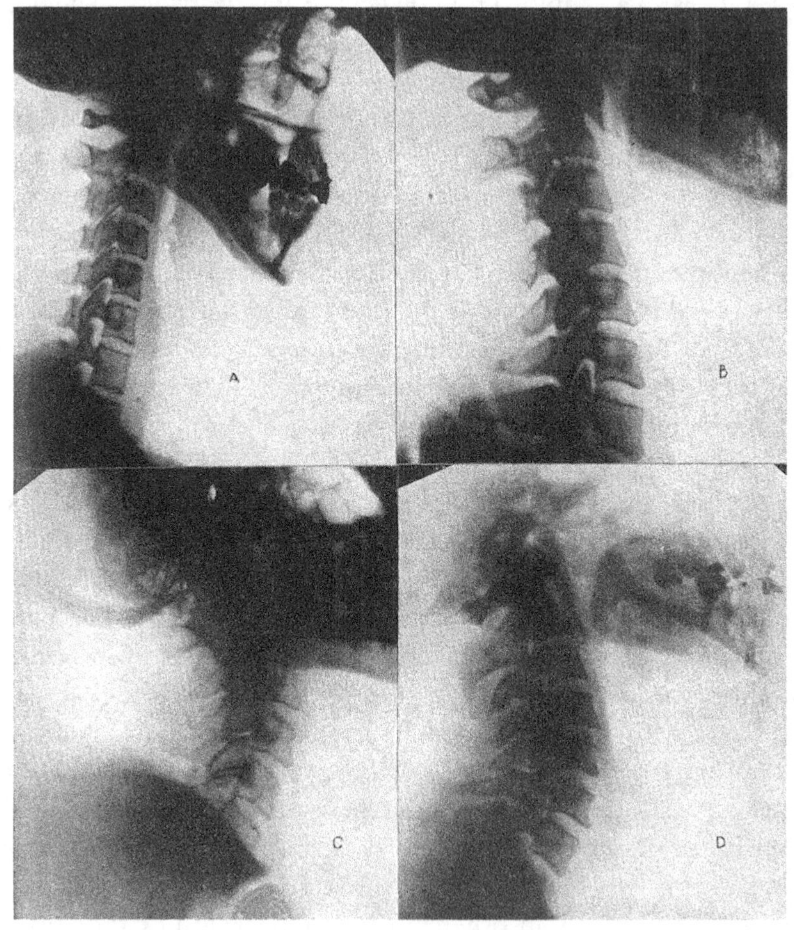

FIG.19. Roentgenograms of cervical spines, showing different types of structure and also the different levels at what curve in extension 'may take place. (A) Slender type. (B) Stocky type. (C) High cervical curve. (D) Low cervical curve. In both C and D extensive bony overgrowth occurs about the margins of the vertebrae and about the intervertebral foramina. Degeneration of the intervertebral disks and forward displacement of the vertebrae occur also.

enters a foramen in the transverse process of the seventh cervical vertebra and emerges on the superior surface of the transverse process of the first cervical vertebra or the atlas. The upper two cervical vertebrae differ from the others in shape and in their methods of articulation. Greater mobility in the cervical spine makes possible greater degrees of position and, in consequence, greater degrees of strain and the accompanying irritative processes. Just as in the low-lumbar region, referred pain, as sciatica or lumbago, with atrophy of muscles of the thigh, may occur in cases of long-standing lordotic curves and strain, so, in the cervical region, similar faulty mechanics and strain may lay the foundation for symptoms in the head, the neck, the shoulders, the chest, the arms or the hands, such as headache, neuritis and weakness.

THE CHEST

Ribs. The ribs differ markedly in shape in the different anatomic types. Their function is to form not only a protective cage for the chest and the abdominal organs but also, and perhaps of more importance, a framework for the attachment of the muscles of respiration. Therefore, the shape of the chest cage is a matter of considerable significance from the point of view of body mechanics. A caliper measurement or a tracing of the chest, taken with a lead tape at the ninth rib, should show that the anteroposterior diameter is about two thirds of the lateral diameter (Fig. 20 A) and that the circumference of the chest at the ninth rib is greater than in the axillary region. The sternum in the erect posture should be convex anteriorly, with the lower end considerably anterior to the upper; the subcostal angle in all anatomic types should form a right angle or more than a right angle.

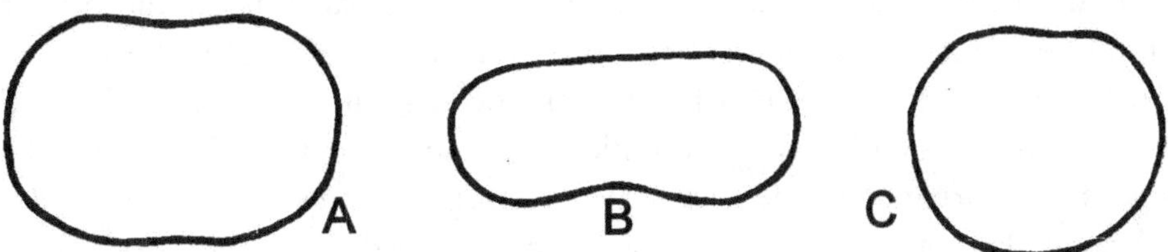

FIG. 20. Tracings of the chest, taken at the xyphoid process with lead tape. (A) Good body mechanics- the depth is about two thirds of the width. (B) Poor body mechanics—the funnel-type chest. (D) Poor body mechanics—-the pigeon-breast chest.

In their downward inclination, the ribs should form an angle with the spine from the horizontal of about 30° less than a right angle (Fig. 21) and, at the sides of the chest, should have space between them. Because of the different shapes of the ribs in the various anatomic types and the differences in the costovertebral and the costotransverse articulations, the shape of the chest in faulty body mechanics varies greatly.

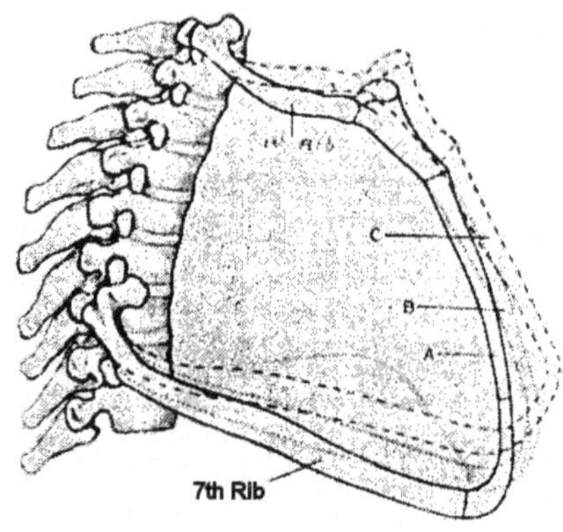

FIG. 21. Lateral view of thorax showing the sternum and the first and seventh ribs. The ribs have a downward inclination of about 30° from the horizontal. Note the movement of the sternum upward and forward in inspiration. Note also the angle formed by the ribs and the spine. (Gray: Anatomy)

In the long-bodied, slender type, the costotransverse articulations are such that when the dorsal spine becomes more rounded, and the head droops forward, causing an increased cervical curve, the chest settles down, the sternum may become perpendicular, and the ribs may point almost straight downward instead of being at nearly an angle of 30° to the spine. At the sides of the chest the ribs may be so close together as to override each other; there also will be a varying amount of rotation in each rib. The subcostal angle may become very narrow, at times not admitting a finger immediately below the xyphoid (Fig. 22); the length of the chest becomes much greater, and its circumference changes, so that it is smaller at the ninth rib than at the axillary line. Depending on anatomic structure, sometimes the funnel-chest or gutter-chest, and sometimes the pigeon-chest type of deformity occurs with faulty mechanics. The former is found chiefly in the slender type of child with faulty posture. The chief factor in its development is a disturbance in the mechanics of respiration associated with a low position of the diaphragm. The pigeon chest also occurs chiefly in the slender type of child but here the mechanical features are reversed.

In the stocky type, the chest, because of the articulations of the ribs and the transverse processes, takes an entirely different shape in the drooped position. When the dorsal spine becomes more rounded, the head comes forward, the upper part of the chest and the sternum become more vertical, and the lower ribs flare outward, both laterally and anteriorly. The relatively short torso makes it possible for the ribs on the sides to be found on the level or even below the crests of the ilia, even though the sag of the chest as a whole is not so great as in the slender type. They may be so close together as to override, and they may be found also at the level of the ilia or even below their crests. The ribs never are as straight downward as in the slender type, the subcostal angle is not as small, and the chest is never as long.

Drooped Chest. These changes in the shape of the chest cage are important because of their effect on the muscles attached to the chest wall. When the chest droops downward the abdominal muscles are relaxed because their origins (the sternum and costal margin) and their insertions (Poupart's ligament and the pubis) have been brought closer together, thus making the function of these muscles less efficient. The diaphragm is affected similarly because the low chest has brought the origin and the insertion of the diaphragm closer together, thus interfering with its proper action.

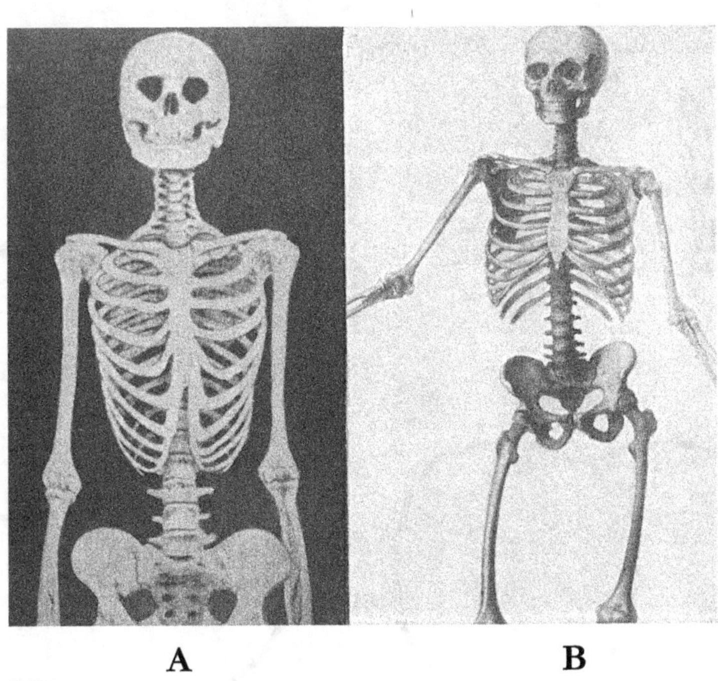

A   **B**

Fig. 22. (Left) Slender-type skeleton, showing the long thorax smaller in circumference at the ninth rib than at axillary line very narrow subcostal angle. This skeleton shows many signs one would expect from long faulty body mechanics. (Right) Stocky-type skeleton. Note the difference in subcostal angle and shape of thorax

The effect of the drooped chest on the action of the diaphragm can be shown in fluoroscopic tracings (Fig. 23); these should be taken in the standing and the lying positions. In correct body mechanics in the standing position, where free motion of the chest wall is possible, the total excursion of the diaphragm between full inspiration and full expiration is greater than in the lying position. In faulty body mechanics the reverse is true. The explanation is largely mechanical; in the correct standing position with the chest held up, the diaphragm is also is held up and its full motion is possible. In the lying position in good body mechanics, on the other hand, the chest, being held up by the pressure of the table on the ribs, cannot change

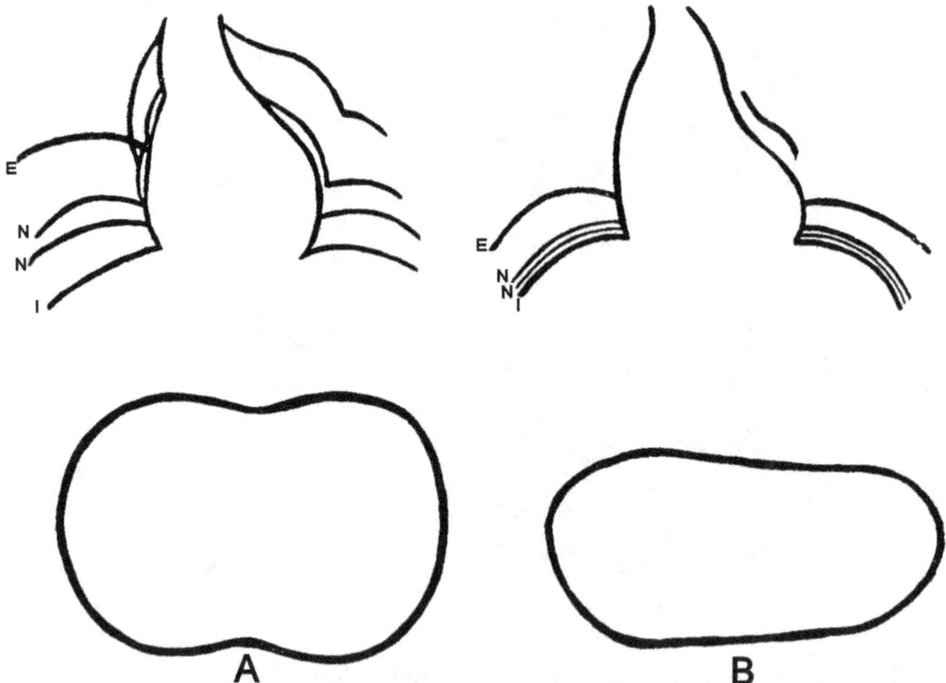

FIG. 23. Fluoroscopic tracings of heart and diaphragm and tracing of chest circumference at the ninth rib. (A) Good body mechanics: I, position of diaphragm at full inspiration. E, position of diaphragm at full expiration, N, N, position and total amount of excursion in ordinary respiration.
(B) Poor body mechanics: I, position of diaphragm at full inspiration. E, position of diaphragm at full expiration, N, N, excursion of the diaphragm in ordinary respiration. Note in B that the ordinary respiration takes place practically at the lowest position of the diaphragm.

its shape as much as in the standing position, and thus the amount of diaphragmatic motion must be less. In the lying position in faulty mechanics, the pressure of the table makes possible a longer excursion of the diaphragm by raising the chest to a higher point than that which is habitual in the ordinary standing position and preventing the drag of the abdominal organs. It is interesting to note that the excursion in ordinary or natural breathing is affected in the same way as is the function of any muscle when its origin and insertion are too close together.

The ordinary breathing excursion in good body mechanics occurs at a point near the middle of the extremes of excursion, thus leaving a factor-of-safety motion which can be drawn upon at any time, as in singing. In faulty body mechanics, where the origin and the insertion are too close together, the ordinary or natural respiratory excursion in the standing position occurs at or very near to the point of full inspiration, so that there is little or no factor-of-safety motion left. It will be noted also that the ordinary or natural breathing excursion of the diaphragm in faulty body mechanics is much less than that found in good body mechanics. With improvement in body mechanics, stamina and endurance are much improved through better function in the diaphragm. An increased and more forceful excursion of the diaphragm is the natural response of all good physical training.

The flabbiness and the easy fatigability of many young people, who seem to be well otherwise, are often the result of a greatly decreased excursion of the diaphragm. While great strength and endurance cannot always be secured, all persons can have improved staying power by improving the function of the diaphragm.

The respiratory action of the diaphragm is not its only function. It also has a definite effect on the great abdominal and thoracic veins which are attached to and pass through it. As the diaphragm descends in contraction and ascends in relaxation, all the organs and the blood vessels attached to it must also descend and ascend. As can be seen at operation on the posterior abdomen, the inferior vena cava is lengthened and shortened with every excursion of the diaphragm. This increases and decreases the size of the vein and, in consequence, the amount of blood present. Because of this, every excursion forces the blood onward and upward into the right side of the heart, where it is pushed onward once more. Therefore, if the excursion is very small, the venous circulation must have lost one of its most valuable aids and there is reason to expect congestion of the abdominal and the pelvic organs, as well as back pressure in the legs, as is seen in varicose veins. This failure of the diaphragm to pump the blood to the right side of the heart is also a possible explanation of the fact that some people invariably faint when they try to stand at attention for any length of time.

Drag and Pathologic Conditions. Another factor to be considered is that the low position of the diaphragm, with its accompanying habitual small excursion, also must mean a drag on the heart, the suspensory ligament of the diaphragm (Fig. 24) and the nerves which come to the heart, the stomach and the diaphragm, such as the vagus and the phrenic and the sympathetic nerves. (Fig. 25) Since the phrenic nerves which innervate the diaphragm arise

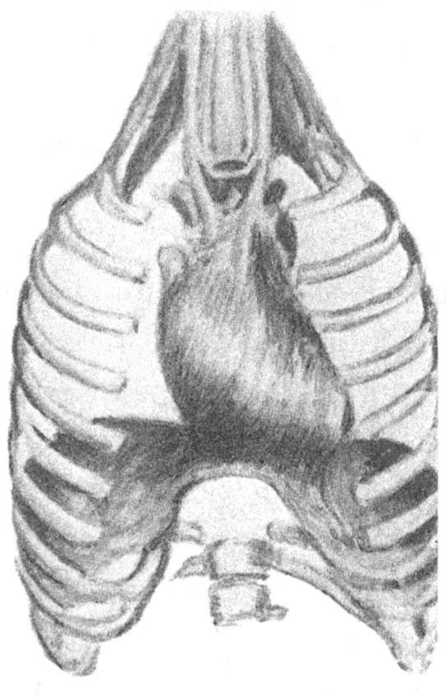

FIG. 24 A plate from Spalteholz Anatomy showing the suspensory ligament of the diaphragm, which is a continuation of the cervical fascia

from the fifth and the sixth cervical nerves, and since the nerves running to part of the shoulder and the arm also come from the fifth and the sixth cervical roots, the reason is clear why pathologic conditions in the gall bladder or the stomach or the heart, by a drag on the phrenic nerves, may cause symptoms in the shoulder and the arm. Conversely, one sees the reason that a forward-drooped position of the shoulder or a markedly flattened chest, with a marked lordotic curve of the cervical spine, may cause pain in the region of the heart or the abdomen; also, the reason that abdominal conditions, such as gas on the stomach, may cause symptoms referable to the heart, owing to sudden changes of position or pressure on the diaphragm, causing stimulation of the vagi or the sympathetic nerves. If such results can arise from sudden changes, the application over long periods of time of lesser stimuli through the habitual faulty use of the diaphragm is a possible cause of subsequent pathologic changes in these organs.

The abdominal and the pelvic organs can also be greatly affected by low position and faulty action of the diaphragm. With the relaxed abdominal wall which may accompany faulty body mechanics, muscular actions, such as coughing or lifting heavy weights, which are accomplished commonly by pushing the diaphragm still farther down, may cause unaccustomed and uncompensated strains in the lower abdominal and the pelvic regions. Inguinal and femoral hernias are believed to come from congenital weaknesses in the fascia and aponeurosis of the lower abdomen. Trauma and increased pressure from the downward displacement of the organs cause strain and overstretching of the fascia. If this continues, an opening develops at the weak area. Omentum or intestine can be forced through this opening. When a hernia is already present, correction of the body mechanics of the lower abdomen lessens the tendency of the viscera to be displaced through the opening in the fascia. Improvement in body mechanics before operation for hernia gives greater assurance that the hernia will not recur. Such strains (and pressures) are a possible cause of hernia in men and of pelvic congestion or malposition of the pelvic organs in women. In the treatment of these conditions it is essential not only that the local abdominal or pelvic condition be given attention but also that the fundamental faulty body mechanics be corrected. Frequently correction not only has obviated the necessity of local surgical treatment but also has relieved many cases of dysmenorrhea. According to the studies of Miller, dysmenorrhea can be caused by the congestion of, and pressure upon, the uterus as seen in faulty body mechanics. Unless maldevelopment of the pelvic organs or infection is present also, improvement or complete relief of the dysmenorrhea follows improvement of the body mechanics.

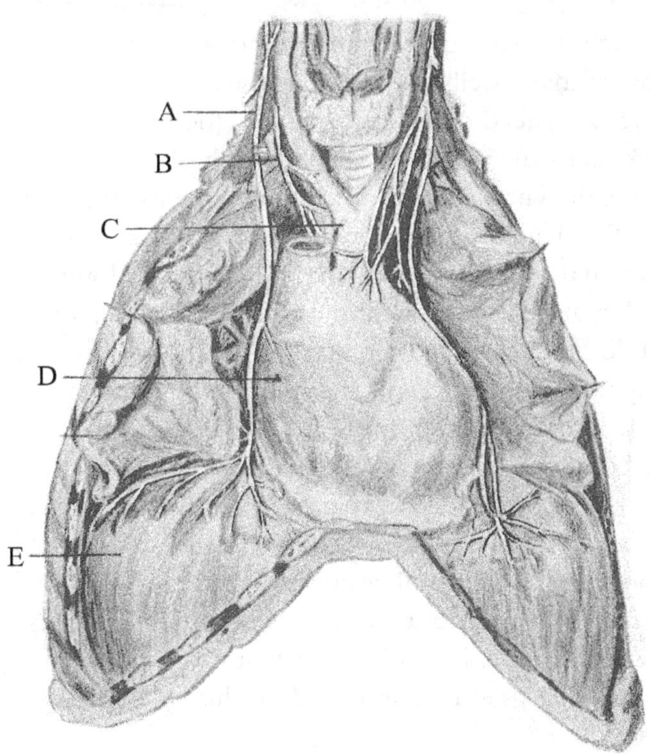

FIG. 25. Sketch of thoracic cavity showing: (A) Right phrenic nerve, (B) right vagus nerve, (C) superior vena cava, (D) heart and pericardium, (E) diaphragm. This picture suggests the way in which ptosis of the heart and the diaphragm may affect these nerves and muscles.

Effects of Faulty Mechanics. The effects of faulty mechanics on the abdominal viscera are understood more easily if considered in connection with what has been said concerning the diaphragm. In the first place, it is necessary to realize that there is no one position that is absolutely essential for the function of each of the abdominal organs, but that, within a given range, there are certain positions which must be considered normal or best for the health of the individual. The stomach, whether of the transverse or the tubular type, should be in the upper part of the abdomen, above the umbilicus. The liver also should be in the upper part of the abdomen, and its main axis should be horizontal. Of necessity there must be more or less mobility of these organs, and their position must vary considerably at different times during the day or the night in each individual. In the slender anatomic type with the tubular stomach (which, when sagged, becomes the fishhook type), the lower border of the stomach is farther down in the abdomen than in the stocky type. However, it should be realized that, with the extreme sag of the stomach, such as occurs in the fishhook or J stomach, there must be sagging of the other abdominal organs as well. For example, the liver may sag downward and rotate so that the long axis is vertical instead of horizontal, with the right border at or below the crest of the ilium. This can occur only when the diaphragm has sagged, leaving little or no space under the ribs. Therefore, the vital factor is not so much the exact position of the stomach or the other viscera as it is the shape of the cavity in which these organs are located (Fig. 26).

Shape of Abdominal Cavity. In good body mechanics the abdominal cavity is large, broad and deep in the lower-rib region, the epigastrium is full, and, on palpation, there is considerable firmness. The lower abdomen is less prominent than the upper abdomen and is in the same vertical plane or slightly posterior to it. This means that the internal shape of the abdominal cavity is that of a pear with the larger end upward. The anterior wall is largely muscular; the lateral walls are mostly bony, for example, the ribs and the ilia; and the posterior wall is made up of the ribs, the muscles, the lower dorsal vertebrae and the lumbar vertebrae and the retroperitoneal fat surrounding the kidneys. Because of the larger size of the lumbar vertebrae and the normal forward convexity of the lumbar curve, because of the smaller size of the dorsal curve and because the top of the diaphragm in good body mechanics is at the level of the eighth or the ninth dorsal vertebra, it can be seen that the abdominal organs have a definite shelf on which to rest and that they are supported on this shelf by the firm lower abdominal muscles

It is interesting to note the changes in the shape of the abdominal cavity in faulty body mechanics. Here the cavity is elliptical or pear-shaped, with the larger end downward. The chest having drooped downward, the lower ribs become crowded together. The anteroposterior and the lateral diameters change, so that at the same vertebral level there is less depth and more width, or possibly more depth and less width, than is found in good body mechanics. The

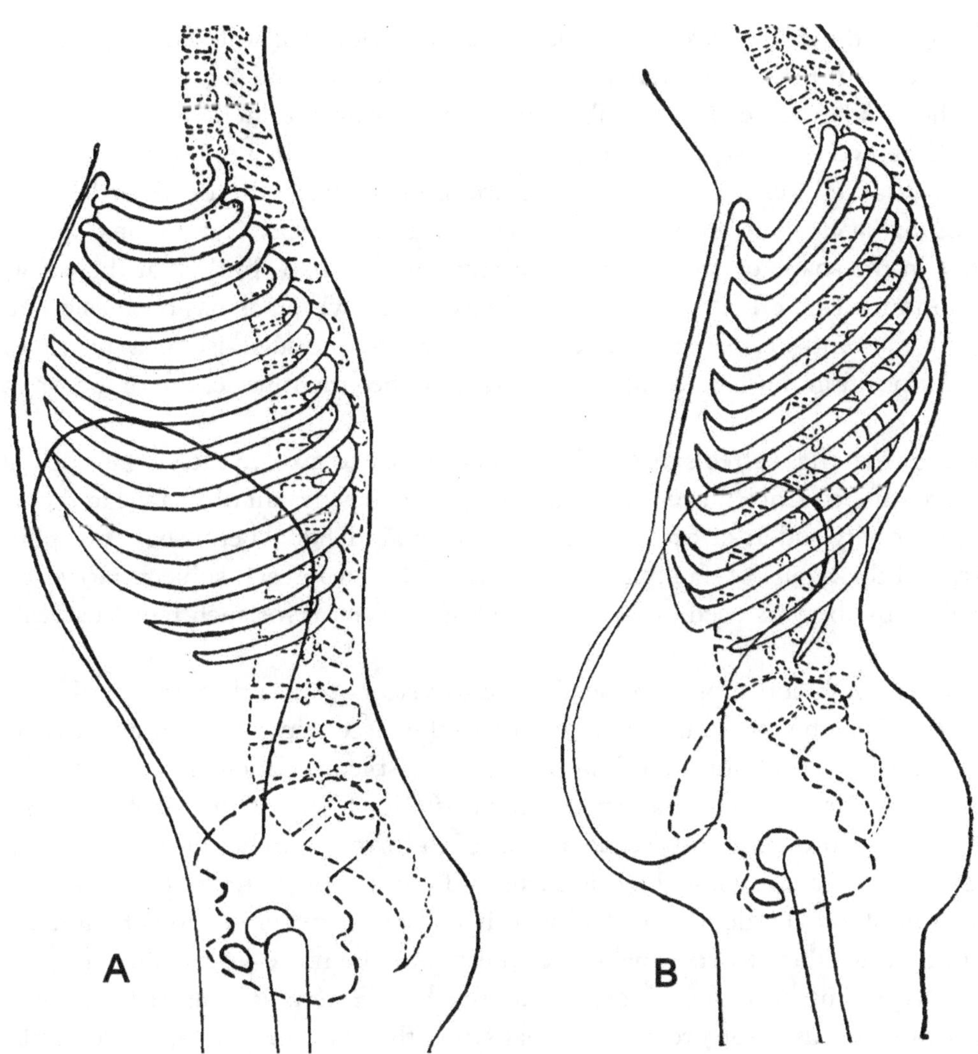

FIG. 26. (A) Diagram of the thoracic and abdominal cavities in good body mechanics. Note how the diaphragm arches upward and forward from the spine, and that the upper abdominal cavity is the deepest part. (B) Diagram of thoracic and abdominal cavities in faulty body mechanics. Note increase in vertical length of thorax and decrease in depth, that the ribs are much closer to the ilium and are farther posterior and more nearly vertical. The abdominal cavity has completely changed its shape, being larger in its lower part. Note the changes in the shape and position of the diaphragm. Note the change in the spinal curves and the contour of the body as a whole, as well as the inclination of the pelvis.

lowered position of the chest makes possible a relaxed abdominal wall, an increase of the posterior convexity of the dorsal and the dorsolumbar curve and an increased anterior convexity of the lumbar curve. The possible good effect from the increase in the posterior abdominal shelf caused by these increased curves is counteracted by the low position of the diaphragm, the lessened vertical height of the abdominal cavity, the decreased lateral or anteroposterior diameter of the upper abdominal cavity and the relaxed abdominal wall.

This change in the shape of the abdominal cavity comes on so slowly that there may be very little or no immediate effect on the enclosed viscera. However, as has been said before, such a change is a potential cause of trouble, since the long-continued use of a muscle or an organ in a faulty position must be compensated for in either the muscle, the organ or some other part.

In considering what these effects may be it is not necessary to take up each organ separately. A general picture will be sufficient. As has been said before, the amount of change in the shape of the abdominal cavity and its effect must vary with every individual because no two persons are built alike, and the habits of faulty mechanics are different in each subject. However, of whatever build, if the body is used incorrectly, the compensation for such faulty use will fail sooner or later.

Arterial System. The blood supply to the abdominal viscera comes through the abdominal aorta. The celiac axis is the most important branch to the viscera in the abdominal cavity, for through it comes the blood supply of stomach, liver, spleen, pancreas, duodenum, and omentum. This vessel leaves the aorta between the posterior fibers of the diaphragm as they arise from the sides of the spine and ascend and cross to form the arch under which the aorta passes (Fig. 27). Immediately below the celiac axis and crossed by it are the pancreas and the transverse portion of the duodenum. In faulty body mechanics, where the diaphragm and all the organs attached to it are forced downward, there must be more or less dragging on the celiac axis, with pressure on the pancreas and the duodenum. In this region and also surrounding the celiac axis is the great abdominal sympathetic nerve plexus, the solar plexus. One of its chief functions is a controlling action on the circulation. The effect of a severe blow on the solar plexus may produce all the symptoms of shock. It is well recognized that to avoid surgical shock in operations on the upper-abdominal region extreme care must be used to prevent undue stretching or pulling of the mesentery or the viscera. The possibility of drag or pressure on these vessels and nerves is very great in faulty body mechanics, with the accompanying changes in the shape of the abdominal cavity, the faulty use of the diaphragm and the lowered position of all the organs.

Venous System. Since the anatomic arrangement of the venous system in this region is somewhat similar to the arterial system, the conditions which affect the one must cause a disturbance to the other. Interference with venous circulation will cause congestion of the organs from which the veins come. With the present belief that chronic passive congestion

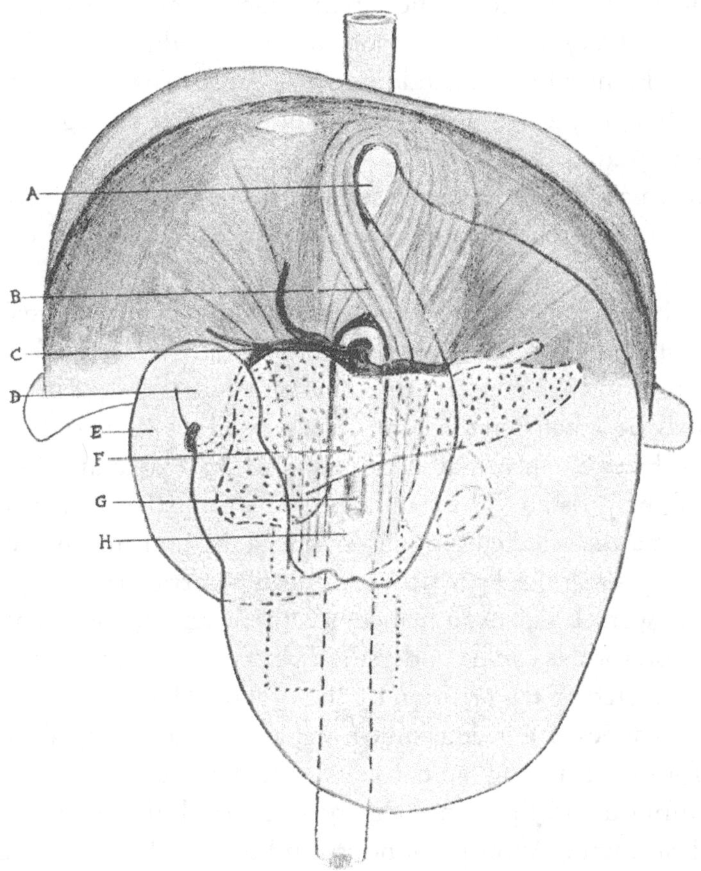

FIG. 27. Sketch of diaphragm. **(A)** Opening in diaphragm for cardiac end of stomach. Note how the fibers of the diaphragm surround this opening. **(B)** Crura of diaphragm crossing above the aorta as it enters the abdominal cavity. **(C)** Celiac axis coming from aorta just below the crura of the diaphragm. Note the branches to liver, spleen, stomach and duodenum. **(D)** First part of duodenum. **(E)** Second part of duodenum which is retroperitoneal. **(F)** Pancreas. **(G)** Superior mesenteric artery emerging from abdominal aorta behind the pancreas. **(H)** Abdominal aorta. From this diagram it can be seen that ptosis of the stomach and other abdominal organs may easily cause interference in the arterial or the venous circulation to the pancreas or other viscera in this region.

and chronic irritation are two of the factors that may lead to malignant changes, the potentialities of faulty body mechanics in the abdomen are serious when it is realized how commonly malignant disease is found there. The same factors may also be reasons for much of the indigestion and the symptoms in the epigastric region which are the fore-runners of gastric or duodenal ulcer.

The conditions which result in congestion in the stomach are likewise a cause of congestion in the other abdominal organs, the liver, the spleen and the kidneys, and the small and the large intestines. Congestion in the kidneys is undoubtedly a cause of the condition called orthostatic albuminuria, in which albumin is found in the urine collected during the daytime but not in that collected at night or after resting.

The congestion which also must be present in the large intestine probably is one of the causes of constipation, so often the latter is relieved by exercise and the correction of faulty body mechanics.

The congestion which may occur in the abdominal viscera with habitual faulty positions of the body naturally will tend to occur also in the pelvic organs, the same factors existing in both regions. The congestion and the constant irritation which must occur in the male pelvis under similar conditions may be a factor in the congested prostates seen in older men when no other cause can be found. Here again it may be a factor in the explanation of the frequency of malignant disease of the prostate. The female pelvis, with its larger size, its large organs and greater blood supply, may be affected seriously by the faulty body mechanics. In some women's colleges where carefully supervised physical education is carried on, the painful menstruation so common in young women has been helped greatly by an improvement in the habitual use of the body. The reason for this can be understood when one realizes how much the circulation in the pelvis can be affected by the position of the organs. Much of the gynecologic disability and long periods of weakness following some pregnancies can be explained on the theory that the compensation for long-standing faulty body mechanics has been broken by the burden of pregnancy and parturition and that, once this has occurred, the body is unable to regain its compensation and strength. A proper understanding of the correction of faulty body mechanics would avoid much of this trouble. The pelvic organs in the female are one of the most common sites of malignant disease, and here again, even more than elsewhere, are the same factors of chronic congestion and irritation.

4

Developmental Deformities

Many deformities develop throughout the growing years. Sometimes these arise from diseases of the bones or of the muscles; however, a large number are simply the result of prolonged faulty use of the body. The skeletal framework invariably grows in a definite manner, and outside influence can wholly change its inherent tendency to assume a certain shape. To some extent, however, the normal development and the size of the bones are dependent on the pressures and the stresses of normal function. The normal growth and development of a bone are dependent upon the inherent tendency of the bone to grow in a certain manner and upon the stresses and the pulls that come upon the bone. A lack of these is seen particularly well in the pelves and the lower extremities of children who never have walked. In those deformities recognized as the result of disease of the bone (for example, rickets), the sole effect is a softening of the bone; its bending and ultimate shape are dependent entirely on mechanical factors. In the same manner, permanent muscular weaknesses lead to failure in the normal support of a portion of the body, the position which it assumes depending on gravity, muscular imbalance and the general alignment of the entire body.

THE HEAD

Deformities which appear about the head are noticed readily because the pairing of ears and eyes and the position of the nose, the mouth and the chin make such asymmetries apparent. One of the most common of these is a tilted position, either in the lateral or in the anteroposterior plane. When the head is allowed to slump, not only is there a forward or a lateral flexion, but there is usually a twist also. The latter is in many cases the result of mild abnormalities in the cervical articular facets, the pedicles, or the transverse and the spinous processes that can be found on close search in almost every skeleton. The head assumes this position habitually, if no effort is made to hold it erect, since it is the easiest one to take. After a short time contractures develop in those muscles the origin and the insertion of which have been brought closer together. This then becomes a fixed position, and the features of the face, the bones of the skull and the cervical spine adapt themselves to it.

The most evident of these changes occur in the face itself (Fig. 28). One eye may be at a higher horizontal plane than the other; one malar bone may be more prominent than the other, causing a fullness over one cheek and a flattening on the opposite side; the nose may tilt sidewise, or one corner of the mouth may be higher than the other. In the maxilla and the mandible alterations in growth may lead to malocclusion of the teeth. In the early stages such malocclusion improves with correction of the faulty body mechanics. While such alterations are taking place, changes occur in the skull, usually in the form of prominences in the region of the occiput or in the temporal region. Occasionally these deformities lead to obstruction in the upper air passages or in the accessory nasal sinuses; they are chiefly the result of altered muscular pulls. There may be faulty occlusion of teeth at the sides or in the front, resulting from a distortion of the mandible.

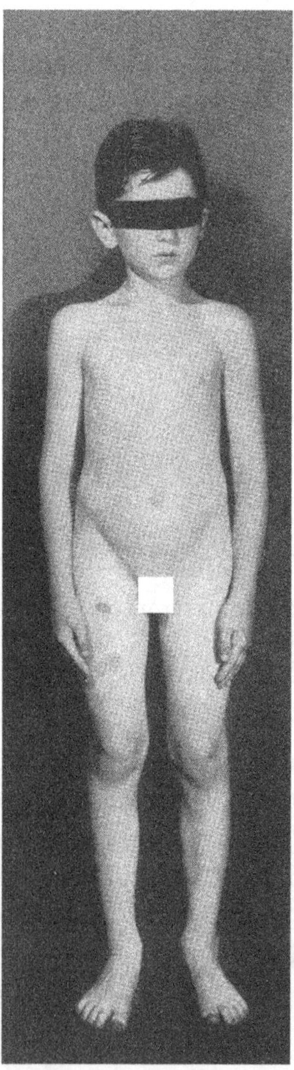

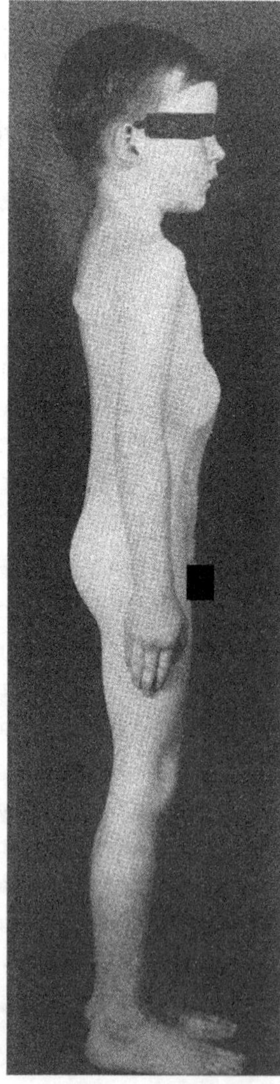

F1G. 28 (Left). There is asymmetry of the face; the right side of the face is broader, and the nose twists to the right. The right shoulder is broader. The legs show internal rotation with pronation of the feet.

FIG. 29 (Right). The chest is flat, and the shoulders are far forward. There is a depression in the lower part of the chest (Harrison's groove), with outward flaring of the lower ribs.

THE THORAX

The thorax is modified by every breath, and its habitual shape, as has been mentioned in an earlier chapter, is largely determined by the carriage of the body. With every inspiration, each rib is lifted upward and rotated outward, while the sternum is pushed upward and forward. If a relaxation of the accessory muscles of respiration is long continued, the chest becomes fixed in that position. At first it is flat. The traction of the diaphragm upon the anterior wall of the thorax is then directly inward instead of upward. This pulls the sternum inward and tends to produce a transverse groove in the thorax anteriorly, a deformity generally known as Harrison's groove (Fig.29). If there is associated with this condition a weakness or a softening of the ribs, a much greater deformity develops, with an outward flaring of the lower part of the chest.

With the anteroposterior flattening of the chest which comes with faulty body mechanics, other deformities can occur easily. There first develops a downward sagging of the entire thorax and its contents (Figs.30 A and 30B). The neck appears longer, and the shoulders assume a lower, sloping and more forward position. This leads to changes in the clavicle and in the shoulder girdle. There is frequently an increased forward curve in the midportion of the clavicle.

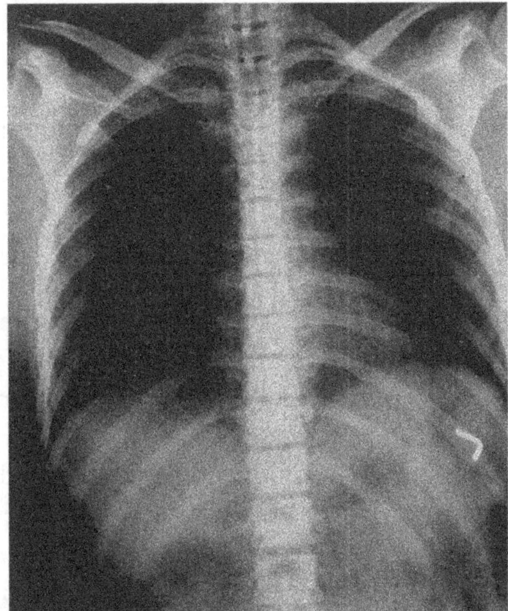

FIG.30 A. Chest of a young adult with faulty body mechanics. The scapulae and the clavicles are low, with a marked sloping of the first and the second ribs.

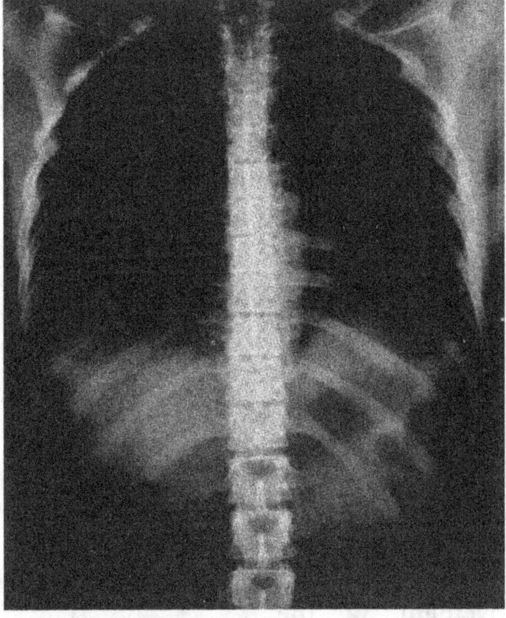

FIG.30 B. After correction of the faulty body mechanics. The scapulae and the clavicles are much higher, and the marked sloping of the first and the second ribs has been corrected.

The scapula rotates outward and downward. With this, the glenoid assumes a position in which it no longer can provide a shelf on which the head of the humerus may rest. This leads to relative instability of the shoulder joint and, when long continued, leads to changes in the coracoid and the acromion. Both these project farther downward than the normal. The body of the scapula itself follows the configuration of the posterior chest wall, its contour becoming changed from that of a fiat blade to that of a more rounded one, in order that it may fit the surface of the ribs posteriorly.

Funnel Chest. One of the most obvious, as well as most distressing, deformities of the chest is the condition known as funnel chest (pectus excavatum) (Fig.31). This may be congenital or, more commonly, developmental. While the corrective measures described in later chapters will be helpful in improving either type, we shall limit our discussion here to the developmental one. For its normal development the chest requires a proper distribution of pressures and muscular pulls from within and from without. Changes in muscular action or disturbances in the function of the lungs can change the shape of the thoracic cage, as shown in children who have had an empyema or who exhibit a permanent weakness in the thoracic muscles. Faulty body mechanics alone produce a downward and inward displacement of the sternum and an internal rotation of the ribs at the costovertebral joints. Within the chest there is a downward movement of the thoracic viscera, due to a relaxation of the mediastinal ligaments and a lowering of the diaphragm.

With this lowering, the action of the intercostales externi in expanding the horizontal diameter of the chest is lost. The anterior fibers of the diaphragm also pull almost horizontally toward the central tendon, retracting inward the lower portion of the sternum and the attached ribs. With long continuance of such disturbed function, funnel chest develops. At the same time contractures which add to the difficulty of later correction develop in the substernal ligament.

Pigeon Chest. A forward projection of the sternum, known as pigeon chest, likewise may be either congenital or developmental. It is seen more commonly in children where the costovertebral joints do not permit much downward inclination of the ribs. It may occur in faulty body mechanics from pressure on the sides of the chest or from weakness of that portion of the lateral thoracic musculature

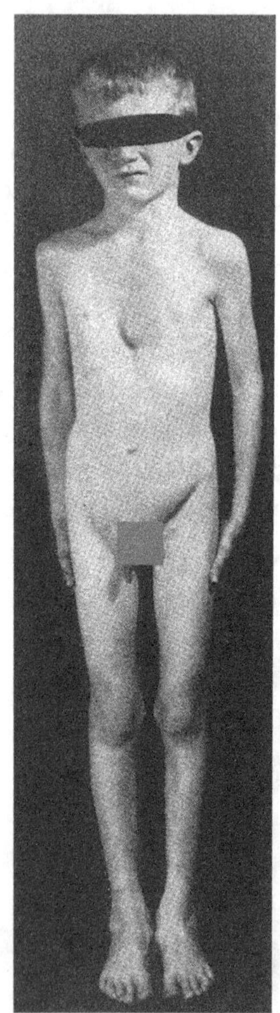

FIG. 31. Extreme funnel chest deformity associated with faulty body mechanics. An improvement in the deformity has occurred since through the partial correction of the faulty body mechanics.

which assists in inspiration. This deformity, as well as the asymmetric distortion of the chest with local elevation or depression of a portion of the chest wall, will develop more rapidly if there is any disease present which makes the bones less resistant to changes in shape.

THE SPINE

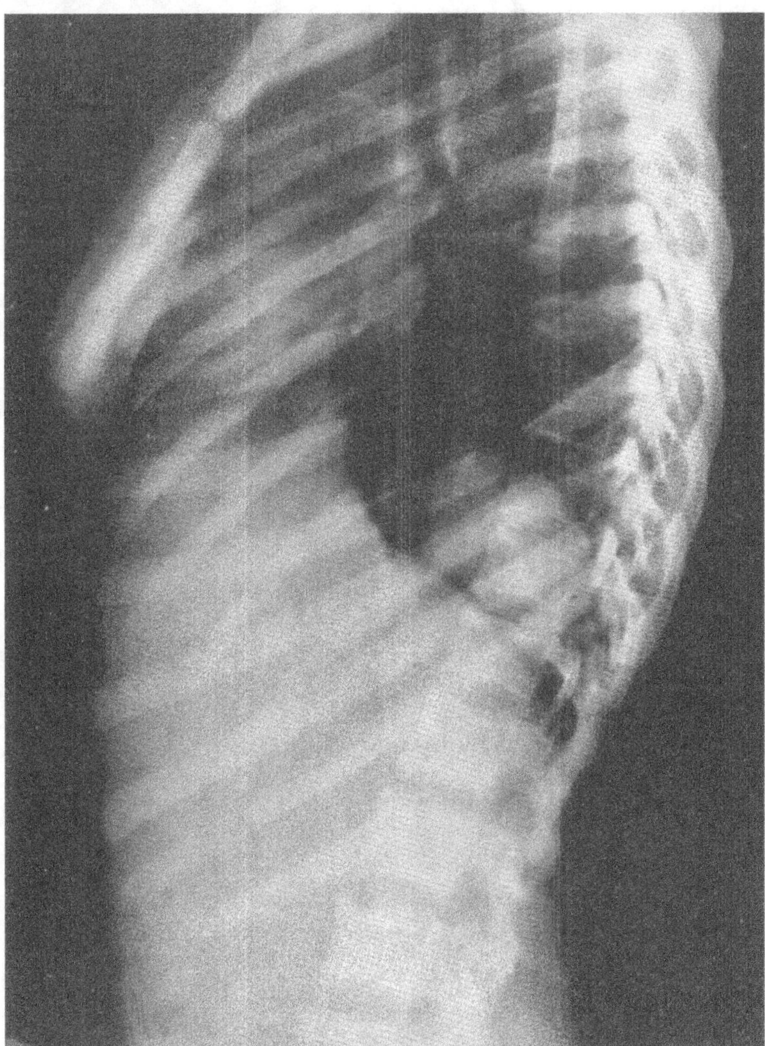

Fig.32. Lateral x-ray film of the spine of an 18 year old girl. There is anteroposterior wedging of the vertebrae in the mid-dorsal region.

Deformity in the spine and contractures of its supporting muscles occur early if there is a sag of the body which increases the anteroposterior curves. With the rounding of the dorsal spine, unusual pressure comes upon the anterior margins of the vertebrae. Should this continue throughout the growing period, a lasting deformation may occur. It shows itself as a mild anteroposterior wedging of the vertebrae at the apex of the curve (Fig.32);. This cannot be entirely corrected after full growth has occurred. A more serious vertebral deformity, called spinal epiphysitis or adolescent juvenile kyphosis, takes place if a disturbance in the epiphyses is also present.

In the lumbar spine a different type of vertebral deformity occurs. Here with faulty body mechanics, an increase in lumbar lordosis takes place which, with growth, causes a posterior narrowing or wedging of the vertebrae.

Changes also take place in the articular facets and spinous processes, most commonly as an alteration in the angle or inclination of the former. Often there is an over riding of the spinous processes or impingement, which causes thickening of the intraspinous ligaments and a bulbous flattening of the spinous processes. In the dorsal spine, with forward flexion, these processes may be bent downward markedly so that full correction of the forward flexion in adults cannot be obtained..

Scoliosis. Through faulty body mechanics, lateral curvature of the spine may develop, progressing to serious deformity and lasting changes in the vertebrae, ligaments, and ribs. This comes about more slowly than do the anteroposterior deformities of the spine. An increase of the anteroposterior curves of the spine and a relaxation of the supporting musculature occur first. A lateral curvature develops from this when there is an inequality in the supporting musculature supporting musculature occur first. A lateral curvature develops from this when there is an inequality in the supporting musculature on the two sides of the body. If, as is very common, there is an anomaly of the spine, making it less stable on one side, it often leans to the less stable side, or the pull of the muscles on one side may be less efficient. After a lateral curvature has begun it never corrects itself spontaneously. The force of gravity leads to increase of the curves with greater deformity in the spine and the thoracic cage, and with ligamentous contractures and disturbance in muscular function (Fig. 33).

Bowing of Sacrum and Coccyx. In the lower end of the spine a developmental deformity sometimes occurs in the sacrum and the coccyx. With the forward inclination of the pelvis in faulty body mechanics, there is an increase in the pull of the muscles attached to the sacrum and the coccyx because of their attempt to maintain the balance of the body. The result is a gradually increased forward bowing, a deformity seen only in roentgenograms. (Fig. 34) It leads to no serious disturbance in function except in women, where it occasionally results in difficulties in childbearing. In the development of the vertebrae from several ossification centers there may be failure of fusion. In the lower lumbar region failure of ossification of the pedicles may lead to forward slipping of the vertebral body. Such forward slipping (spondylolisthesis) is encouraged, and symptoms develop quickly, with lordosis and increased forward inclination of the pelvis (Fig. 35).

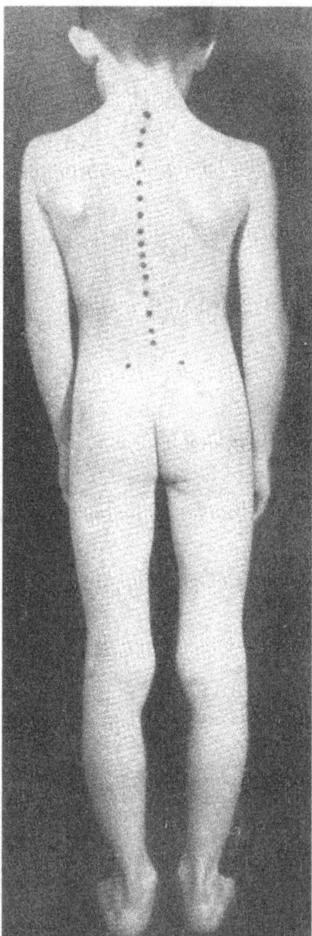

Fig.33. lateral curvature the spine associated with faulty body mechanics. There is a curve of the entire spinal column with convexity to the left. The left shoulder is higher, There is a twist of the tibiae with pronation of the feet.

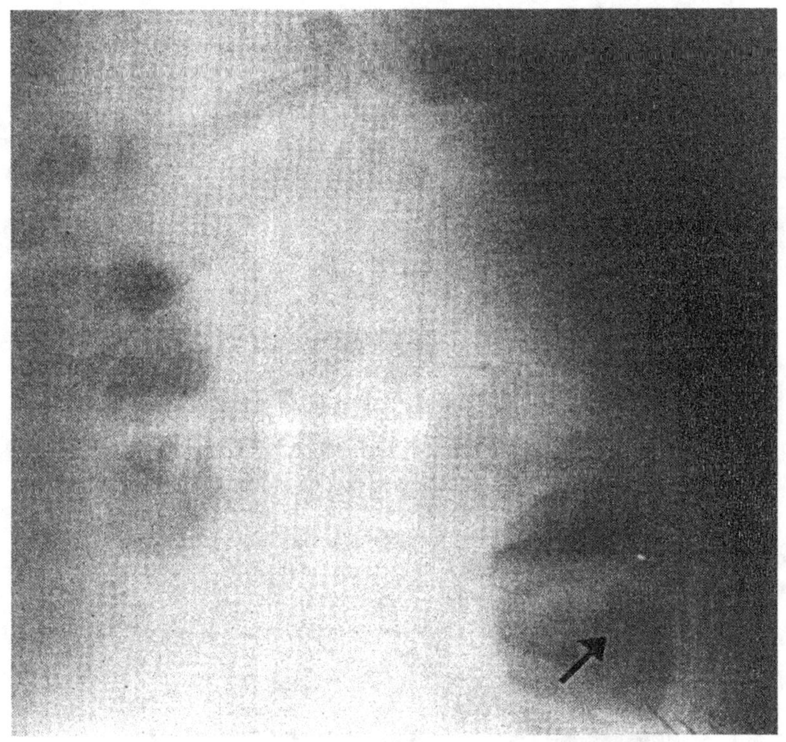

Fig.34. Lateral roentgenogram of pelvis. the sacrum is curved forward sharply in its midportion (arrow). this was caused by faulty body mechanics with increased forward inclination of the pelvis during growth.

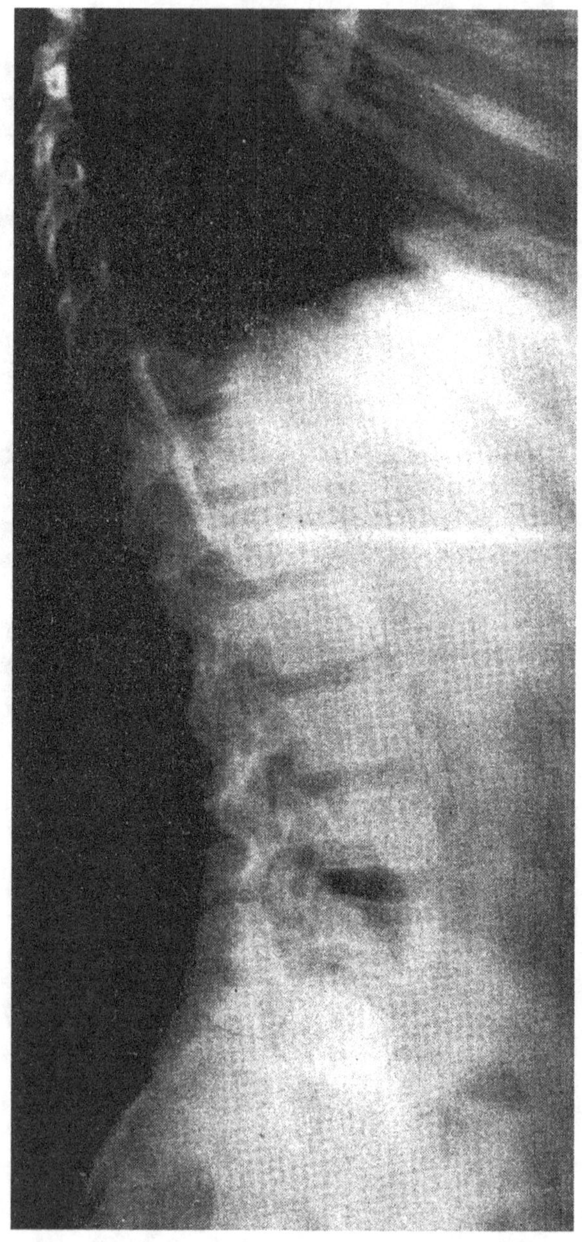

Fig.35. There is forward displacement (spondylolisthesis) of the fifth lumbar vertebrae on the sacrum in a 7 year old boy. The lumbar lordosis encourages the forward displacement and decreases the stability of the fifth lumbar vertebrae.

THE EXTREMITIES

Upper Extremities. In the upper extremities developmental deformities are seldom serious. and usually lead to little if any disability in childhood. We have already mentioned the deformities of the scapula. In the shoulder joint, relaxation in the supporting capsule and instability of the shoulder joint may occur with forward and downward displacement of the shoulder. with this there gradually develops a contraction of the internal rotators of the arm. contractures in the flexors of the forearm may also take place. these, while interfering little with function, result in strains and in bursitis and arthritis at the shoulder in later life.

Lower Extremities. In the lower extremities a number of deformities occur with faulty body mechanics. The pelvis may show changes from the alteration in the weight thrust and muscular pulls. The rami of the pubis and the ischium may project farther forward, resulting in the deformity known as ischium varum or valgum. The superior and the posterior margin of the acetabulum may be altered by the constant forward inclination of the pelvis, which also leads to a relative instability in the hip joint. the muscles about this joint are attached in such a manner that in normal function their contraction tends to pull the head of the femur into the acetabulum. When this pull is changed, as occurs when the pelvis tips forward, the action of the muscles in stabilizing the hip is lost, resulting in irritation and later arthritis at the hip joint.

Changes take place in the neck of the femur during the period of growth. With the forward inclination of the pelvis and the subsequent internal rotation of the femur in order to bring support under the changed center of gravity, there comes a tortional stress on the femoral neck, which tends to produce a coxa vara and an anteversion. A twist or an outward bowing may also appear in the shaft of the femur. These changes develop more rapidly and to a greater extent if any conditions which weaken the bones are present.

At the knee, with faulty carriage of the body, the weight is thrust more to the inner side of the joint, leading commonly to a knock-knee deformity. Distortion in growth of the epiphyses may also occur, as has been shown in experimental animals by Anderson. The tortion of the femur may be carried into the tibia, the changed thrust of weight leading to a twist or bowing in this region (Fig. 36). With the change in the origin of the hamstring muscles resulting from the forward inclination of the pelvis and the relaxation and later contracture of the iliopsoas group of muscles, a flexed or hyperextended knee is found when the patient is standing. Long continued, this condition leads to deformity in the articular surfaces of the knee joint. In middle age it is the usual cause of villous arthritis of the knee joint, as has been demonstrated by Stump.

The foot is one of the commonest sites of deformity in faulty body mechanics, the deformity most commonly seen being a valgus of the os calcis and an eversion of the forefoot. It aries chiefly from three causes: (1) The internal rotation of the leg to support the forward displacement of the center of gravity cannot occur at the ankle joint and must consequently do so in the tarsal joints. This cause a valgus of the os calcis, an inward projection of the mid-portion of the foot, and an eversion of the forefoot. (2) The faulty weight thrust projected upon the inner side of the foot tends to roll it inward, with increasing valgus. (3) With the change in the origin of the supporting muscles of the pelvis, thigh, and tibia, adequate support of the foot by the muscles is no longer possible. Contractures occur in the muscles and ligaments about the ankle joint. Changes take place in the tarsal bones, in the fore part of the foot., and in the great toe, progressing more rapidly if faulty footwear is worn.

In adults these changes take place more slowly than in childhood, and are more commonly the result of contractures than of changes in the bones.

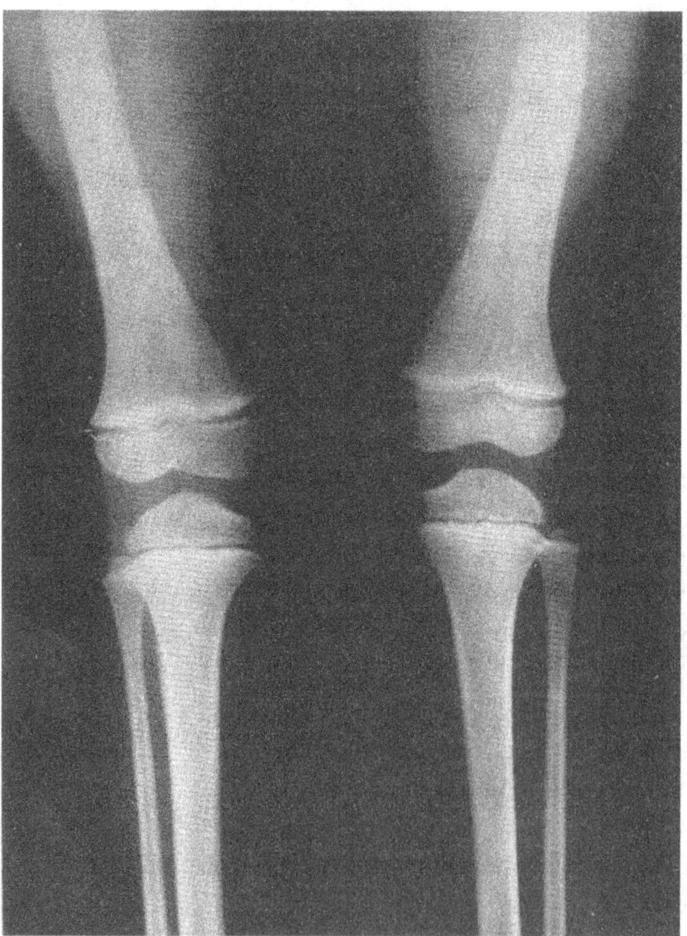

Fig. 36 X-rays of the legs of a child with knock knees and faulty body mechanics. There is an overgrowth of the lower femoral epiphyses.

5

Backache and Other Spinal Sprains

BACKACHE

The problem of backache is so extensive that it is impossible to discuss or even mention its many possible causes. Therefore this chapter is limited entirely to the mechanics of the body as a whole. An understanding of the conditions present in the back when the body is used in the position of faulty mechanics and a knowledge of how to correct this will be found to be of great benefit not only in the prevention of backache but also as a part of its treatment no matter what the cause.

In adult life, at least, backache, in one form or another, is the cause of more lessened efficiency and discomfort than is any other chronic condition. It is so common that the large majority of people, especially those of advanced age, expect to have a tired, aching back whenever they do certain things. Hence, backache is looked upon commonly as a natural misfortune of age for which nothing can be done. It is only when it lasts long enough or becomes acute enough to interfere with work or pleasure that a consultation is sought. One has only to consider the wide variety of treatments for backache, ranging from drugs to manipulations and from braces to surgery, to realize that no one of these procedures touches the fundamental cause. Nevertheless, there must be a basic cause, the proper understanding of which would tend to simplify the treatment in the same way that specific therapy has simplified the management of such conditions as typhoid and diphtheria.

Basic Mechanics. In this discussion no attempt will be made to classify the types of backache, such as lumbo-sacral, sacro-iliac and dorsolumbar, nor will the differential diagnosis between the various kinds be considered. Neither will a distinction be made between acute and chronic backache. Suffice it to say that the location of the pain is a matter of chance, and that the difference between an acute back condition and a chronic one is largely a matter of time and degree, the basic condition behind both being the same. Such conditions as tuberculosis or pyogenic osteomyelitis or organic disease of the spine also will not be discussed, for these are relatively rare compared with the so-called acute and chronic backaches. However, it is well to remember in treating these diseases that the same basic mechanical conditions may be present as are found in acute or chronic backache.

Recognition of Types. In the preceding chapters special emphasis has been laid on the fact that no two individuals are built alike or use their bodies habitually in similar ways. One has only to stand on a street corner and watch the crowds go by in order to see how differently people walk. One can realize then that every spine at every step is receiving a heavy or a light jar of the body weight from the ground. Each person has become accustomed to his own way of walking and, be it heavy or light, has more or less compensated for the strain thus caused. Therefore it is fundamental to recognize the type of individual that one is examining. By such recognition the physician is enabled to form a fundamental conception of the structure of the spine, as well as of the muscular, the nervous, the circulatory and other systems of the body. Without a knowledge of the structure of the body, by which is meant the shape of the vertebrae, the articular facets, the viscera, and so forth, it is impossible to understand the way in which the habitual use of these bones and joints in faulty mechanical positions may be a cause of strains and their accompanying symptoms.

Evaluation of Symptoms. Too often, when a patient comes to a doctor complaining of backache, an attempt is made to trace the symptoms to one specific cause: the orthopedic surgeon looks at the spine, the gynecologist, at the pelvic organs; the neurologist considers the backache a form of neurosis, the internist, a symptom of improper visceral function, and so on. However, when the patient is examined from the point of view of body mechanics, it is realized very quickly that even though the predominant symptom may be backache, the faulty mechanical condition present must affect not only the back but every other organ or system to a greater or a lesser extent. Therefore, to treat only the back or the pelvic organs or the nerves or the intestinal tract is to envisage only a small part of the picture. Of necessity, the emphasis here is laid mostly on the correction of the spinal mechanics, but, as has been said previously, what is done to correct the spinal mechanics also will correct the faulty mechanics of the rest of the body. In order to explain all this more fully, a typical case of backache is cited.

Case History. A man of fifty had suffered off and on for years from an aching and tired back, which developed after every unusual effort. Gradually, the back became really painful, with occasional attacks of sciatica, occurring, for no reason known to the patient, first in one leg and then in the other. At first, the attacks were infrequent and occurred only when he was tired or after he had remained in one position too long. As time went by the attacks became more common, until the patient was unable to ride in an automobile, or to lift anything, or at times to lean over to put on his shoes, without getting a catch in his back. Many forms of treatment, varying from medicines to surgery, had been advised. From the point of view of body mechanics, it was essential to inquire into the patient's history and to find out about other conditions which might or might not be present. In other words, it was necessary to realize that a man with a backache was being treated, and not just a backache. Of equal importance in this case was a long standing history of indigestion, constipation, extreme headaches and nervousness, for all of which hospital and sanatorium treatment had been given. Of course, knowledge of these symptoms immediately revealed that the backache was only a part of the trouble, and that associated with it was a general run-down condition, with poor functioning of all the systems of the body. The patient himself, being unusually intelligent and mentally stable, realized that his condition was entirely due to long hours of overwork, with an unwise amount of exercise. Like so many people, he had thought that plenty of exercise was an antidote for the sedentary nature of his work. Therefore, any constructive treatment had to take into account all these factors.

THE PHYSICAL EXAMINATION was entirely negative from a pathologic and medical point of view but, from a physiologic and functional aspect, was extremely illuminating. Fig. 37 shows (l) that the patient was of the slender anatomic type and (2) that he was using his body at the extreme of faulty body mechanics. The motions of the spine were without any protective

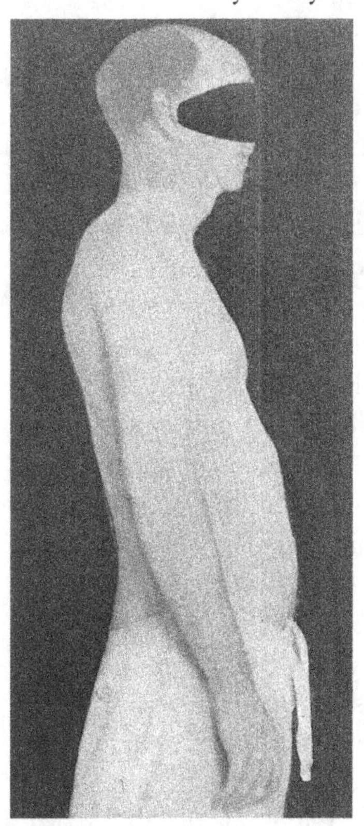

muscular spasm except at the extreme of flexion. In the habitual standing position there was no motion in extension in the low-lumbar spine, and attempts at such motion caused discomfort. In the forward flexed position there was tenderness over the interspinous ligament between the fifth lumbar vertebra and the sacrum; probably it was due to an occasional impingement of the spinous processes which must have occurred in the habitual position in which the back was used. There was also some tenderness immediately below the posterior-superior spines of the ilia, which sometimes is considered to be due to sacro-iliac strain. Limitation of straight leg raising was present, with pain referred to the back as well as to the thigh and the leg. The latter findings suggested sacro-iliac strain as a cause of the trouble, and undoubtedly there was strain on these joints because it is difficult to see how any spine, and particularly one in a slender type of individual, could be used in habitually faulty mechanics without causing at least some secondary strain to the sacro-iliac joints. The hip motions were free and without any muscular spasm so long as there was no motion of the pelvis or the lumbar spine.

FIG. 37. Patient of slender type, with backache, showing extremely faulty body mechanics. The habitual faulty posture shows that, in the standing position, the low back is used at the extreme of extension, as must occur when the chest and the upper part of the body are carried so far posterior to the hips. Of necessity, with this curve comes increased dorsal curve, drooped chest and prominent lower abdomen. Forward head and increased cervical curve are natural accompaniments of faulty posture. The outwardly flared lower ribs show that faulty posture has been present habitually for years.

Examination of the spine was made not only in the standing but also in the sitting, the prone and the knee-hand positions. The latter position was advantageous because it took the weight of the upper body off the vertebrae and thus gave information on the freedom of motion not only of the spinal joints but also of the ribs and their position in relation to the transverse processes. It also made possible an examination of the tone of the abdominal muscles and the determination of their condition and position. Further examination in the standing position revealed, as was to be expected from the faulty mechanics, that the chest was used habitually in a position approximating full expiration: in other words, the ribs were crowded together at the sides, the subcostal angle was narrow, and the vertical length of the chest in relation to its circumference was extreme; the lower ribs were flared outward at the costal margin, and the latter deformity was not correctable in full inspiration. Breathing in the standing position consisted of very shallow respiration, with most of the motion occurring in the lower part of the abdomen below the umbilicus; also, there was an occasional deep sighing respiration in which the whole chest cage was considerably raised as well as changed in shape.

Examination in the standing position showed the upper abdomen to be relatively shallow and small and the lower abdomen, protuberant, with no muscle tone. The upper abdomen allowed easy palpation of the posterior abdominal wall and the great vessels. Palpation of the lower abdomen showed the abdominal viscera to be very heavy and situated mostly below the umbilicus. When the lower abdomen was compressed suddenly by the examiner's hand, there was a marked expulsion of air from the mouth because of the sudden upward movement of the diaphragm when relaxed at its lowest position. This indicated that not only the abdominal muscles but all the abdominal viscera were relaxed and were being used at or near one extreme of their possible positions. The heaviness of the viscera could be explained by congestion due to the slowing of the circulation, which was necessarily present when all the organs and the muscles were used in such faulty mechanical positions. In the standing position it was possible to note how great was the downward inclination of the ribs and how long the chest was in relation to the total body length. Bimanual palpation of the abdomen at the costovertebral region revealed the presence of very little substance, and, in the lying position, there was so little musculature and retroperitoneal fat that even close to the transverse processes the fingers of the two palpating hands practically touched, with nothing but the two layers of skin between them. Palpation of the epigastrium, in the standing position as well as in the lying position, showed a marked crease or hollow, and the abdominal aorta could be felt easily. In other words, the viscera which should have been in the epigastrium, and the retroperitoneal fat which should have given them support to stay there, had been pushed or dragged out of position.

Examination in the standing position from the rear showed that the gluteal or buttock muscles were small and flabby and that there was little or no capacity for active muscle contraction. This lack of tone was due to the fact that in the habitual standing position these muscles were mechanically so relaxed that they could not function easily, and so other muscle groups had taken up their work. The feet showed faulty statics, as was evidenced by more or less pronation and sagging of the arches. Such pronation means lack of spring and elasticity, resulting in increased strain on the knees and the back.

The patient also showed other effects of fatigue and strain. The eyes looked tired, and the sclera had lost its glistening appearance; the skin of the face looked heavy and had a poor color; there were lines under the eyes; the circulation of the hands and the feet was poor, as evidenced by congestion, coldness and clamminess.

X-ray examination of the spine showed no anatomic abnormality, but there was definite evidence of a generalized atrophic condition of the vertebrae, as shown by the contrast between the shadows of the bodies of the vertebrae and the soft parts. This is a very common condition in the slender type where there is a long-standing story of fatigue. This can be considered as an evidence of faulty physiology which has not yet reached the stage of organic pathology.

Fluoroscope tracings of the diaphragm and the heart, taken in the standing, as well as the lying position, added one more factor in the picture of a tired individual with poor body mechanics. The diaphragm was very low, and the excursion was less than in lying: the position of the diaphragm in ordinary respiration was at or near that at full inspiration. The position and the shape of the heart were also interesting. Being of the slender type, it was more nearly vertical than transverse, and in standing its location was two or more vertebrae lower than in lying. As would be expected with a low position of the heart, there was an equally low position of the arch of the aorta. This well might mean a more acute angle of the aortic arch, which possibly could affect the ease of flow of the blood stream and exert some reflex effect on the blood pressure. These mechanical differences, which were due to the ptosis of the diaphragm as well as of the heart, well may have been one of the associated causes of the general run-down condition of the patient which led to his symptoms.

With the picture suggested by such a history and such an examination, it is evident that the back symptoms were only a part of the story and that sooner or later the faulty body mechanics must of necessity have led to a breakdown somewhere in the body. With this patient it was the back which gave the most prominent symptom at the time of examination, but the other symptoms were of equal importance.

With such an understanding of the ordinary case of backache, it is easy to understand that the treatment must be planned not only to relieve the back symptoms but also to include the rest of the body.* Therefore the patient was put to bed, even though at first it seemed that this aggravated all the symptoms, because the only sure way to take all the strain off the back was to put the spine in a horizontal position, and thus to take the weight off the vertebral bodies and the articular facets.

It can be understood easily that for a less severe case the form of treatment described can be modified to fit the circumstances so long as the fundamental principle of acquiring good or better body mechanics is carried out.

Treatment. When such a patient is put to bed, and the legs are allowed to stretch out flat, the lumbar spine is held in extension because of the pull of the iliopsoas and other anterior muscles of the thigh. This represents a position of strain. Therefore the hips and the knees must be flexed by a sufficient number of pillows to relieve any strain (Fig. 38); in this way the spinal joints are put in to a neutral position or one in which the strain is relieved. The same principle is applied to all sprains and fractures, namely, to put the joints, bones and the ligaments in the best anatomic position possible.

With the patient in the lying position, exercises are begun immediately. These are not planned primarily to strengthen the muscles but to teach the patient how to use his muscles with the body in the correct position and to maintain this position during the exercises and in everyday life. These are begun early because, as is well recognized, any muscle which is used properly becomes stronger, While a muscle which is used in a faulty position. anatomically and mechanically must compensate for the faulty mechanics before it can function properly.

The kind of exercises and the method of progression which have been found to be useful are explained in Chapter 11. In giving them one must be governed by the general condition of the patient and by the amount of correction that can be done without causing an increase of the symptoms.

When the patient gets up and begins to walk it is not to be expected that the faulty habits of a lifetime can be corrected immediately nor that the muscles, now beginning to be used in a different way, will be strong enough to hold the body in the correct position. Therefore, a support should be fitted so that it will help the patient to hold himself correctly. It should be added that no brace possibly can hold any patient in a good position without his co-operation.

The kind of brace to be used is of no importance, provided that it enables the patient to use his body in better body mechanics. Experience has shown that to accomplish this it is necessary to understand certain fundamental anatomic and mechanical principles, the exact operation of which varies in the different types of anatomy. The brace should have a firm hold of the pelvis and should be long enough in the back to give some pressure on the lower end of the sacrum. From this point it should be extended upward far enough to give a forward push to the lower ribs and the spine; otherwise there is a tendency for the patient to lean backward over the top of the brace. The back support is fastened by straps to an anterior pad made of leather and felt on a steel frame and large enough to fill the space between the anterior superior spines, the umbilicus and the pubis. The pad is held in place by perineal straps. With women, the brace is supplemented by a corset which is fitted with the same purpose of flattening the back and holding in the lower abdomen.

A brace and corset properly fitted not only hold in the lower abdomen but tend to change the curves of the back so that the lumbar curve is lessened, and the dorsal spine and the chest are carried more upward and forward. This, of course, brings the weight of the upper body and the abdomen on the lumbosacral and the sacro-iliac joints into a much better mechanical

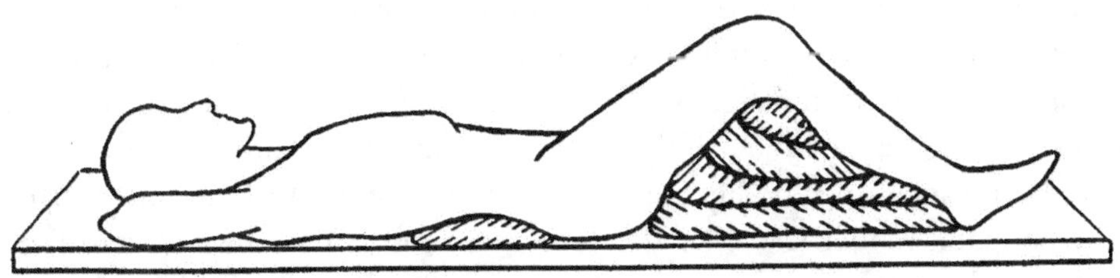

FIG. 38. Diagram showing the position in which a patient with an acute, painful back is placed in bed. The pillows under the knees flex the hips and relieve the strain on the lumbar spine. The pillow under the lower lumbar region also helps to relieve strain on the spine.

position. Special care should be taken that no pressure or constriction arises in the region of the lower ribs or the epigastrium. Whatever pressure is applied to the abdomen should be exerted upward from the pubis, never inward or downward. When a brace is employed it should be explained to the patient that it is only a temporary aid to help him get the feeling of the correct way of holding his body, and that as soon as he does so the support can be abandoned.

The end result from the point of view of body mechanics in the case reported above is shown in Figure 39. From the patient's point of view, not only was the ache entirely relieved but also the indigestion, the headaches and the nervousness. Easy fatigability disappeared, so that he was able to resume his work and to play golf and to enjoy them both.

OTHER SPINAL SPRAINS

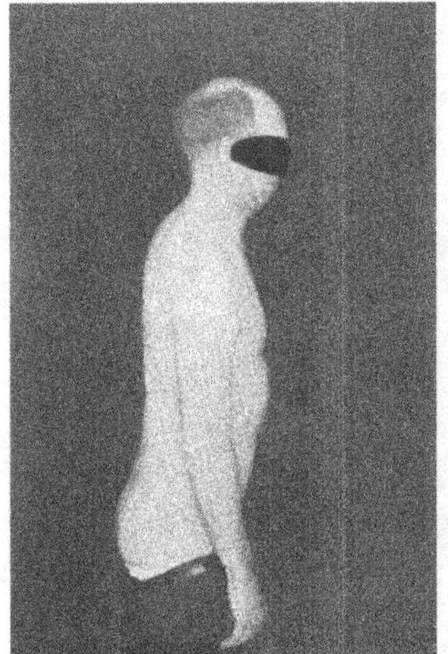

Cervical Spine. What has been said thus far in connection with backache and spinal symptoms has had to do chiefly with the lower part of the spine and the pelvic mechanism. while this region is undoubtedly the one most commonly affected, the rest of the spine must be considered also, for between every vertebra are true joints that may be strained under voluntary use or as a result of violence. There are special regions which are more likely to show symptoms because of the natural way in which the body is used, but any of the joints may cause trouble. Since the cervical spine is held

FIG. 39. Same patient as in Figure 37 after education in body mechanics. Full correction was not obtainable because of deformities from long-continued faulty use. Clinically, there was complete relief of symptoms. Note that the weight of the upper body is now over or slightly in front of the hips, which means, of course, that the lumbar spine no longer is being used at the position of full extension. The abdomen is flat, and the lower rib region, or epigastrium, has much more depth and fullness than in the original posture, Figure 37

normally in a position of moderate extension, only slight relaxation of the body will suffice to increase this position to one of complete extension, thus rendering it liable to strain or irritation. In this position the foramina, through which the nerve roots pass, must be narrowed, and pain referred to the cervical or the brachial plexuses is not difficult to understand.

Sprain of the muscles and the ligaments, as well as irritation of the intervertebral joints, can lead to local pain, tenderness over the vertebrae and to muscular spasm. Referred pain from irritation of the cervical nerves can arise from several causes. In faulty body mechanics alone, with cervical lordosis, the neural foramina may become narrowed. In later life bony overgrowth occurs about the vertebrae and their joints. This limits movement and narrows still further the neural foramina. With faulty posture and repeated mild traumas, the intervertebral disks may degenerate, bringing the vertebral bodies closer together. This usually leads to crowding and irritation of the cervical nerves (Fig. 40). If the irritation occurs chiefly in the upper cervical spine, the referred pain is usually in the occipital region, following the course

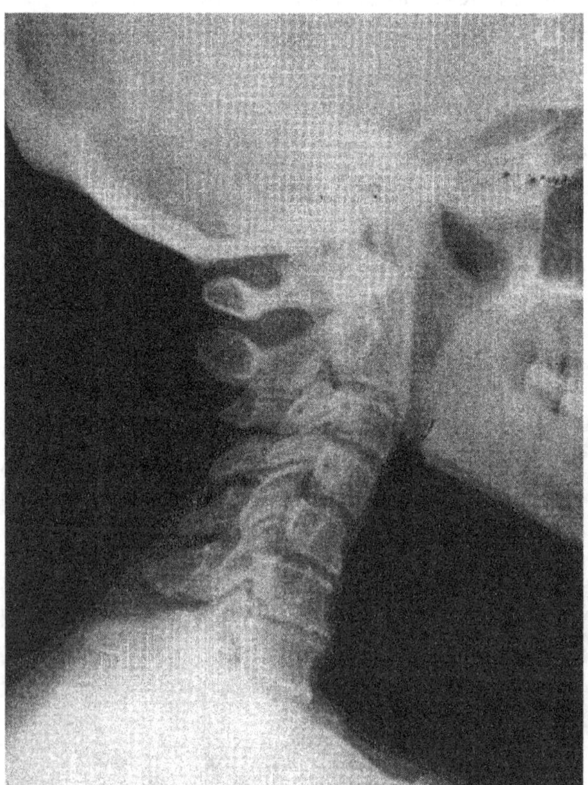

FIG. 40. Faulty body mechanics. The lower cervical spine is flat. There is extension at the third cervical vertebra. There is degeneration of the intervertebral disk between the sixth and the seventh cervical vertebrae. There is extensive hypertrophic arthritis about the margins of the vertebrae. The neural foramina are narrowed.

of the greater occipital nerve. If the deformity and the irritation are in the lower cervical region, the referred pain may be felt in the upper back but more commonly over the shoulder and in the arm. Such pain frequently leads to an erroneous diagnosis of sprain or bursitis about the shoulder.

Thoracic Spine. The thoracic spine is susceptible to strain in any of its joints. The cervicodorsal region, with marked rounding of the upper dorsal spine as a part of poor body mechanics, is very commonly the seat of trouble. Pain may be referred locally down the arms; at times there may be virtual paralysis of the different groups of muscles. With increased forward bowing in the mid-thoracic region, pain often is found in the interscapular region. This is usually muscular strain from excessive pull upon the trapezius muscles, particularly their attachments to the thoracic spinous processes. With severe thoracic kyphosis and round shoulders, a bursitis may develop beneath the scapulae. Because of the marked flexibility of the spine at the dorsolumbar juncture, this also is strained frequently. Here pain is referred to as kidney pain. In many cases this is due to joint strain, but equally often it is caused by the sag of the last rib against the transverse process of the first lumbar vertebra. Furthermore, it requires special attention on account of the articulation of the ribs, since it is in this region that many patients have symptoms, and from it that pains are referred commonly. In addition to the spinal joints there are 44 separate joints associated with the spine and the rib mechanism; hence this topic merits special consideration.

Rib Joints. There are 24 joints, called the costo-vertebral joints, formed by the juncture of the heads of the ribs with the sides of the spine. Beside these there are 20 joints, the costotransverse, formed by the angle of the ribs and the outer part of the transverse processes of the upper 10 dorsal vertebrae. Each of these 44 joints involved in the mechanism of the thorax is a true joint and is as liable to disease or injury as are others, with the added disadvantage that, while most other joints after periods of activity have periods of rest, the rib joints, unless they become ankylosed from disease, never are completely at rest so long as life lasts.

The costovertebral joints for the upper 10 dorsal vertebrae are so placed that part of the articulation of the head of the rib is with the vertebra above, and part with the vertebra below. The intervertebral disks lying between the two vertebrae are just in front of the costovertebral joints. The two lower ribs form their articulation with the sides of the eleventh and the twelfth dorsal vertebrae and do not override the intervertebral disks.

The costotransverse joints usually are placed with their articular surfaces on the anterior part of the transverse processes but at times they are actually on top of them; all possible variations between these two extremes occur (Fig. 41). If the rib articulates on the top of the process, the articular surface is at times horizontal, at other times, oblique. Sometimes the location of the costotransverse joints varies in the same individual. Several of the vertebrae, usually those in the middle section, have their articulation on the upper part of the transverse processes, while others have it directly in front of them.

Another feature of considerable importance in the mechanics of the function of the rib joints is the length of the transverse processes. Sometimes they are very short, at other times long. The difference which the length of a process makes in the degree of leverage exerted by the main part of the rib on the costovertebral joint is obvious

The range of motion in the rib joints is limited by the anatomic structure and by the muscles and the ligaments, the extreme range being enough to allow a movement of the thorax in full respiration yielding from 3 to 5 inches difference in chest circumference. To ensure the normal use of these joints, the body should be so held that the neutral position is about midway between that at full inspiration and that at full expiration. To obtain this position the ribs should slope downward from the spine' at an angle of about 30°.

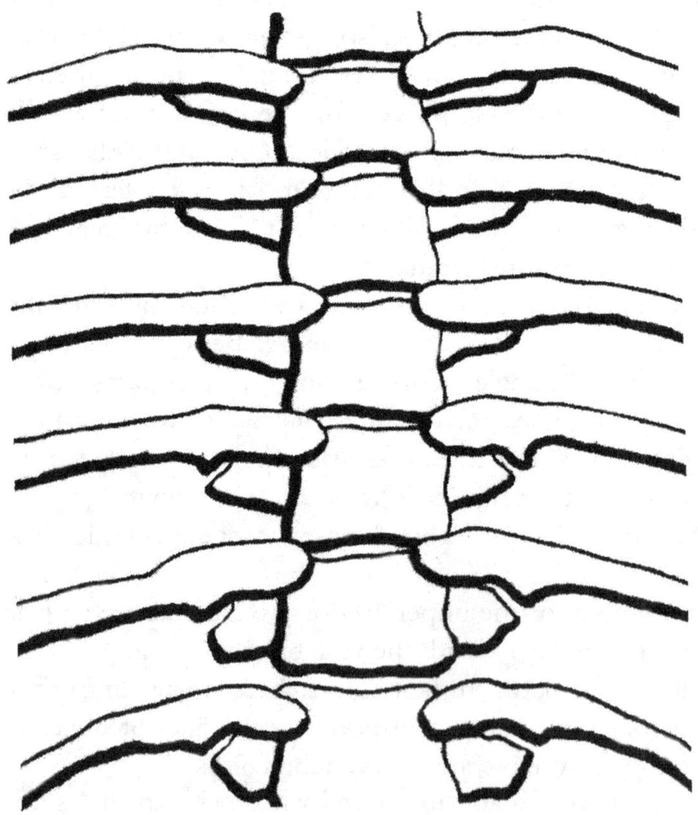

FIG. 41. Sketch of the rib joints. There are two joints for each rib— one between the rib and the vertebra, and another between the rib and the transverse process. These joints can be sprained readily when there is increased downward inclination of the shaft of the ribs.

Sprain and Strain. As the body often is used, the chest is sagged, and the head and the shoulders are rounded forward, so that the ribs hang below the normal low point of rib function. This means that the muscles and the ligaments are out of balance, and the inevitable strain, if continued for any length of time, must result in weakness and joint irritation. When the chest is lowered the position of any one rib depends to a considerable extent on the position of the costotransverse joint, for if the articulation is on top of the transverse process, sagging of the rib must result either in rotation of the head out of its normal position, or the rib may act as a fulcrum and pry it above that position. However, whether the costotransverse articulation is on the top of the transverse process or in front of it, the rib, in sagging, must use this joint as a fulcrum and either twist the rib and thus rotate the head abnormally or actually force it into an abnormal position. With the rib joints, as with any of the others, these faulty positions, if long maintained, must cause irritation, together with changes in structure—a true arthritic condition (Fig. 42).

With such a condition, the symptoms resulting from the mechanical strain may be referred to the region of the costovertebral joints at the back or along the sides of the chest. The latter strain is due to the fact that each intercostal nerve trunk leaves the spine at the level of the corresponding costovertebral joint and passes along the rib. Irritation of the nerve root causes symptoms to be referred to its distribution.

Referred Pain. Today very few cases of pain referred to the back of the leg, a condition formerly called sciatica, are treated with reference to the leg symptoms; instead, most of these cases are recognized as being due to abnormal conditions in the low back. Likewise, many cases of pain referred to the chest wall, or around the body at the different levels, with nothing showing in the chest examination, are explained easily by the irritation of the intercostal nerves at the costovertebral joints.

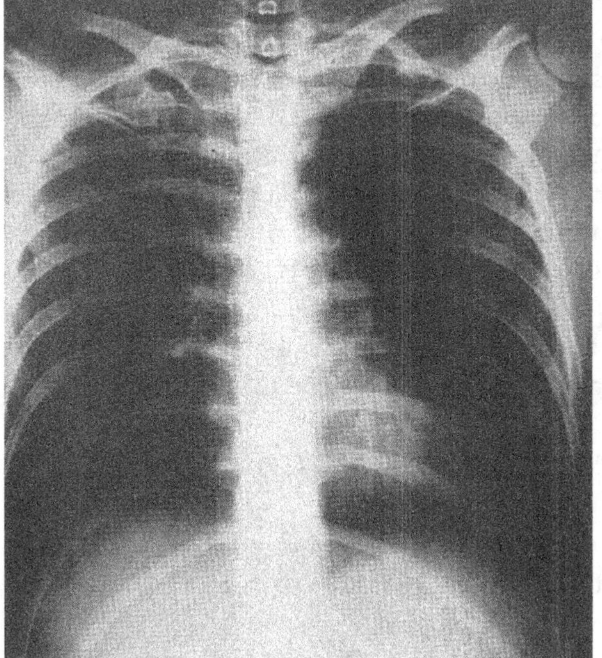

FIG. 42. Anteroposterior roentgenogram of dorsal spine, showing the costovertebral and the costotransverse joints. Spur formation can be seen at the costovertebral joints in the upper dorsal spine.

The circulatory disturbances which are seen many times in connection with the irritation of these joints may be explained when one realizes that adjacent to the costovertebral joints there are not only the roots of the nerves supplying sensation and motor control, but also the ganglia of the sympathetic system which are connected with the other nerve cells of that system.

Commonly, the disturbances in the rib joints are gradual in development, and all the symptoms are subacute or chronic. At times, as the result of a wrench or an injury, the irritation becomes much more marked and represents a true acute joint strain, with intense suffering and an actual displacement of the head of the bone. In these cases the effect on the sympathetic ganglion is much more marked, and with the change in the general superficial circulation, flushing or pallor of the face is greatly enhanced.

When these joints are visualized as true joints subject to strain from overuse or violence as is any other joint, it will be understood why they are equally liable to disease or injury.

Treatment. Once the condition and the proper mechanics are understood, treatment first consists in having the body so used that the neutral position is with the ribs midway between the positions of full inspiration and full expiration. To obtain this, mechanical supports often are needed until the joints have recovered from their irritation or until the muscles have been so developed that the neutral, normal position is possible.

If there is extensive disease of the joints, so that ankylosis is probable, it becomes important that the neutral position be obtained. In this position the effort that must be placed on the diaphragm when thoracic movement has been eliminated will be less than would be the case if the chest were markedly sagged.

The so-called floating ribs, two on each side, are freely movable and naturally produce marked strain to the rib joints and much greater possibility of irritation of the nerve roots and trunks; there is no costotransverse articulation to limit the motion of the main joints, and the ribs are not supported in front by the costosternal cartilage. The posterior position which these ribs frequently assume must mean not only a marked backward position of the ribs themselves, with strain on the joints, but twisting of the ribs as well. Pain caused by irritation of the nerve roots which are adjacent to the floating ribs will be referred to the side of the abdomen from the pubic bone to the crest of the ilium. It is this irritation that undoubtedly explains the so-called abdominal pain; mentioned in the writings of the late Dr. Carnett, of Philadelphia.

OPERATIVE TREATMENT OF BACKACHE

If, after treatment designed to obtain proper balance of the whole body, as well as the spine, not relieved or recurs quickly, The patient should be studied carefully to determine what should be done further. In most instances it will be found that the patient has not yet learned how to use the back habitually in good alignment, the muscles and the ligaments are not sufficiently

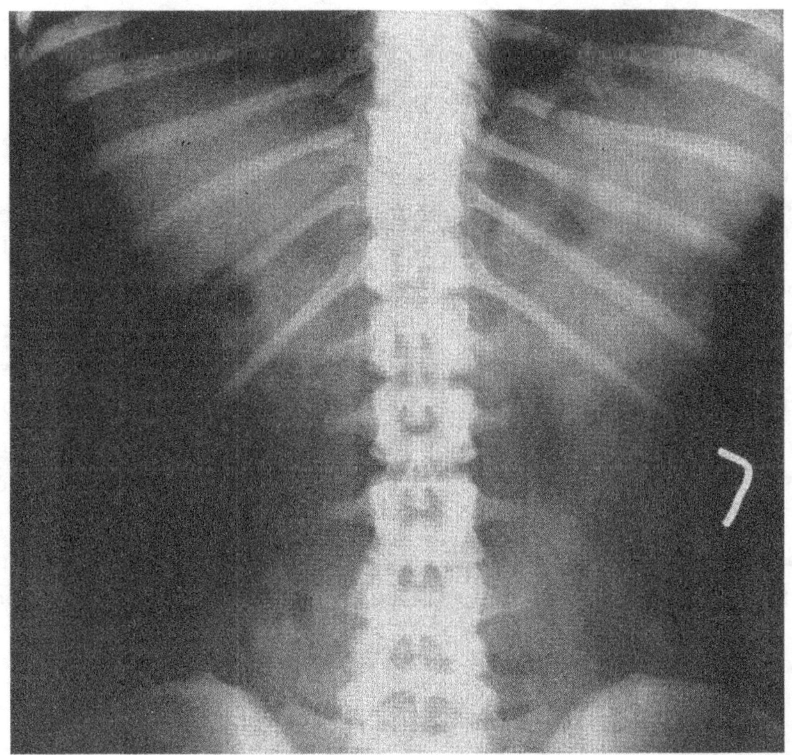

FIG. 43. Roentgenogram of low-dorsal spine, showing marked downward displacement of the ribs, with a sag at the costovertebral and the costotransverse joints.

strong, or an unusual sprain has come on a certain area of the back. Here, the backache usually subsides as the back becomes better aligned, with the weight borne evenly on the vertebral bodies and the intervertebral disks and with retraction of the sagged portions of the body.

When symptoms persist or recur soon after such treatment, more radical measures may be necessary. Usually a fusion, an operative stiffening of the unstable portion of the back, is considered. Fusion operations are indicated when lasting stability of the back cannot be secured because: (1) a congenital deformity makes the back permanently so weak that it cannot be held in good alignment, (2) disease has so changed the vertebrae or their supporting structures that deformity occurs, and the spine cannot be well aligned, severe lasting weakness is present in the supporting musculature.

When a permanently unstable portion of the spine requires fusion, it is necessary that it be kept in good alignment while the vertebrae are fusing. Otherwise, severe sprain will come upon the spine and the pelvis immediately above and below the fused portion. If operation does not achieve good mechanics, as well as relieve instability, the later condition of the patient may be worse than before.

There may be a gradual adaptation of the contents of the spinal canal. In such instances symptoms may subside spontaneously. However, in most instances treatment is required to relieve the spinal symptoms and the referred pain. Many of the patients with lesions of the intervertebral disks can be relieved by correcting the faulty body mechanics. This provides the greatest possible dimensions in the spinal canal and in the neural foramina. If, in addition, a spinal brace is used to hold the back in good alignment and to avoid further sprains, the patient recovers in most instances through gradual adjustment within the spinal canal. Often such treatment must be pursued for several years. However, the patient usually can return to his activities after a few weeks but must continue with a spinal support for a long time (Fig. 44).

When little if any relief follows such treatment, operation is considered. This usually consists of partial laminectomy and removal of the disk substance. In most instances, all of the nucleus pulposis is removed. While the removal of the intervertebral disk alters somewhat the depth and the alignment of the interspinal joints in the area operated upon, the spine adjusts quickly to this, usually without symptoms. In most instances, the vertebrae adjoining the ruptured intervertebral disk tend to become stiffened, and in some instances bony fusion takes place. Because mobility in the back is restricted permanently somewhat by the operation, good body

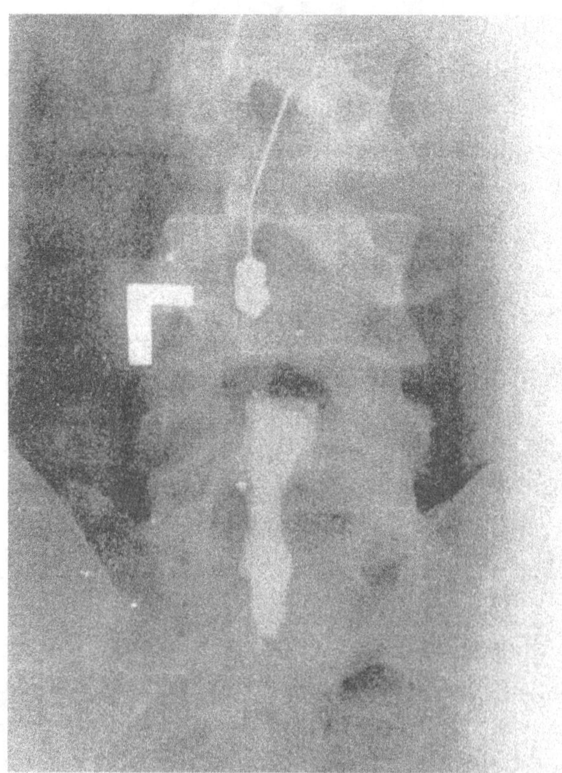

FIG. 44. Myelogram of the lumbar spine. The pantopaque shows a filling defect on the right side at the lumbosacral vertebral interspace. At operation, a large rupture of the intervertebral disk was found to be pressing on the root of the fifth lumbar nerve.

mechanics is even more important after operation than it was before. If the spine is very unstable, a fusion of the spine in the operated region may be required, but this never should be done without correction of the alignment of the spine.

Occasionally, after operative removal of a ruptured intervertebral disk, the patient still complains of back pain and also of referred pain. While in a few instances such pain may be the result of further herniation of adjacent intervertebral disks, in most instances it is due to sprains resulting from use of the body in bad alignment. We have observed a gradual disappearance of all symptoms in most of such patients after the mechanics of the spine had been corrected as fully as possible.

LESIONS OF THE INTERVERTEBRAL DISKS

When the body is used in bad alignment degenerative changes follow sprains and deformities rapidly. Evidences of these degenerative changes are found frequently in the vertebrae and in the intervertebral disks. Some of these changes are found in all older individuals, as Schmorl has shown, but they are much more extensive and appear at an earlier age when there is faulty body mechanics and fixed spinal deformity. The fibrous capsule, the annulus fibrosis, of the intervertebral disk becomes weakened and thin. Then it is easy to produce a herniation of the central jellylike portion (nucleus pulposis) of the intervertebral disk. This herniation of the central portion of the disk can occur into the vertebral body, where It produces no symptoms but is seen as a rounded opacity within the vertebral body. When the substance of the disk is displaced posteriorly it frequently presses upon the spinal cord or upon a nerve root. This is seen most often at the lumbosacral region, less commonly in the lower-cervical spine. If such herniation occurs suddenly, as is seen sometimes in younger patients after severe injury, symptoms may appear at once. The most common symptom is pain along the cutaneous distribution of the nerve root which is pressed upon. Less common, are weakness, paralysis or disturbances in sensation. Usually, there are local symptoms in the back, pain on motion, local tenderness, muscular spasm and restriction of motion. In older individuals there is often a gradual degeneration and herniation of disk substance, and symptoms usually appear gradually and are frequently not so severe.

6

The Circulatory System

The circulatory system merits serious consideration in any treatise upon body mechanics, since its functions are influenced greatly by the other organs of the body and by the external environment. The circulation is governed by the same laws that control the flow of liquids in a closed system of cylindrical tubes. The heart changes its shape and position with each breath. The movement of the ribs and the change in the elastic portions of the lungs are essential to the proper functioning of the pulmonary circulation. Proper muscular tonus and retraction of the abdominal wall are important for the return flow of the venous blood.

The circulatory system serves two great purposes: (1) the alimentation of the tissues and (2) the removal of waste products. Any disturbance in cardiac function injures tissues, among them the cardiac muscle itself, either by gradual malnutrition or by slow intoxication. In Chapter 3 the way in which faulty body mechanics could disturb the circulation was shown; the factors

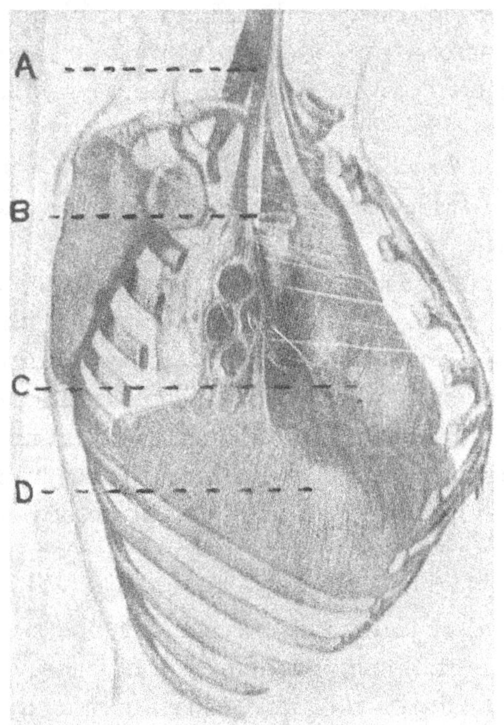

FIG 45. Lateral view of thoracic cavity showing the suspensory ligament of the diaphragm. This extends downward from the deep portion of the cervical fascia around the heart and is attached to the anterior part of the diaphragm. Any position of the head or of the cervical spine which lowers the cervical fascia, A, such as a head held forward or an increased cervical lordosis results in a sagged position of the heart, C, the diaphragm, D, and the great vessels, B.

responsible for this interference are complex and varied. In this chapter we shall describe only the simpler ones which are seen frequently and are observed easily.

THE HEART AND THE DIAPHRAGM

When the body is held badly the shoulders and the ribs droop, flattening the chest anteroposteriorly. With this, the diaphragm assumes a lower position, carrying with it the heart, the aorta and the great vessels (Fig. 45). The heart functions to distribute blood, and the diaphragm assists the venous return. Damage to cardiac structure or interference with the normal excursion of the diaphragm is more serious for the well-being of the individual than is involvement of the branches of the circulation, with the possible exception of the larger cerebral and cardiac vessels. Both the heart and the diaphragm function automatically and are regulated by the sympathetic nervous system. The latter can be contracted voluntarily but usually functions automatically through the phrenic nerves.

Return of Blood to the Heart. A number of observers have noted the importance of proper functioning of the diaphragm for the return of blood to the heart. Mettenlieter states that venous blood is drawn to the right side of the heart by the increase in negative thoracic pressure in inspiration and by the downward movement of the diaphragm. Sir Arthur Keith considers the movement of the diaphragm the most vital factor in the filling of the right side of the mammalian heart; the thoracic segment of the inferior vena cava lengthens in each inspiratory downward excursion of the diaphragm. A marked increase in blood flow from the inferior vena cava was observed by Turner with each inspiratory movement of the diaphragm, this increase being augmented as the excursions became greater. This action of the diaphragm in returning blood to the right side of the heart is partially or wholly lost with the downward sag of the diaphragm in faulty body mechanics (Fig. 46). This leads to splanchnic congestion and partial stagnation of the blood in the lower extremities.

Shape of Pericardium and Thoracic Cavity. The change in the shape of the heart and in the size of the thoracic cavity because of faulty body mechanics impairs the function of the heart (Fig. 47). Nature has made provision for this to a certain extent by the difference in shape and position of the heart in the slender type of individual, where displacements can occur more easily. However, in any anatomic type serious interference with the heart's action may result from a long-continued stooped position, with compression of this organ, as has been shown by Herz Podaminsky found that occupations in which the body was bent forward produced a diminution of the minute volume, a decrease in blood pressure and an enlargement of the transverse diameter of the heart at the expense of the left ventricle. An exaggerated form of the compression and the displacement caused by faulty body mechanics is observed in severe scoliosis. Here, there is increased pressure in the pulmonary circulation, failure of the right side of the heart and finally, complete heart failure. Stoll observed that improvement

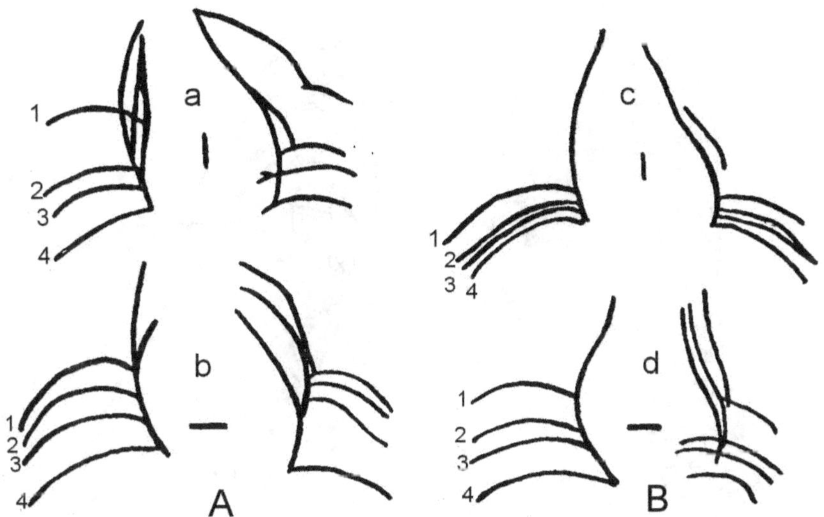

FIG. 46. Tracings of the diaphragm (fluoroscopic). (A) Good body mechanics: a, standing; b, lying. (B) Poor body mechanics: c, standing; d, lying. (See text.) 1. Position of diaphragm at full expiration. 2. Position of diaphragm at normal expiration. 3. Position of diaphragm at normal inspiration. 4. Position of diaphragm at full inspiration. Note that in good body mechanics the total excursion of the diaphragm is greater in the standing position, a, while the reverse is true in faulty body mechanics, c. In good body mechanics, A, the normal excursion, 2-3, of the diaphragm should be about midway between the extremes of inspiration, 4, and expiration, 1, while in poor body mechanics, B the normal excursion of the diaphragm is habitually near the extreme of inspiration, 4.

in cardiac function followed an increase in the anteroposterior diameter of the chest. Similar findings were obtained in the remedying of functional cardiac disturbances in recruits during the First World War.

Displacement of the Heart. Cardiac function is disturbed-also by the downward displacement of the heart, the pull of which narrows the lumen of the aorta and the arteries from the aortic arch. The displacement interferes mechanically with contraction. The stretching and the displacement produce increased pressure against which the heart must work not only in the vessels arising from the thoracic aorta but in the pulmonary venous circulation as well (Fig. 48). Experimental animals usually die within 2 days after constriction of the pulmonary veins. Animals held upright for prolonged periods often die from the displacement of the heart and the increased resistance against which it must work. This is seen sometimes in sheep held upright during shearing. In man, Nature has provided a much greater reserve, and the effects of such displacement and increased resistance are not immediately serious. Long continuance

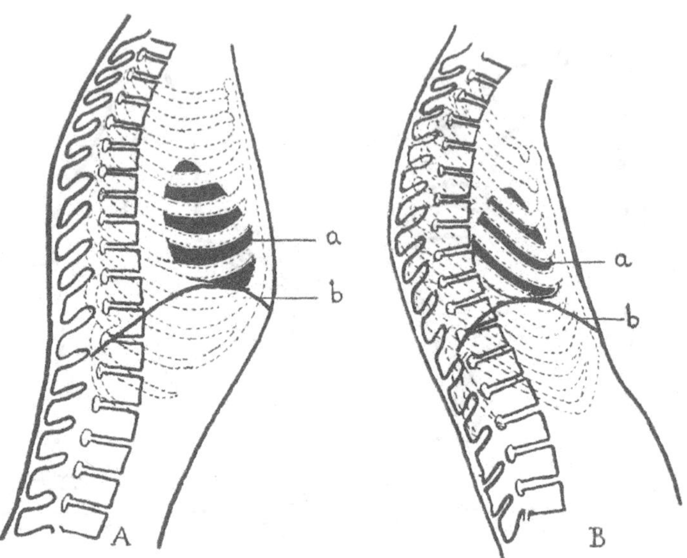

FIG.47. Lateral diagrams of thoracic cavity showing changes in the shape of the thoracic cages and the position of the heart and the diaphragm. (A) Good body mechanics. (B) Same individual with bad body mechanics; a, heart; b, diaphragm. Note that in good body mechanics, A, the diaphragm is higher anteriorly under the heart than at its attachment to the spine. In bad body mechanics, B, the anterior part of the diaphragm has sagged so that it is at the same level as the attachments posteriorly. With this sag the depth of the chest has decreased, so that the posterior mediastinum has been practically obliterated. The change in the shape of the diaphragm, B, must produce a change in the shape and the position of the liver, with resulting interference with the portal circulation.

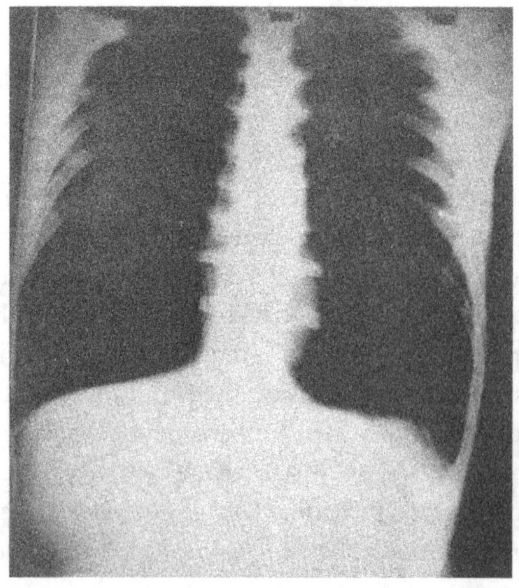

FIG. 48. Roentgenogram of chest, taken in the standing position, showing the vertical or "droplet" heart. The aortic arch is at the level of the fifth rib anteriorly instead of the second rib. The heart is in the mid-line. The diaphragm is very flat instead of being dome-shaped and is at the level of the eleventh rib on the right and the twelfth rib on the left. With this position there may be considerable strain on the great vessels. This picture shows only the change in the thoracic cavity. There must be equally marked and important changes in the abdominal organs.

of this downward displacement of the heart leads to incompetence of the right ventricle and the gradual development of decompensation.

The cardiac muscle is a very efficient type of musculature, showing signs of fatigue only after greater exertion changes than that required by the function of ordinary striated muscle (the diaphragm excepted). It has a very efficient blood supply in order that its nutrition may not be impaired, and this supply is increased readily 4 or 5 times during activity or with lowered oxygen saturation of the blood. However, with excessive strains, the heart reacts much as do other muscles. With long-continued overwork, it hypertrophies. There is a limit to hypertrophy, however, and once it is passed further strain leads to atrophy and degeneration, as in any other muscle. Scarring occurs after injuries and infections. Repair may take place to a certain extent in lesions of the musculature, as has been shown in cardiac surgery.

Cardiac Strain. Strain of the cardiac musculature develops either when the ventricles are required to eject blood against a higher resistance or when, weakened from any cause, they must work against the normal resistance. In such cases there is a gradual reduction in systolic dilatation and a higher initial tension. If this overload comes gradually, thickening of the heart wall and enlargement, particularly in the left ventricle, develop. If strain is thrown on the heart too rapidly, the tonic and elastic reaction of the ventricles is gradually lost, and dilatation develops. An increased residue then remains in the cardiac chambers, less blood leaves the heart, and there is congestion, seen particularly in the pulmonary bed and in the liver. The peripheral circulation becomes less and less efficient, and cardiac failure begins. All normal hearts have reserve power which is not utilized under ordinary demands. If this reserve is called on gradually, the constant increased tension to which the heart fibers are subjected stimulates them to increase in size and to hypertrophy. Hand in hand with this goes an increased capacity for work, known as hypertrophic compensation. The limit to which the heart can increase its work under demand is soon reached. Heart failure may develop at any level of activity which has previously been satisfactory. This gradual development may be initiated by the mechanical changes resulting from faulty body mechanics.

Chronic Valvular Disease. Chronic valvular disease of the heart is very common. Statistics are incomplete, but such data as are available suggest that it is one of the most common causes of death. Even more serious than the shortening of life is the role of organic heart disease in the production of chronic invalidism. Valvular disease is serious only in so far as it decreases the heart's efficiency in pumping blood. When valvular lesions are accompanied by enlargement of the heart they usually are classified as organic disease of that organ, in which it has less ability to repair or to improve its functional efficiency. While complete functional integrity often cannot be restored, no cardiologist will deny that invalidism and death may be postponed in almost every case by wise management of the patient and his activities. It has been our experience that the correction of the mechanics of the body helps greatly in reducing the peripheral load, in lessening cardiac strain and in increasing the patient's usefulness.

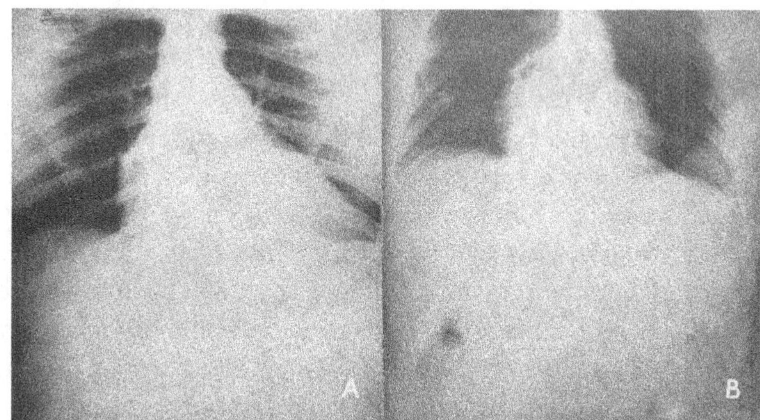

FIG. 49. (A) Roentgenogram of a patient with an enlarged heart associated with very faulty body mechanics and signs of cardiac failure. **(B)** Roentgenogram of the same patient taken 5 weeks later. All signs of cardiac failure had disappeared; there was no cardiac murmur. Note the change in shape and size of the heart. Treatment consisted of the correction of the faulty mechanics of the whole body, beginning with rest in bed in correct position. No drugs were used.

If this improvement in body mechanics can be secured early, when the valvular lesion and the cardiac enlargement are not considered to be serious, functional efficiency of the circulation often may be preserved indefinitely with the individual at full activity. Figure 49A shows a roentgenogram of the chest of a patient with marked enlargement of the heart and beginning heart failure. At the time this photograph was taken the patient was unable to make the slightest exertion without symptoms of cardiac distress. Rest and correction of the faulty body mechanics were the only treatment employed. No digitalis or other medication was given. Figure 49B shows the roentgenogram of the chest 5 weeks later, when the heart returned to normal size. All the symptoms disappeared, and the patient has remained well for 15 years.

Chronic Cardiac Disease. In any study and treatment of chronic disease involving the circulatory apparatus, all the factors which affect the efficiency of the circulation must be taken into account. If these are recognized early, and if proper treatment is instituted, cardiac disease may be prevented. Chronic cardiac disease rarely develops in the presence of good body mechanics. Most students of such disease state that cardiac failure has its origin in a vast number of causes, some of them unknown. Sir James MacKenzie wrote:

"It is necessary to- know the life history of such diseases from their onset to their termination in death or recovery. The investigators must have the opportunity of seeing such disease in all stages that they may detect the circumstances that favor or induce their onset; can watch the phases from the early stages when the symptoms are limited mainly to feelings of ill health on to the later stages when the agents of disease have damaged the tissues and produced physical signs."

In cardiac disease Sir James recognized 4 stages: a predisposing, an early, an advanced and a final stage. While much study has been made of the advanced stage, the prodromal stage has not been investigated so that faults and minor strains may be found and eliminated, thus preventing later damage to the circulatory system.

In any appraisal of circulatory efficiency the adequacy of the heart to carry on the circulation is of more importance than the appraisal of any single physical sign, no matter how alarming. False emphasis has been placed on instrumental investigation at the expense of clinical observation and the judgment of the patient himself. Electrocardiographic study, while helpful in determining the amount of damage to cardiac musculature, has no direct value in prognosis. Some repair and recovery of function will take place if Nature is given an opportunity to heal and if every possible hindrance to circulatory efficiency is removed. Fortunately, not all cardiac disturbances are considered to be significant, but all must be evaluated. The experience of medical officers during the First World War and since has shown that a number of cardiac disturbances, among them certain murmurs, do not represent pathologic change in the heart. **Functional Disturbances.** In studies of cardiac function the shape and the position of the heart have received too little attention. Alterations therein often have a vital relationship to the so-called functional disturbances. This and other investigations of the heart must be considered in relation to the physiologic adequacy of the body as a whole. None of the usual cardiac tests gives adequate data for prognosis. The last century has given us clinical observation on the course of the common cardiac lesions where treatment was given with full acceptance of all the patient's disabilities. These have led to gradually increasing circulatory failure and death. Only recently have attempts been made to remove such disabilities, mechanical or otherwise. They have shown that many disturbances in circulatory function can be relieved and that they need not be the cause of chronic disease.

Obesity and Cardiac Dysfunction. Obesity is related closely to degenerative changes in all of the tissues and is a common accompaniment of many cardiac disturbances. Increase in the anteroposterior curves of the spine and circumferential enlargement of the body occurs. Obesity in middle age usually follows excessive intake of food and lessening of physical activity. The sagged, prominent abdomen shifts the center of gravity forward; to compensate for this, lumbar lordosis is increased. This is followed by increased forward bowing of the thoracic spine and flaring of the lower ribs (emphysematous or barrel-chest deformity). The upper chest tends to be flat. There is forward inclination of the head, with increased cervical lordosis. The shoulder girdle is forward, and the knees are often slightly flexed. The diaphragm assumes a lower position in the thoracic cavity. Respiration is interfered with by the shape of the chest, by the low position of the diaphragm and by the greatly increased amount of fat in the upper abdomen. There is a considerable decrease in tidal air. Dyspnea is a common complaint, often without exertion.

The circulation of venous blood is slowed. Circulation time is prolonged. It always is improved in recumbency, since in this position, the thoracic shape is improved, the diaphragm is higher, and the pull of abdominal fat and heavy abdominal viscera is eliminated partially. Both breathing and circulation are improved by loss of weight and by a spinal support which also lifts up and supports the heavy abdominal viscera. Exercises must be prescribed gradually in this type of patient.

THE VASCULAR SYSTEM

Angina Pectoris. This is a disturbance usually associated with lesions in the coronary arteries, which supply blood to the musculature of the heart. There is a decreased flow through these arteries, and this leads to ischemia of the musculature, resulting in cramp like pain. This pain sometimes is felt locally in the chest and sometimes is referred through the sympathetic nerves to the left shoulder and the left arm. The condition may come on suddenly, owing to the lodging of a thrombus in one or more main branches of the coronary arteries, or more slowly, as in arteriosclerosis or in chronic insufficiency of the aortic valve, occasionally with lesions about the aortic valve. Death may occur, or collateral circulation may be established. In the recovery from this lesion, rest and the gradual correction of the faulty body mechanics are extremely helpful measures. With adequate support to the abdominal cavity, the return circulation is improved; the heart fills more adequately; the coronary circulation is augmented. By lessening weight, by correcting postural deformities and by good abdominal retraction, the anginal pain usually is alleviated.

Pseudo-angina. In many instances there is a similar distribution of pain, and a diagnosis of angina is made wrongly where there is no disturbance in the circulation to the musculature of the heart. The electrocardiogram shows no evidence of such disturbance. This condition has been recognized by Carnett, Gunther and others as being a pseudo-angina. Here the cause of the pain is the irritation of the lower-cervical and the upper-thoracic nerves. This is brought about by faulty body mechanics through pressure on or pinching of the nerves, either at their foramina of exit or at the costovertebral joints. This is produced through the increased flexion of the spine, the downward displacement of the ribs and the overstretching of spinal muscles and ligaments. Impingement of the nerves can occur much more easily if there is an arthritis about the spinal joints. Careful examination of such patients in the standing position with X-ray and electrocardiographic tests will save this type of individual from constant fear and from a life of lessened activity, often of invalidism. Pseudo-angina can be cured by avoiding the strain of faulty body mechanics.

Blood Pressure. The normal blood pressure varies widely, but a definite normal difference is found among the various anatomic types. The stocky type has a higher blood pressure than the intermediate type or the slender type. The range of normal systolic blood pressure is usually from 120 to 145 mm. of mercury, and that of diastolic pressure between 60 and 80 mm. If a slender individual had a constant systolic blood pressure of 145 mm., or if a stocky individual had one of 120 mm., it would be more significant than if the conditions were reversed. It would suggest that the individual was not in the best of health and lacked stamina. Taking blood pressure readings and pulse rates in the standing and the lying positions is useful in determining endurance. Modifications of this procedure, as in the Turner and the Schneider tests, are employed in athletics and in the Army to test physical fitness and staying power. It has been observed that the pulse and the blood pressure change little in standing and lying after body mechanics have been corrected.

Hypertension. Arterial hypertension is the result of an increase in the peripheral resistance to the flow of blood. We speak of hypertension when the systolic pressure is constantly above 160 mm. of mercury. It is found commonly with arteriosclerosis and is considered to be both cause and effect. There are many causes of increased peripheral resistance; it may be due to circulating stimulants and hormones which act on the vasomotor system. Eventually changes occur in the elasticity and the muscular tonus of the blood vessels, and, in Nature's attempt at repair, calcium and cholesterol are laid down in the arterial walls. Vascular accidents, most commonly cerebral hemorrhage, can take place easily when these changes have occurred in the arteries. The interference with blood flow resulting from a low diaphragm and from peripheral congestion helps in bringing on this condition. We have found that marked elevations in the blood pressure can be decreased by removing the congestion and decreasing the strain on the blood vessels through improvement in the mechanical use of the body as a whole.

Hypotension. Arterial hypotension is seen most frequently in individuals of the slender type. It is diagnosed commonly when the systolic blood pressure falls to 100 mm. of mercury or below. Here there may be a decrease in the peripheral resistance, with failure of the vasomotor system and lack of tone in the arteries. Often there is a weakness of the musculature of the whole body, including the heart. There are symptoms of fatigue, dizziness, and lack of stamina and occasionally syncope. The extremities are cold and clammy, and increased sensitiveness to heat and cold is usually present. These conditions probably are not entirely the result of the hypo-tension but are produced by the same causes. When we come to study the underlying causes we generally find a weak individual with bad mechanical use of the entire body. Faulty body mechanics has been observed commonly in this condition; its correction usually has brought about improvement in symptoms and correction of the hypotension.

Extremities. There are a number of disturbances which produce local alterations of the circulation in the extremities. Occasionally one sees lack of tone in the arteries, with dilatation. More often a local dilatation occurs from weakening of the arterial wall. Constrictions and closures of the vessels sometimes occur. The most outstanding of these conditions are found in Buerger's disease, Raynaud's disease and arteriosclerosis. Here local exercises and mechanical increase and decrease of pressure on the limb have been found to be helpful. Much more improvement occurs if the general circulation of the whole body is stimulated and aided through exercises which correct the faulty body mechanics, particularly those which improve the function of the diaphragm.

Arteries. The arteries are the elastic distributing system for the blood. They have smooth musculature within their walls, which can contract and expand with the changes in pressure accompanying each beat of the heart and also can contract through the action of the sympathetic nervous system. The external coat of the arteries is a modified part of the general connective tissue, with which it is continuous. Because of this the arteries share in many of the diseases of the surrounding tissues. A number of chronic diseases attack the arteries from within, however. The arteries are affected by infections and by the wear and tear which comes with increasing age. Infections sometimes weaken the arterial wall locally and may lead to rupture of the vessels and hemorrhage. The usual effect of disease is to produce a constriction and a thickening of the intima, the inner layer of the vessel wall, with an increase in connective tissue. Later, fatty degeneration and the deposition of lime salts take place.

What relation can be established between disease of the arteries and faulty body mechanics? First, much of such disease is believed by most internists to be preventable. The causes are thought to be those added stresses of long-continued pressure that may arise when the heart is working under unusual strain or when the vessels are inadequately protected by the surrounding tissues. In addition, the action of circulating chemical substances and disturbances in the innervation of the arteries play a part. The influence of faulty body mechanics on the body as a whole has been shown in the preceding chapters. There are effects on the heart, on the blood pressure, on the nervous innervation and on the tissues surrounding the blood vessels. Removal of these disturbances leads to less strain on the arteries. While much can be done to improve arterial disease after it has developed, much more can be accomplished by early treatment before pathologic changes have occurred.

Peripheral Circulatory Disturbances. This case illustrates the complexity of diagnosis and treatment involved in many chronic cases.

Case 1. This patient, a woman of 69 years of age, was seen in November, 1930, having been referred from her family physician in New York City. Her symptoms consisted of pain referred to the feet and the lower legs, chiefly the right foot. At one time the pain was so severe that an exploratory incision was made, but no abnormality was found, and no relief was obtained. The condition had been present for 12 years, gradually increasing in severity, and had grown rapidly worse in the preceding few weeks.

On examination, the patient was seen to be very slender in anatomic type. She weighed 105 pounds. The mechanics of the body were extremely poor, with a very flat chest, a low position of the ribs, a marked sagging of the abdomen and a marked pronation of the feet. There was disturbance of circulation in the feet, so severe on the right that when the foot was placed on the floor it became completely livid; at other times it became completely blanched. This was associated with much pain. When the patient was lying down the circulation improved but was not normal. In the other foot it was poor, and the foot was livid when dependent. Pulsation could be felt in the anterior vessels in both feet but, in the posterior vessels, it was difficult to detect. There was also some pain referred to the arm, with distinct tenderness over the coracoid process.

Naturally, the patient had received much treatment from many different specialists, but she had grown steadily worse. She was taken to the hospital and was put to bed for special treatment with exercises and positions. These were instituted in order to raise the diaphragm and to increase its action and thus to improve the circulation in the legs. A plaster-of-paris cast that could be removed easily for bathing was applied in order to hold the foot in a good position as the patient lay in bed. Fomentations were applied to the back so as to stimulate the peripheral circulation, with the expectation of stimulating that in the sympathetic nerves and thus improving the superficial circulation in general. The pain was so severe that at first deodorized tincture of opium was used for relief.

The patient remained at the hospital for about 2 months and in that time showed marked general improvement; the circulation in the feet was also distinctly better. Supports for the feet were adjusted. One toe, which had been stiff and in the hammer-toe position, was manipulated under nitrous- oxide anesthesia. After this, the patient was able to walk about her room with little pain. At this time the pulsation in the vessels of the feet had improved slightly, and she was allowed to go home. She returned from time to time for observation, and there was found to be a steady improvement in all the symptoms referred to the feet and the legs; she was able to walk about fairly freely, leading a relatively normal life for one of her age.

Veins. The veins are more frequently the seat of obvious pathologic changes than are the arteries. This is due chiefly to the slower rate of blood flow and the differences in anatomic structure. The veins have thin, less elastic walls and they are not so well supplied by musculature and nerves. They have valves at frequent intervals along their course which prevent the back flow of blood, particularly in the upright position. Acute inflammation of the veins may be caused by sudden mechanical or chemical injury or by infection; infection commonly occurs when there is a stagnation or a slowing of the flow of blood. Lesions in the veins are seen in all anatomic types. In the slender type inflammatory changes and varicosities are observed in early life, while in the stocky type these changes occur in middle and later life, when the increased weight and sagging of the abdominal viscera make the return flow of blood more difficult. Associated with infections in the veins (phlebitis), there is sometimes a coagulation of the blood within the vein, commonly called thrombophlebitis. This occurs most frequently after operation or illness when the body is permitted little or no motion. It can be prevented by measures which improve the circulation, since thrombosis does not occur when the rate of blood flow in the veins is normal.

Varicosities. Varicosities in the legs are common in the presence of faulty body mechanics (Fig. 50). They are seen often during and following pregnancy, where their cause is admitted to be the mechanical interference with the return venous flow through the external and the common iliac arteries. Downward displacement of the organs has a similar effect on the venous return. Deformity or poor muscular tonus in the lower extremities, as seen in faulty body mechanics, may lead to local stagnation and enlargement of the veins, since the massaging action of the skeletal muscles is lost. However, the principal cause is the interference and the stagnation which occur in the abdominal cavity. Here, congestion results; (1) from the loss of normal tone in the veins and the viscera when the support of the well-retracted abdominal wall is lost; (2) when the diaphragm is low, its pumping action in returning blood to the right side of the heart is markedly impaired or lost. Varicosities which result from overstretching and loss of competency in the valves, most commonly in the superficial veins but also in the deep veins and in the communicating systems, can be prevented by the habitual good mechanical use of the body. The predisposing causes can be removed, and improvement

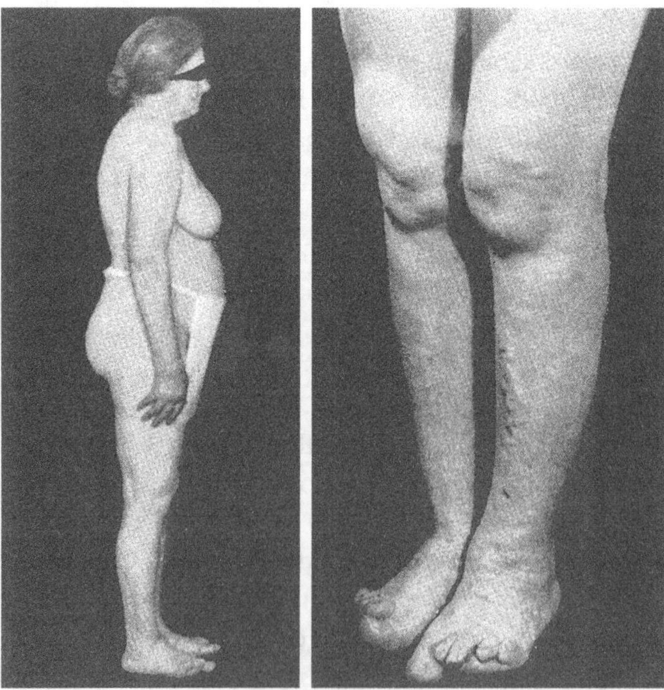

FIG. 50. (Left) There are large varicosities along the calf and the thigh. The feet are strained, the chest is low, and the abdominal musculature is flabby. (Right) Enlargement of a section of A to show the varicose veins in thigh and calf.

brought about, even after the full development of varicosities. There is some shrinking of the wall of the vein, with improvement in tonus. This is often greatly helped by the temporary use of an elastic bandage. The frequent reports of the recurrence of varicosities after surgical ligation or obliteration by injections suggest that local measures are inadequate and that such disturbances involve more than the limb itself. We have observed frequent relief from varicosities where the only treatment was the correction of the faulty body mechanics.

Senile Arteriosclerosis. Arteriosclerosis is identifiable pathologically and to a lesser degree clinically, in three main forms: (1) arthrosclerosis, a patchy degeneration of the intimal coat of the large arteries, (2) Monckeberg's degeneration in which calcification of the medial coat of the artery is observed and (3) arteriosclerosis, a diffuse thickening of many arteries, seen to a certain degree in all people over middle age. Both atherosclerosis and diffuse arteriosclerosis are components in what we term senile arteriosclerosis. With rapidly advancing hypertension, the degeneration and the subsequent fatty proliferation is found chiefly in the internal coat. With the slower processes of advancing age, the degenerative processes are more diffuse and involve all of the arterial layers and the capillaries as well. The vessels are more tortuous; they are rigid, and their elasticity is lost. Many of these features can be observed in older individuals. Later, changes take place in the various organs from diminution of blood supply. With increase in the process, the blood pressure may increase, calcification of the vessels may be observed in roentgenograms, and changes may be found in the retina. The most important clinical feature is disturbance in function of the central nervous system, the viscera and the voluntary muscles. It should be obvious that much of this change in the arteries cannot be healed, and that normal texture and elasticity cannot be restored to the arterial wall. For these reasons, treatment must be directed to improving the blood flow to the various organs, in this way improving their efficiency. In this program of treatment, exercise, rest, diet and drugs all play a part. Good hygiene must be practiced. The activities of the individual and his rest should be compatible with his age. Because the elasticity of the arteries is lessened, the arterial trunk cannot store the load of cardiac systole, and blood pressure rises. The amount of blood going to the organs is lessened from the labored cardiac function and from decrease in the actual and the potential lumen of the blood vessels.

If there are no obvious symptoms, all that is required usually is reduction of obesity and elimination of unnecessary strains, both physical and mental. The body should be brought into as good mechanical alignment as possible. Most helpful is good diaphragmatic excursion, and retraction of the protuberant abdomen.

Improvement in the disturbances of the central nervous system is slow indeed, but gradual subsidence of headache, vertigo and temporary confusions has been observed through correction of the faulty body mechanics. The extreme forward position of the head and the tremor of the hands is helped also. More help can be expected in the extremities. Color is improved, and the warmth of the extremity is increased. If there is pain on activity, or cramp, rest is given first, with the limb (usually the lower extremity) a few inches below heart level. Diaphragmatic exercises are begun at once. Buerger exercises and special foot exercises to aid the return flow of blood are helpful also but are less effective than improving the functions of the heart and the diaphragm.

7

Angina Pectoris and Postural Emphysema Related to Obesity

By WILLIAM J. KERR, M.D., F.A.C.P.*

CAUSATIVE FACTORS

Obesity is probably the most important underlying cause of pathologic old age. The manner in which atherosclerosis, diabetes, and other metabolic diseases are related is not clear. However, the effects of obesity on posture and the mechanics of the body are, in general, well understood. We recognize the distortion of the normal spinal curves as the girth increases. Girdle obesity results from excessive intake of food coupled with decreased physical activity in middle life. The readjustments in the spinal axis lead to a series of local changes which produce symptoms. Many of these symptoms are due to injuries resulting from a combination of maladjustments between the interrelated functions of the spinal axis and its attachments and supporting structures, and the organ-systems which have a normal range of efficiency.

The protuberant abdomen moves the line of gravity forward. To compensate for this shift in the load, the normal curves of the spinal axis are exaggerated. Lumbar lordosis is increased. The lumbar vertebral bodies are widely spaced ventrally and the sacrum assumes a more horizontal position when the subject is erect. The thoracic spinal curve is increased dorsally and the pressure on the ventral portions of the disks and bodies of these vertebrae is augmented. The lower ribs are elevated and flared as in the inspiratory position. This distortion of the lower ribs causes a stretching of the diaphragm and is one of the factors which lead to an increase in the size of the thoracic cage (the barrel chest).

The upper ribs are collapsed ventrally because of the forward movement of the upper thoracic spine. The cervical spine shows increased lordosis and the head is carried forward, causing the patient to present a stooped appearance (Fig. 51). The deformity is so great that most persons with this syndrome have difficulty in securing a properly fitting collar and due to the increased lumbar lordosis the coat hangs free behind supported entirely by the kyphotic

Professor of Medicine, University of California Medical School; Physician in Chief, University of California Hospital; Member, American Board of Internal Medicine; formerly President, American Heart Association, American Rheumatism Association, and American College of Physicians.

upper thorax. These subjects when erect must always look upward to meet the horizon and for this reason may suffer from strain of the extra-ocular muscles. The shoulder girdle is carried well forward and the arms hang in front of the normal position.

The subject usually stands with the knees slightly flexed to "get in under" the load. The local changes resulting in injuries to bones, cartilages, and supporting structures are discussed elsewhere. The symptom-complex designated as radiculitis is closely allied to the postural disturbances in obesity but is not limited thereto. The relaxation of the fascial sheet which extends from the cervical region through the mediastinum and pericardium to the diaphragm and the lumbar spine also interferes with normal respiration.

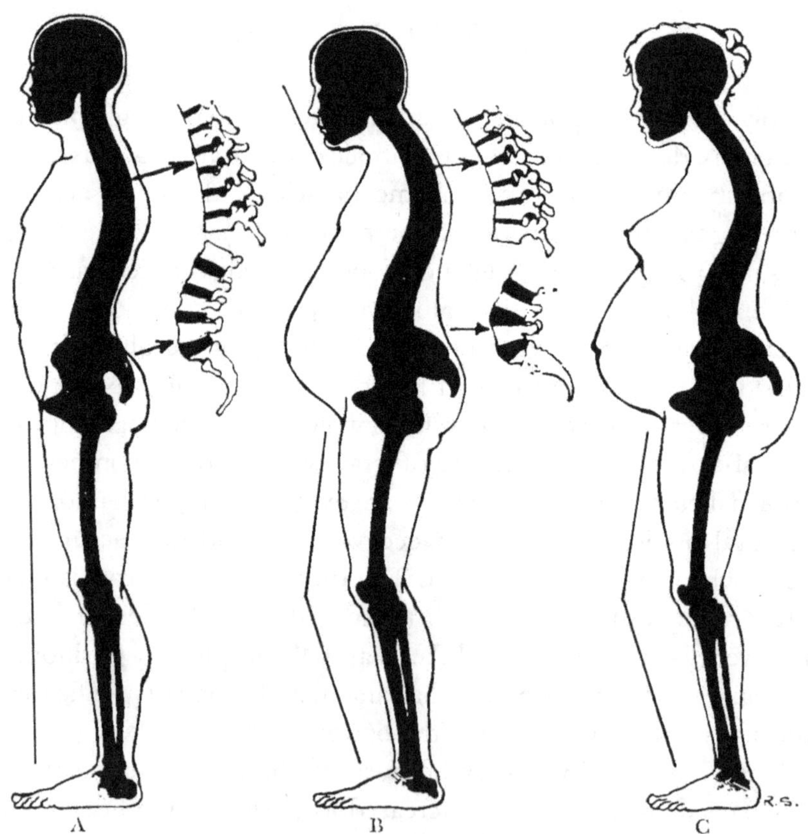

FIG. 51. Types of posture showing effects on spine. (A) Posture, spinal curves, and intervertebral disks normal. (B) Relaxed posture with accentuated spinal curves resulting from a pendulous abdomen. (C). Postular changes late in pregnancy, similar to those in B, but which never persist long enough to affect the intervertebral disks. (Courtesy, Annals of Internal Medicine).

The great increase in intra-abdominal fat in structures such as the omentum, the stomach, the intestines, and the mesenteries, suspended in part from the diaphragm, serves as an added handicap to normal respiration when the subject is erect but may actually assist in respiration when he is supine. Observations made with the aid of the fluoroscope or roentgenogram show that, due to the pull of the suspended counterweight, the diaphragm stands at a lower position in the chest and the range of movement is greatly limited in the erect, but is more normal in the supine, posture (Fig. 52).

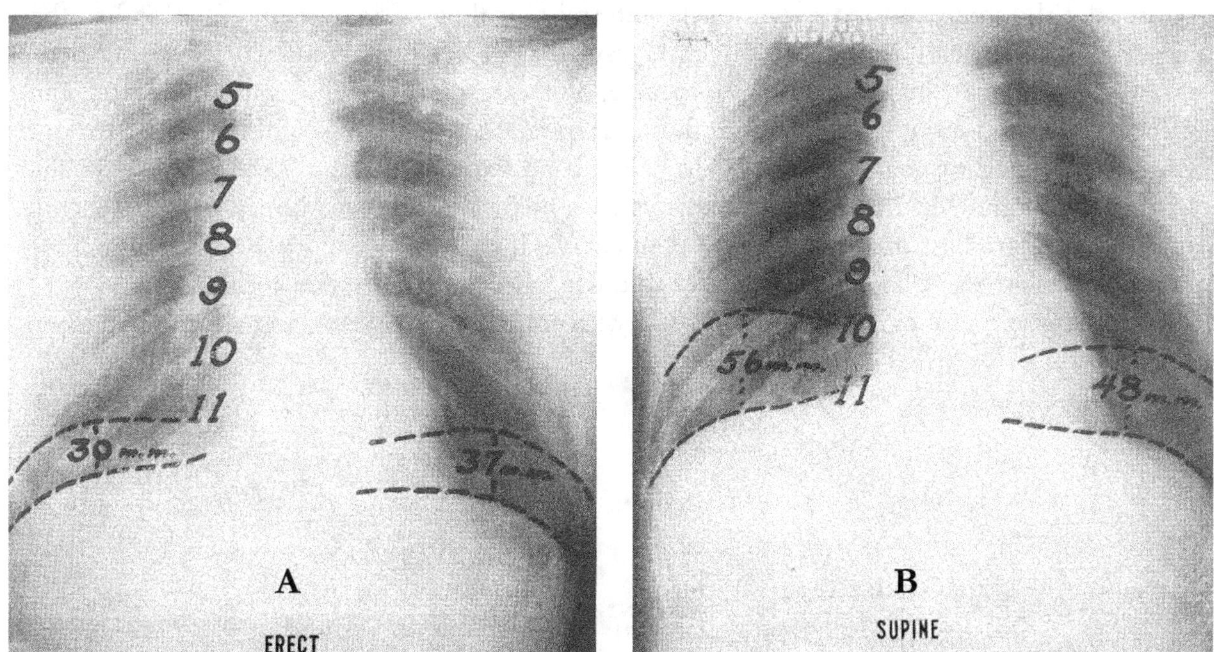

FIG.52. Position of diaphragm in A, erect posture and in B, supine posture.

The respiratory functions are restricted, as may be seen from a comparison of the components of the air breathed by patients and by normal subjects. The chief variation occurs in the tidal air, which is diminished in this syndrome. Changes in vital capacity do not occur until late in the course of the disease. Most of the patients complain of dyspnea when erect and during exercise—a peculiar type of dyspnea different from that usually experienced in cardiac failure. We have designated it as "orthostatic dyspnea" because it is observed only when the subjects are in the erect posture and not when they are supine, as is the rule with the dyspnea of cardiac failure (orthopnea).

There is evidence that the blood on the venous side does not return normally to the heart when the subject is erect. Circulation time is usually prolonged but may return to normal when an elastic abdominal support is employed. The output of the left ventricle is probably impaired.

100

This change is observed only when the subject is in the erect posture, and is not apparent in the supine posture or when an elastic abdominal support is worn. The fall in blood pressure and pulse pressure and the inadequate rise in cardiac rate probably indicate a faulty cardiac output. We have not found any reliable tests for cardiac output which can be employed to substantiate this hypothesis.

The diaphragm acts in part as a venous heart or boosting station for the return of blood to the heart from the abdomen and lower part of the body. The alternating variations in pressure within the abdomen and thorax aid in the intermittent flow of increments of blood to the right side of the heart against the force of gravity, while the blood from the head and neck and to some extent the arms, aided, of course, by the force of gravity, is more passive. The effect of reduced intrapleural pressure during inspiration is probably significant in returning the venous blood through the superior vena cava and particularly from the arms. The hiatus of the diaphragm acts like a valve in this venous heart and tends to keep the blood in the inferior vena cava flowing forward to the right auricle. It is obvious that these normal functions and relations are disturbed in the obese or in those with marked visceroptosis.

For many years we have observed patients with emphysema, obesity, and a combination of

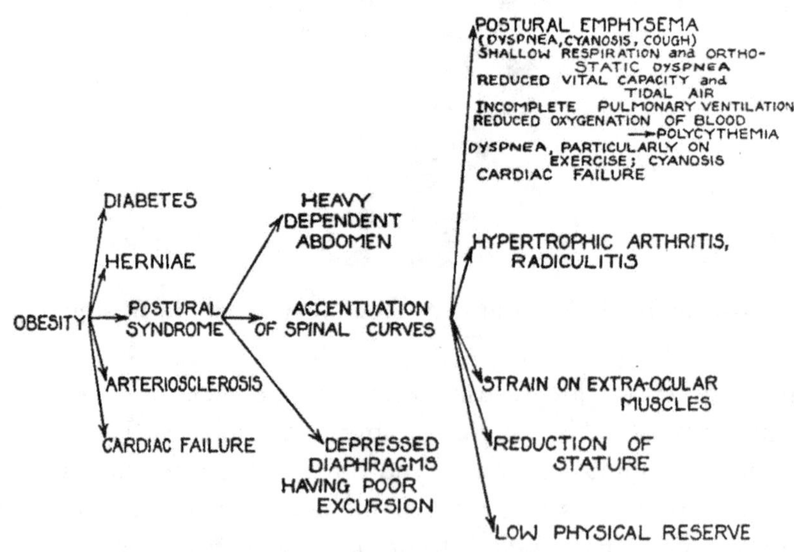

FIG. 53. Schematic representation of the postural syndrome resulting from obesity. From Kerr and Lagen. (Courtesy, Annals of Internal Medicine.)

complaints usually attributed to old age. It was obvious that the cardiac and respiratory symptoms did not respond to the usual methods of treatment for cardiac failure. In 1932, 1933, and 1934 the excellent papers of Alexander and Kountz and Kountz and Alexander directed our attention to the nonobstructive type of emphysema which has been spoken of as senile emphysema but is usually due to the postural defects described. Many years ago, in 1923, Goldthwait gave an admirable description of the symptoms and signs of ptosis of the heart and diaphragm. These and other reports led us to undertake studies on patients with postural emphysema. we found that the complex disturbances could be analyzed in part and that new avenues of approach to some related problems could be explored (Fig. 54).

Alexander and Kountz had described a ptosis belt with a flexible abdominal pad and found it valuable in the treatment of this type of emphysema. We (Kerr and Lagen) modified this

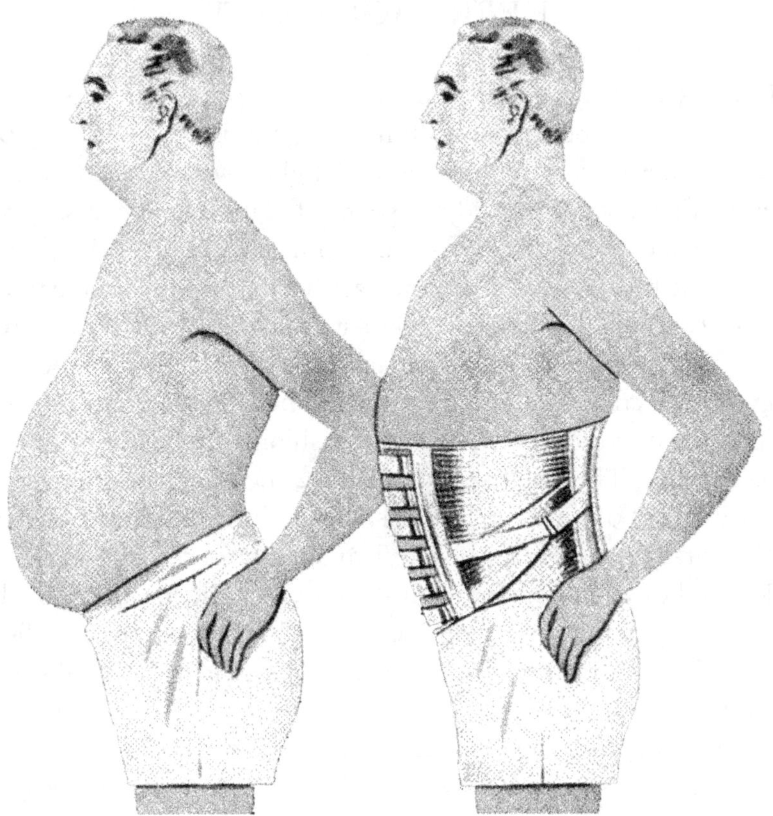

FIG.54. The obese patient with postural emphysema before and after fitting with the Kerr Lagen belt.

belt as described and as shown in Fig. 54. The results of the use of this belt in the treatment of postural emphysema are excellent in the thin visceroptotic person as well as in the obese. The orthostatic dyspnea disappears as the diaphragms move more normally. The polycythemia tends to diminish as the blood is aerated better, and the radicular symptoms are less pronounced as the line of gravity is restored. At this point a careful program of dietary restriction is added in an attempt to reduce the weight to approximately that in the early twenties. With co-operation this reduction may be achieved within a period of five or six months. At some stage postural exercises may be instituted, but it is not reasonable to make the attempt until the size of the protuberant abdomen has greatly diminished. It should be remembered that persons beyond middle life may not have excessive weight for their height but they may have gained in girth at the expense of the tissues of the extremities.

KERR-LAGEN BELT

The belt that we are presenting embodies several new principles. It is constructed with the physiologic function of the abdominal wall in mind, and is designed to supplement and aid the ventral muscles rather than to replace them. A tightly wound cloth binder would support the abdomen more efficiently but would not permit the mobility necessary for respiration.

The supporter is made of coutil, pekin-stripe cloth, and elastic goring, fastened on by skate buckles and hooks. The front sections and the back section are of double thickness. The outer layer is of high quality coutil, the inner of pekin-stripe cloth. The only difference between the two is in the softer and finer quality of the pekin-stripe material, which, being next to the skin, prevents chafing. Both sections are tailored or fashioned. There are three double stays in the back section with a seam at each, which permits fashioning the supporter to fit the contours of the individual patient. The back section is 81/2 inches in height, and the stays are of whalebone. For conditions of extreme lordosis, the cloth section in the back may be extended up to the twelfth thoracic vertebra and have firm aluminum or steel stays incorporated in it. The stays should not, however, be bent to fit the curve of the lumbar spine but should touch the body at only the upper and lower edges of the belt, allowing the middle to span or ridge the lordosed spine. The left front section has the hooks attached to it. The right front section has attached to it the straps.

Patients are taught to put on the belt before arising in the morning, preferably outside the undershirt. If a union suit is worn, the belt can be worn underneath it over a thin garment. The patient should be in the supine position when he puts on the belt, and the belt should be tightened from below upward. This is important in order to move the abdominal fat and viscera upward rather than to compress them in the lower abdomen. The unusual feature of the belt is the width and height of the elastic side sections, particularly the width. This is obtained by making the front narrow and thus permitting the elastic side sections to extend farther forward on the abdomen where the elasticity is much more beneficial than if it were placed toward the back. The increased elasticity permits expansion of the belt during inspiration, aids rather than suppresses abdominal breathing, and prevents limiting respiration to the thorax, as is seen in obese states naturally or when a firm, inelastic belt is applied. The increased elasticity also aids in expiration and overcomes the prolonged expiratory period seen in these patients with depressed diaphragms due to abdominal ptosis or emphysema. The diaphragm more readily assumes the expiratory position and is ready to descend with the next inspiration. There is no decrease in the supportive effect during the inspiratory expansion.

ANGINA PECTORIS

In the course of treating patients with postural emphysema, a number of them complained of typical attacks of anginal pain. This did not surprise us because in this group we have always encountered these attacks as well as other vascular crises, such as apoplexy and gangrene of the extremities. However, when these patients began to report that their pains had disappeared under treatment, we took some note of it. As the result of subsequent studies we have made reports on a large series of such cases. We have also made observations on a group of patients with cardiac irregularities and on another group with cerebral symptoms which appear to be related to the same mechanism. In all of them treatment similar to that used in postural emphysema has given spectacular results. In a series of almost 300 patients with anginal pain, the attacks have been prevented almost uniformly. Many sufferers have been restored to an active business or professional life. Many probably have avoided an untimely death from coronary occlusion or other serious cardiac accidents by timely treatment.

The method of treatment is the same as has been described for postural emphysema (Fig. 55). The elastic belt acts as a means of artificial respiration. It is applied snugly and holds the diaphragm in a higher position even if the patient is in the erect posture. In order to secure the greatest excursion with respiration, it may be necessary to adjust the tension of the belt fluoroscopically. When the diaphragm starts from a higher position in expiration, the positive contraction of its muscle sheets increases the intra-abdominal pressure and the elastic parts of the belt are extended. With relaxation of the diaphragm the elastic parts of the belt exert an external pressure which brings the diaphragm back to the expiratory position. The changes in intrapleural pressure are largely passive and reciprocal. The heart fills more adequately from below the diaphragm and presumably has a better output. If the output is better the coronary circulation is augmented and consequently the supply of oxygen to the cardiac muscle is not greatly reduced. This, in short, is an explanation of the mechanism which has been disturbed by obesity and has caused postural defects resulting there from. The consequent disturbances in function of the lungs and heart result in anginal pain. Other factors are operative in some cases of anginal pain. For example, anything that increases the work of the heart (increased rate) or decreases the amount of oxygen-carrying capacity of the blood may bring on pain in the absence of postural emphysema. In some instances, these factors may augment each other. Since the diaphragm serves a most important function in returning blood to the heart, any fixation of the leaves of the diaphragm may interfere with cardiorespiratory function. This interference is seen when subdiaphragmatic factors, such as tumors, enlarged organs, fluid, or gas, fix the diaphragm at a high position. Deformities of the spine or rib cage likewise may interfere with this important function.

The statement of some authors that angina pectoris is not related to obesity is probably not based upon careful observation. In our experience most patients who complain of anginal pain in their forties or fifties are or have been much overweight. Those who complain of anginal pain only after the age of 60 years are more likely to be of slender build and will prove to be of the visceroptotic type.

Cerebral vascular accidents such as thrombosis or hemorrhage are commonly seen in the obese with the syndrome described. Attention to dietary restriction, abdominal support, and postural exercises are also of prophylactic value in these cases.

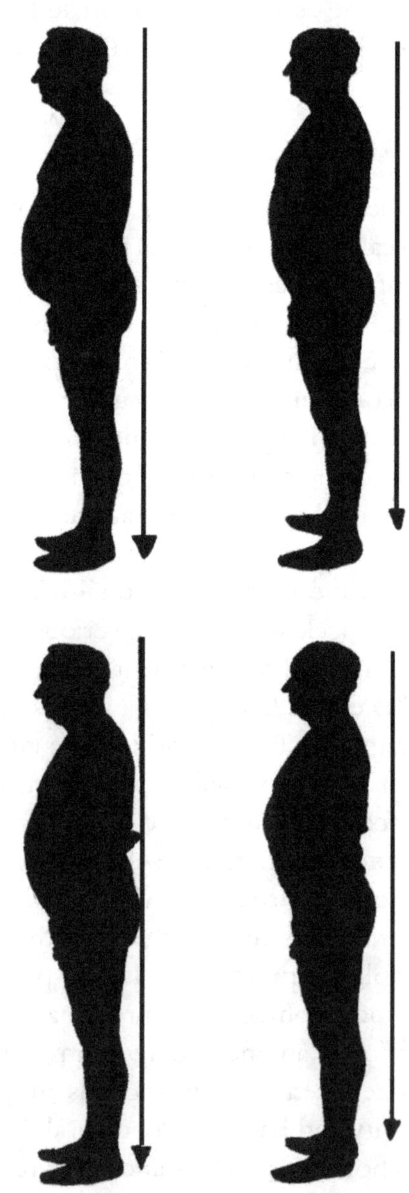

FIG.55. Upper figure without belt.Left hand figures made on first visit of patient, right hand figures taken three months later.It must be emphasised that these are natural poses; no attempt was made by the patient to exaggerate his posture. (From Kerr and Lagen. Courtesy Annals of Internal Medicine.)

8

Diseases of the Abdominal Viscera

The dependence of function on normal position and proper support is exemplified well by the abdominal viscera. Serious disturbances in function can occur in faulty body mechanics. Usually such disturbances come slowly, and pathologic changes in the organs appear only after years of faulty posture. The appearance of degenerative changes probably could be delayed if the added strain on the organs were removed. At least, many functional disturbances could be prevented or relieved, as will be shown in this chapter.

POSITION OF THE ORGANS AND THE VESSELS

All the organs used for the digestion and the assimilation of food are in the abdominal cavity. They are fitted into a space immediately under the diaphragm and are protected by the lower ribs, except in a small area in front, the epigastrium (Fig. 27). The liver, together with the gallbladder and the stomach, lies close under the diaphragm and is attached to it, rising and falling with every diaphragmatic motion. The other organs in the upper abdominal cavity are the spleen, the 2 kidneys, and the 2 suprarenal bodies, the pancreas and the duodenum. Other structures located in this region are the abdominal aorta and its chief branches, such as the celiac axis, the renal arteries and the superior mesenteric artery, also the great abdominal veins, the vena cava and the portal vein. Closely surrounding the celiac axis and its branches is the splanchnic sympathetic nerve plexus-the so-called solar plexus (Figs. 27 and 56). All these organs and vessels are held in position by the diaphragm above and by the basketlike curve (Fig. 56) of the ribs at the sides and the back. Posteriorly is the lumbodorsal region of the spine, with the 2 deep lateral cavities formed by the backward curving of the lower ribs. The posterior muscles, such as the psoas, as well as the posterior wings of the pelvis and the normal curve of the lumbar spine, form a shelf which supports the upper-abdominal organs from below, and with the aid of the abdominal muscles (when properly used), tends to keep these organs in the proper position for their best functioning.

In the epigastrium, the pancreas lies across the aorta and the vena cava at the level of the first lumbar vertebra, immediately below the celiac axis and above the superior mesenteric artery. To the right of the pancreas and below it are the second and the third parts of the duodenum. Anterior to the pancreas is the solar plexus (sometimes called the "great abdominal sympathetic brain") , which has been mentioned above. The mesentery of the small intestine,

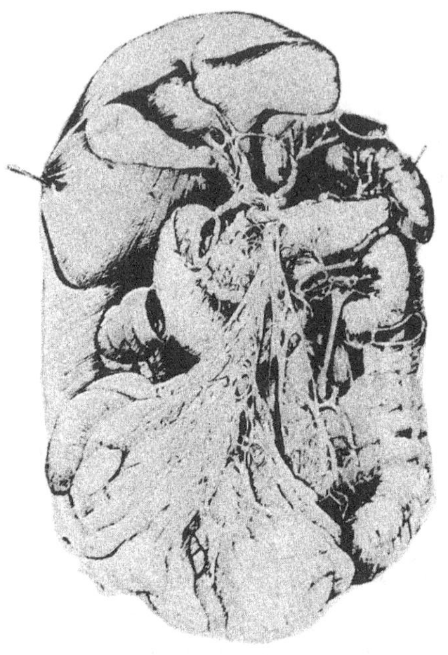

FIG.56. Schematic view of upper abdominal cavity. The liver has been retracted showing second and third parts of the duodenum, the pancreas, the spleen, the left kidney and the suprarenal, with the mesentery of the small intestine pulling downward across the pancreas and the duodenum. Note the tracery of the sympathetic nerves accompanying the blood vessels to all of the viscera in this region. Sagging of these organs must cause drag on the sympathetic nerves as well as blood vessels.

which carries the superior mesenteric artery, veins and nerves, is attached firmly to the posterior abdominal wall and crosses the third portion of the duodenum. As the small intestine, except the duodenum, lies free in the abdominal cavity except for the mesentery, the full weight of the small intestine comes on this narrow band, with its blood vessels and sympathetic nerves, as it crosses the collapsible duodenum.

The large intestine consists of the ascending, the transverse, and the descending colon. The ascending and the descending colon are attached retroperitoneally in the stocky anatomic type, but in the slender type are usually free with a mesentery, as is seen often in roentgenograms. The transverse colon is attached to the greater curvature of the stomach by the transverse mesocolon behind the omentum. Its weight is carried by the stomach and its attachments at the hepatic and the splenic flexures. The large intestine, being attached to the lower border of the stomach, like the stomach is subject to rise and fall with the excursion of the diaphragm.

From this brief review of the anatomic positions of these important organs of digestion it is evident that their position at any one time is dependent upon the position of the diaphragm, to which they are attached. If the diaphragm is down, they are down. Every respiration moves them to some degree. This fact always has been recognized in palpating the abdomen to determine the location of the liver, the spleen and the kidneys. The position of the stomach

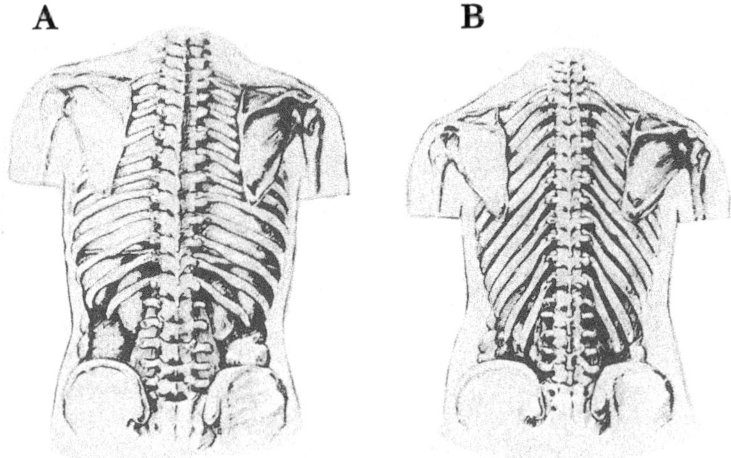

FIG. 57. (A) Posterior view (diagrammatic) of the torso in good body mechanics, showing how the ribs give room and support to all of the upper abdominal organs. (B) Posterior view of the torso in faulty body mechanics, showing the ribs pulled in and crowded together and much more nearly vertical. Ribs in this position can give very little support to the upper abdominal organs.

can be seen to change with respiration under the fluoroscope.

Changes in position in the other viscera are also commonly observed. Their habitual position is dependent upon the tone and retraction of the abdominal wall, upon the extent of the lumbar lordosis and the associated forward inclination of the pelvis, and upon the position of the diaphragm.

THE DIAPHRAGM

It has been shown in that the position of the diaphragm and its excursion are dependent upon the shape of the chest and the abdomen (Figs. 22 and 58). The drooped attitude of faulty mechanics lowers the diaphragm; the erect posture, with good body mechanics, raises it and increases its excursion. Therefore, in the drooped posture, the diaphragm being low and almost at complete inspiration, the liver, the spleen, the kidneys and the stomach, with the attached transverse colon, are also low. The effect of this is important.

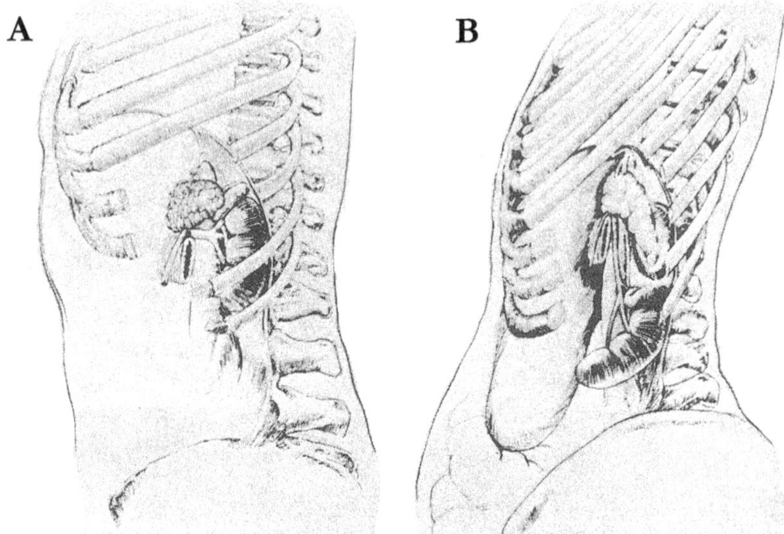

FIG. 58. (A) Lateral view of the abdominal cavity in the position of good body mechanics. Note that the diaphragm is highest at its anterior attachment, thereby making the greatest possible room for the viscera in the upper abdomen. The lower abdominal muscles are flat. This flat abdomen, combined with the normal tilt of the pelvis, gives upward support to the abdominal organs and makes more secure the shelf upon which the kidney rests. (B) Lateral view of the abdominal cavity in the position of faulty body mechanics. Note the change in the shape of the diaphragm. The anterior portion is much lower, thereby rotating the liver downward and forward, with a resultant change in the axis of the gallbladder. The amount of displacement and rotation varies with the type of anatomic structure. The lower abdominal muscles are relaxed and protuberant, and this, combined with the increased forward tilt of the pelvis, takes away from the viscera the upward support of the abdominal and the psoas muscles. It also lessens the shelf upon which the kidney normally rests. With this sagged position of the abdomen there is less space in the upper abdominal cavity for the viscera which normally should be there.

THE LIVER

The liver, being held by its suspensory ligament, is pressed downward and rotated forward and over to the right. As it rotates in the manner described, the position of the fundus of the gallbladder is changed, so that it is lower than the cystic duct, thereby making free drainage of the gallbladder more difficult; this also tends to produce more of a drag mechanically on the cystic, the hepatic and the common ducts, as well as on the hepatic artery and vein. Chronic passive congestion of the liver and the gallbladder, as well as biliary stasis, is a possible result of such malposition if this is of long duration. Possibly, because of the greater flexibility of the skeleton and the natural mobility of the abdominal organs, the slender anatomic type suffers less from this displacement than does the stocky type. The latter is less extreme in its bad posture but is subject to equal, if not greater, crowding of the abdominal viscera. It is in the latter, the stocky type, that chronic gallbladder and liver troubles are persistent and marked.

THE PANCREAS

The pancreas is fixed in its position. It is attached to the posterior abdominal wall at the level of the first and the second lumbar vertebrae and crosses the aorta between the celiac axis and the superior mesenteric artery. Below it lies the third portion of the duodenum. To the right is the second part of the duodenum; above and anterior to it is the solar plexus; and in front is the pyloric end of the stomach. Below and posteriorly lie the kidneys, which serve partially as a support to the pancreas when the body is used properly. The pancreas cannot be displaced and therefore it is subject to pressure (1) by the celiac axis as it is pulled downward by the stomach and (2) by the stomach itself (Fig. 59). Dissecting-room specimens actually have shown a groove across the body of the pancreas caused by the pressure of the celiac axis. Since duodenal digestion of all foods is dependent on the hepatic and the pancreatic secretions, nutrition may be disturbed when there is interference with the full physiologic function of either organ. If the blood supply of the pancreas is interfered with by pressure, chronic passive congestion may occur. Not only may the external secretions be damaged, but the internal secretion of the islands of Langerhans also may be deranged temporarily or permanently. Such derangement may lead to temporary or chronic glycosurias, the general ptosis from faulty body mechanics being the original cause of such dysfunction. This circulatory stasis, or chronic passive congestion, also must lower resistance to infection and be at least a potential factor in the etiology of some cases of acute or chronic cholecystitis and pancreatitis.

Treatment. With this conception of the potential factors in the etiology of these diseases, the treatment should be planned to improve the circulation of the organs involved, no matter what other forms of treatment are indicated. This can be accomplished by the use of the special positions mentioned in the chapters on treatment, Chapters 11 and 12. The horizontal position, with the chest raised, relieves the downward drag of the abdominal organs and allows the diaphragm to rise to a higher level. This makes possible its greater excursion and, by improving the circulation, decreases venous pressure and congestion. The value of this position cannot be overemphasized, for the diaphragm, through its action on the great abdominal veins, is the chief means of forcing the circulation from the abdominal vessels to the right side of the heart. An improperly working diaphragm, together with the abnormally low position of the organs themselves in faulty body mechanics, can explain local as well as general congestion of various

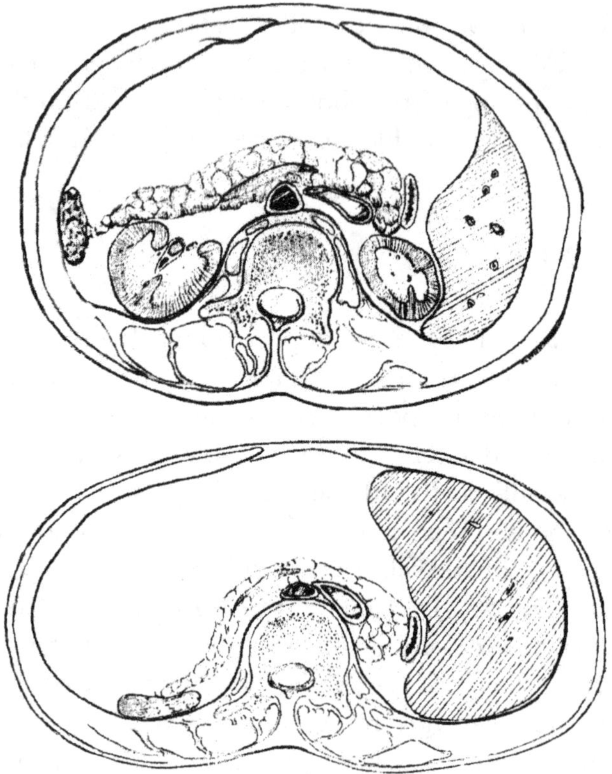

FIG. 59. Diagrammatic transverse sections in the region of the pancreas. (Top) Good body mechanics. Note that the pancreas is in nearly a horizontal position, the head and the tail both being supported by the kidneys and the retroperitoneal fat. (Bottom) Faulty body mechanics. In this position the kidneys have sagged out of place, and the retro-peritoneal fat, upon which the kidney rests, has been absorbed. The pancreas, being fixed to the posterior abdominal wall, has conformed necessarily to the prominence of the lumbar spine. This permits the head and the tail of the pancreas to sag backward, making undue pressure on the whole organ. (See text.)

abdominal organs. It also may account for the impaired function of the organs which are so dependent on their normal blood supply and their balanced sympathetic and vagus stimulations.

CASE REPORTS

Case 1. Apparent Diabetes Mellitus in a Child. A boy 6 and a half years of age was examined first in September, 1920, in an attempt to improve the posture and thus, the general health. He had diabetes and had been given a hopeless prognosis by a well-known specialist in that disease. It was after this prognosis that, in despair, correction of posture was considered. When first examined the child was in extremely poor condition, with the posture as shown in Figure 60 A. There had been a great deal of trouble with the digestion, with much vomiting, and with persistent sugar in the urine in spite of careful dieting. The muscle tone was extremely poor; the ribs and the diaphragm were sagged. The intestines were distended markedly with gas, and the ptosis of all the organs was extreme. As part of the poor body balance, the feet were flat, the pelvic joints were strained, and there was marked sagging of the shoulders.

The child was taken to the hospital, where, because of the poor position of the organs, and because the condition was so grave, a plaster-of-paris jacket was applied with the body hyperextended. By this means the ribs and the diaphragm were raised as much as possible, with the natural drawing up of the abdominal organs.

At first the child was very sick, vomiting was frequent, and feeding was difficult. However, the condition changed gradually, food was taken more easily, the vomiting ceased, and the sugar in the urine disappeared. At the end of 4 weeks the child was taken home to continue the treatment there. At the end of 2 months he was much improved, was eating heartily with no special restriction, the sugar in the urine had not reappeared, and the attacks of vomiting had ceased wholly. The child then was allowed up, wearing a special brace during the day to hold the body properly poised, and wearing the plaster-of-paris jacket at night. At this stage in the treatment special exercises were started, with a gradual increase in the activities.

Following this, there was a steady improvement in general vigor, until the child was able to lead a normal life. The jacket was given up after a few more weeks, but the brace was continued for a longer time. The child has been seen occasionally since then for general guidance in his development. He has matured as a splendidly poised young man, with all the interest and the activities of health. There has been no return of sugar in the urine nor evidence of other visceral disturbances.

In this case the sugar in the urine, as well as the vomiting, were evidently part of the poor mechanics of the body. The drag or the pressure on the pancreas was to be expected if the mechanics of the viscera of the upper abdomen were appreciated. Apparently neither the pancreas nor the stomach was diseased, and once the faulty mechanics of the whole body was corrected, not only were the organs able to function normally but, with the general improvement in the muscle tone, the flat-foot, the round shoulders and the joint strain was corrected also.

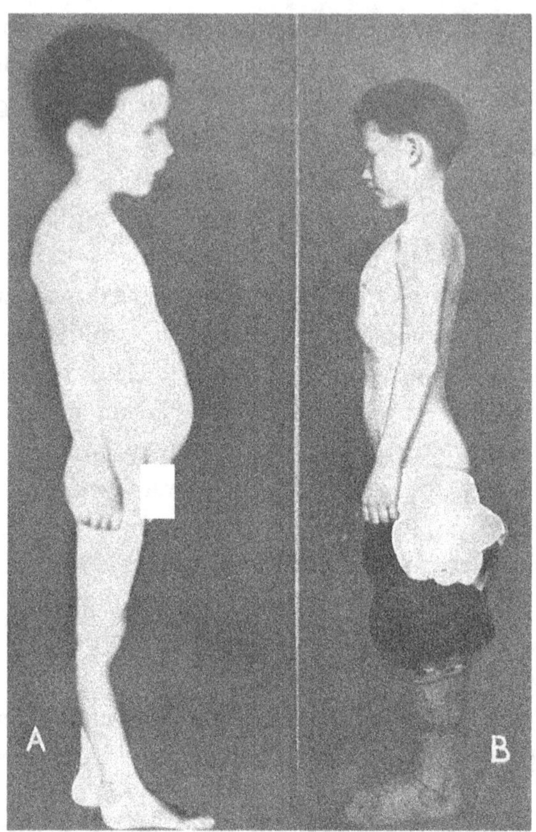

FIG. 60. (A) Diabetes mellitus (Case 1 at age of 6 and one third years). Note the faulty mechanics, as well as the facial expression, and the disproportionate size of head, neck, chest, and abdomen. The chest is very flat. The lower abdomen is particularly large and prominent. The knees are hyperextended. (B) Case 1 at age of 12 years. Note the change in the body mechanics, as well as in the facial expression. There is a change in the proportion of head, neck, chest and abdomen. The body mechanics are not perfect, as evidenced by the hollows under the ribs and the fact that lower abdomen is more prominent than the upper abdomen. The diabetic symptoms had disappeared entirely.

Diabetes Mellitus in an Elderly Woman with Gangrene of the Foot. In contrast with this in point of view of age, the following case, equally serious in prognosis, is presented. the two cases taken together probably represent the extremes of this disease.

Case 2. A married woman, 70 years of age, had been advised to have her left leg amputated for diabetic gangrene. She consulted us in the hope of saving her leg. At that time the circulation in the left foot was very poor, and the pulsations in the dorsalis pedis and the posterior tibial arteries could not be felt. The dorsum of the foot was deep red, with a sharp line of demarcation just above the ankle. A slough with the usual offensive discharge had started at the side of the big toe. Muscular control of the toes was present. The circulation in the other foot and leg was also poor, no pulsation of the arteries at either ankle being felt. The general body mechanics were poor, and the common bed position at the time of consultation was with two or more pillows under the head, so that the body was flexed sharply at the dorsolumbar level. (The constricting effect of this upon the action of the diaphragm must be apparent.) There was one and a half degrees of elevation of temperature, and the pulse was weak and rapid. The sugar content in the urine had been high but had been kept under control with insulin.

Amputation was advised against, and treatment for the faulty body mechanics was begun at once. The patient was kept in bed; all pillows were taken away in order to raise the ribs and thus not only raise the diaphragm but make its function more nearly normal. In her usual position in bed, there had been marked restriction of the action of the diaphragm, as well as of all the organs in the upper abdominal cavity. Exercises to increase the action of the diaphragm were begun, and hot fomentations were applied to the back, with hot mildly antiseptic dressings to the foot.

At first the insulin was stopped, but the diabetic features became worse, so that 5 units were given, and this was increased to 10 for a few days. At the end of 10 days the insulin was discontinued, the sugar in the urine after that never amounting to more than a trace. The general condition improved rapidly, and the circulation in the foot changed more rapidly than had ben expected. The discolouration disappeared except at the base of the great toe, where a slough formed between it and the second toe. This gradually came away, as did part of one of the phalanges of the great toe.

Gradually, with the improvement in the general strength, the exercises were increased, including those commonly given for the circulation in all the tissues. A body support, to be worn with a special corset, and a foot plate were fitted, and at the end of a month the patient was allowed to be up for short periods. The circulation in both legs improved, so that pulsation of the arteries at the ankles could be felt. At the end of six weeks from the beginning of treatment the patient left hospital to carry on at home. At that time the slough had come away, and the wound was healed almost entirely. The patient was walking about the hospital without difficulty. Not only was the circulation in the legs much improved, but the general circulation was normal, so far as one could tell, with the pancreas functioning so that much of the time there was no sugar in the urine, and never more than a slight trace.

Since leaving the hospital the patient apparently has done well, although she has refused further medical supervision. She is active, ding her own housework, and on fairly free diet, such as was begun at the hospital, and the leg has been saved.

In this case it is probable, in the light of the patient's age and the severity of the condition, that the pancreas had received some permanent damage from the long continued faulty mechanics, but the amount cannot have been very great or incompatible with reasonable health. The case was handled from the point of view of correcting the faulty body mechanics, and the results were as expected except that the changes were more rapid. Nature is ready to repair damage if given a chance.

THE SPLEEN

The spleen lies below and in contact with the diaphragm. Its blood and nerve supply come through vessels from the celiac axis and the portal vein. In the drooped posture it is displaced downward with the diaphragm because of the change in the position of the ribs. Such displacement produces a pull on its pedicle and, interfering with the normal blood supply, causes a chronic passive congestion which sooner or later will affect the functional capacity of the spleen. Secondary anemias are not uncommon in the slender anatomic type with habitual poor posture.

THE STOMACH

The stomach must be considered from the point of view of the slender and the stocky types of anatomy. In the slender type, the pylorus is always higher than the lesser curvature, as the stomach is of the "fishhook" shape (Fig. 5A). Any relaxation of the suspensory ligament of the diaphragm, which must occur in the drooped posture, lowers it and the cardiac end of the stomach. In the slender type, particularly, this increases still further the sagging of the stomach, thus retarding its emptying and producing gastric stasis. As a result there may be a train of symptoms such as hypochlorhydria or hyperchlorhydria, hypoperistalsis or hyperperistalsis, cardiospasm or pylorospasm, depending largely on which set of nerves is stimulated or dragged upon by the faulty mechanics. Once the significance of this faulty mechanics is understood, these distressing symptoms can be treated much more logically. It is interesting to note that functional disturbances, such as hyperacidity and gastric stasis, have been considered to be the forerunners of the common chronic organic diseases of the stomach, such as ulcer, gastritis and cancer. It is not inconceivable that faulty body mechanics, with its ptosis and disturbed functions, precedes chronic physiologic derangements and permanent organic disease.

In contrast to the vertical or "fishhook" stomach of the slender type, the stocky type has the "cow's horn" or transverse stomach (Fig. 5 B). In this type the pylorus is not above the lesser curvature, and the stomach is not so movable and cannot be displaced so far downward. Its lower border is usually at about the level of the lower costal margin. Because of this lessened mobility in the abdominal cavity, due in part to the more bulky abdominal viscera, it is subject to relatively greater pressure than is the slender stomach. Consequently, although the faulty posture in the stocky type may not be relatively as great as in the slender type, stasis, abnormal muscular action and abnormal secretions are often present. For the same reason, such symptoms in this type are relieved more easily, and function is restored more speedily by correction of the drooped body.

Cyclic Vomiting, Congenital Visceroptosis, Imperfect Poise, Malnutrition, Etc. In an article by Goldthwait and Brown, entitled "The Cause of Gastroptosis and Visceroptosis" and published in the Boston Medical and Surgical Journal for May 26, 1910, attention was called to a condition seen with the slender type of individual when the body is imperfectly poised. It was pointed out that in many cases not only were the abdominal viscera different in shape from the textbook type, but also the mesenteries were longer, with the result that when the body was poorly poised it was possible for the organs to sag much more than when the textbook type of anatomy existed; The marked stomach seen in later life is a combination of the acquired sag which comes from years of, wrong body position and from the normal low position of the organs. When the body is drooped, the stomach drops to a level much below the normal, so that its lower border is at times in the true pelvis. This means that the pylorus and the first portion of the duodenum are dragging across the fixed or retroperitoneal portion of the duodenum and adjacent structures. This, of course, makes the draining of the stomach more difficult, so that material may be retained there much longer than is normal; sometimes the food of the first meal is in the stomach when the next meal is taken. This delay apparently ends in Nature's emptying the stomach through the mouth, and in a certain number of cases the attacks of vomiting occur with regular periodicity, a condition described in recent years as cyclic vomiting.

The following case is illustrative of this condition. The symptoms are merely an outcome of the bad mechanics of the viscera, in which, for some reason, the stomach rebels more than do the other organs.

Case 3. A boy, 8 years of age, for several years had had much difficulty with his digestion. Every 3 or 4 weeks there was a slowing down of the appetite, followed by a few days of much vomiting; practically no food was taken during this period. In spite of medical treatment the condition continued, with a natural gradual increase in the general malnutrition. The child was a member of the family of one of us, and in the hope of explaining the condition much investigation in the dissecting room at the Harvard Medical School was carried on, with an ultimate understanding of the mechanics of the abdominal viscera. Once this was achieved the treatment was confined virtually to correcting the extremely faulty mechanics, which are shown in Figure 61. This was accomplished by taking special positions and performing certain exercises lying down. In order that the stomach might be drained thoroughly and thus gain its proper tone, the position of hyperextension (see Fig. 99A) was taken after every meal, and this was followed by the prone hanging position (Fig. 62). (In the latter position the lower part of the stomach is raised so that any material that would not be drained naturally into the duodenum drains upward toward it and is passed on rapidly into the intestine.) In connection with the treatment a brace was used to improve the general posture.

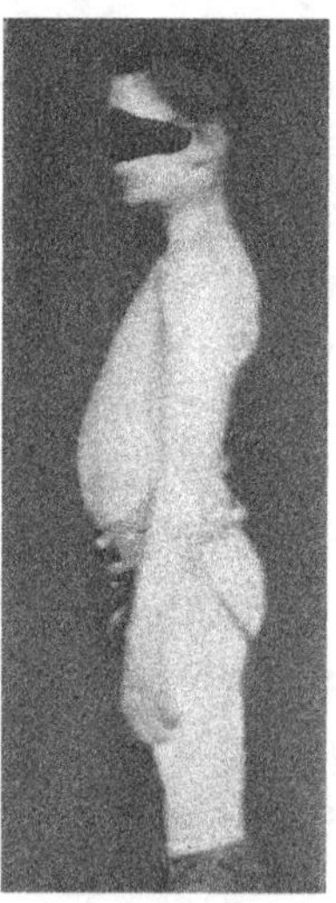

FIG. 61. Case 3, aged 8 years. Diagnosis: cyclic vomiting. Note the faulty body mechanics as evidenced by the flat chest, the forward-drooped shoulders, the large abdomen and the extreme lumbar curve of the spine. The brace seen in this picture does not and cannot correct the faulty body mechanics. It only relieves the extreme sag and thereby lessens the drag on all the viscera. Such a brace must be used only in conjunction with other treatment over a long period of time, as described in the text.

Excellent results were obtained with this procedure, whereas previous to treatment attacks of vomiting were marked, and the child was easily made car sick. Little by little, with the correction of the mechanics and the regular, thorough drainage of the stomach, the condition improved. A year later the child was taken with his family across the country to Alaska and back, with absolutely no difficulty from car sickness or from disturbance of the digestion. He developed into a strong, healthy, well-poised man, still with a slender type of anatomy, but with the mechanics of the body such that there was no disturbance of the viscera.

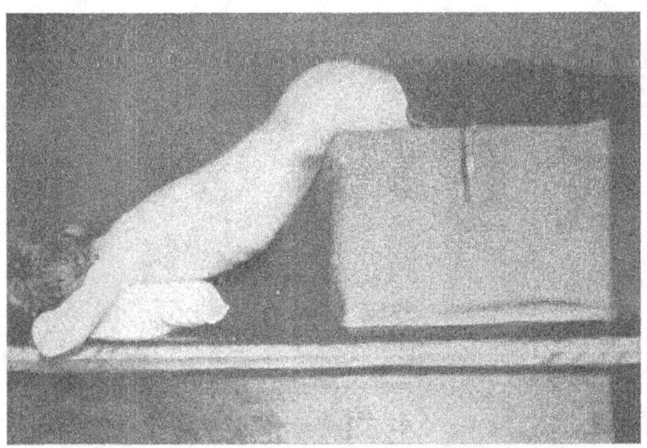

FIG. 62. Prone hanging position. The head and the shoulders are much lower than the hips. This position permits the sagged viscera to fall back into the upper abdomen, thereby relieving the downward drag on their attachments.

Case 4. Abdominal Pain, Floating Kidney, Appendicitis, Postoperative Adhesions, Backache, Congenital Visceroptosis. A woman 32 years of age was examined first in June, 1912. She had been operated on twice, 4 years before, without permanent benefit, once for a floating kidney on the right side, and once for removal of the appendix. She then had refused further treatment by the surgical department of one of our largest general hospitals. She was sent to a sanatorium for nervous diseases, where she remained for 6 months, and from which she was discharged without relief. Following this, after having received much medical treatment, she was examined by one of the best-known internists, who, after careful study, reported that nothing could be done for her except to make her comfortable until she died. It was at this time that the physician in whose family the patient had been employed sought orthopedic advice.

After the orthopedic examination no promises were made, but the extremely poor body mechanics (Fig. 62) were demonstrated, and the hope was expressed that the correction of this would relieve the symptoms. The patient was in poor general condition. For a number of years she had had pain and distress in the abdomen, more on the right side than the left, with an increasing sense of weakness in the abdomen, making it hard for her to sit up. The digestion had been very poor. There had been considerable vomiting. The patient had been seriously constipated, and movements were followed by prostration. There was considerable pain referred to the low back as well as to the left side of the chest. Sleeping was difficult, chiefly because of back pain.

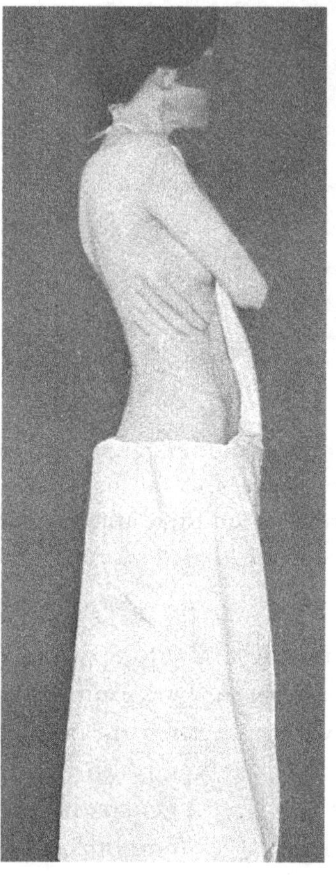

FIG. 63. Lateral view of patient, taken in 1912. Note the extreme slender anatomic type with the marked faulty body mechanics; the chest is very flat and drooped downward, the ribs being very nearly vertical. The epigastrium is very hollow, and the lower abdomen markedly protuberant below the umbilicus. Note operative scars. The spine is used at the extreme of its cervical, dorsal and lumbar curves.

Examination showed extreme visceroptosis of the so-called congenital type, with the ribs and the diaphragm low, the tubular stomach well down in the pelvis, and the transverse colon low, but the hepatic and the splenic flexures fairly high. The liver was low, and the remaining kidney was low and floating, as one would expect with such a low diaphragm. There was very little retroperitoneal fat (Fig.63), and undoubtedly many abdominal adhesions as the result of operations. The general body mechanics were as shown in Figure 64. There was marked chronic strain of the pelvic joints.

The patient was taken to the hospital, and an attempt was made to correct the extremely faulty mechanics. She was kept in bed at first, and everything possible was done to raise the ribs and to draw up the diaphragm in the hope of stretching the abdominal adhesions. Special positions were used, and special exercises, as described in other chapters, were given. The condition was so extreme that a plaster-of-paris jacket, applied in the corrected position, was used.

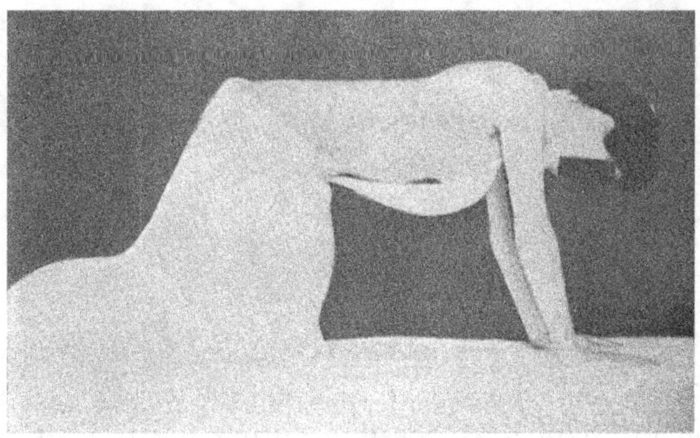

FIG. 64. This shows the position in which patients are examined to acquire information impossible to get when the patient is on his back. In this position the organs fall away from the posterior wall, the abdominal muscles relax, and deeper palpation is possible if there is no inflammatory process present. Note the marked hollow or depression in the loins. This shows almost complete absence of retroperitoneal fat in the region of the kidneys which, of course, makes the so-called "floating kidney" more possible.

Later on a leather jacket (Fig. 65) was substituted, at first day and night, and then only at night. With this type of jacket the patient's sleep was much more restful.

At the end of 5 weeks the patient had improved enough so that a short back brace was fitted, and with this under a special corset, she was allowed to be up for short periods, the leather jacket being worn only in bed. She remained in the hospital for 3 months, during which the gain was marked, with relief of practically all the symptoms and considerable gain in weight.

Following this, the patient was examined from time to time at the office. The apparatus was modified, and the exercises were changed as seemed best, the object being always to make the general body mechanics as nearly perfect as possible. The recovery was complete and has so continued (Fig. 66). During World War I the patient successfully carried the responsibility of the social service work of one of our large hospitals at a time when a shortage of help made such duties unusually hard. The service which she was able to render to her patients was of a very high order, partly because of all that she herself had been through.

In this case, as in many others, the patient's health depended on making possible the functional performance of parts of the body. No actual disease of the organs having been found at any time, the successful result was obtained by correcting the faulty mechanical adjustments and by treating the patient and not the symptoms.

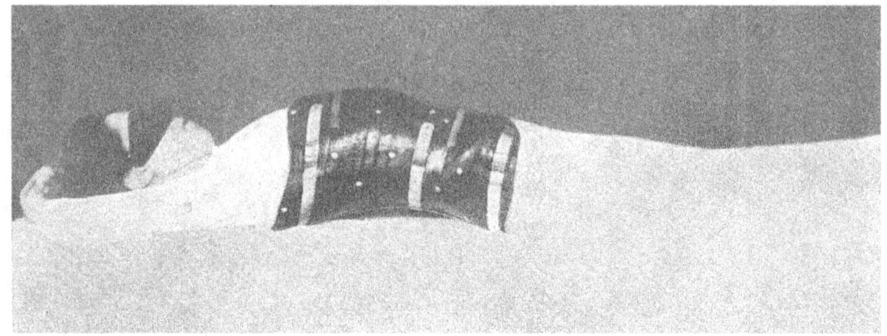

FIG. 65. (Top) This type of leather jacket was used to keep the body in as good mechanics as possible during the time in bed. With this, the patient slept better and was able to compensate for the long-standing fatigue.

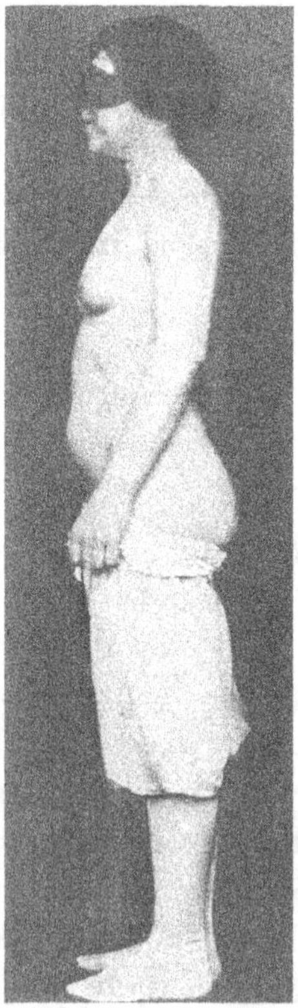

FIG. 66. (Right) The same patient l6 years later. Note marked improvement in general condition, as well as in body mechanics. It was impossible for her to correct fully her body mechanics because of bony deformation due to many years of faulty use. The correction she obtained allowed her body to compensate for the strain and the fatigue of the original position.

Case 5. Chronic Backache, Visceroptosis, Gastric Ulcer, Gallbladder Disease. A man 39 years of age was examined first in October, 1914, having been referred to us by Dr. F. C. Shattuck, in an effort to discover whether the weakness of the back was associated with the abdominal symptoms. The chief symptoms had been pain and distress in the abdomen, with considerable nausea; these had not yielded to treatment. Various diagnoses had been made, among them gastric ulcer and gallbladder disease.

At examination the outstanding feature was the marked sagging of the body. The chest was low, and the abdomen sagged, the lumbar spine was used in the position of extreme extension, and the general muscle tone was poor. The photographs taken in the beginning (Figs. 67A and 67B) well show the apparent general weakness and fatigue. The prominent abdomen does not necessarily represent extreme size or fatness, since the patient was photographed in as erect a position as possible.

The condition was explained to the patient, and special exercises were begun for him to carry on at home. A brace to support the body and to hold the abdomen in better position was planned, and he was seen at the office from time to time. There was a gradual improvement in the condition and a disappearance of the symptoms as the body mechanics became better.

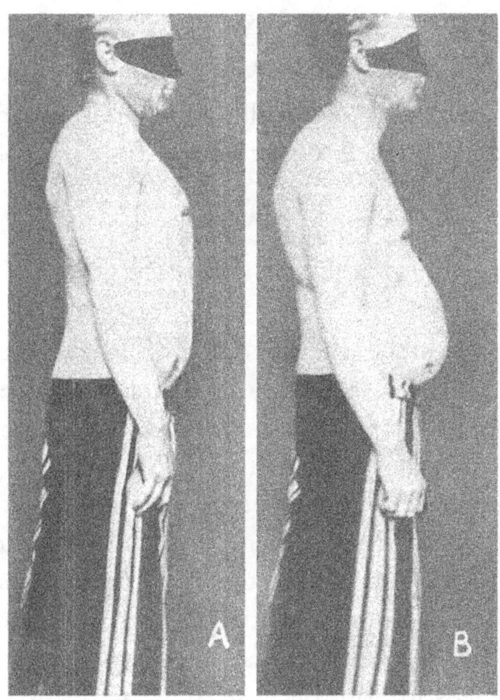

FIG. 67. (A) Case 5. The patient is attempting to pull in the abdomen. The chest is raised without contracting the abdominal muscles. (B) The same patient shown in the habitual standing position with the forward head, the drooped shoulders and the flat chest. Note the prominence of the abdomen in its lower portion.

THE DUODENUM

The duodenum lies about the head of the pancreas. It is retroperitoneal in its second and third portions. Therefore it is subject to pressure and constriction by the mesentery of the small intestine as the latter crosses from the back wall of the abdomen to reach the small intestine. If ptosis is present, the duodenum, being a collapsible tube, may be closed completely by pressure, and duodenal stasis may result. In faulty body mechanics the pylorus is usually a considerable distance below the beginning of the retroperitoneal or second part of the duodenum, which is fixed and immovable (Figs. 1, 5, 6 and 27). This downward displacement may produce a kinking of the duodenum at the junction of the first and the second portions, with all the possibilities of interference with function and circulation which inevitably accompany it.

It is interesting to note that duodenal ulcer, dilatation and stasis occur most frequently between the pylorus and the second portion of the duodenum. It is conceivable that duodenal stasis and dilatation of the first portion of the duodenum may obstruct the hepatic duct, giving rise to symptoms of duodenitis, pancreatitis or biliary stasis (Fig. 68).

THE SMALL INTESTINE

The small intestine varies greatly in the slender and the stocky types (Chap. 2), not only in length, but in secretions, mobility and assimilation. The slender type has a small intestine, often a third or a fourth as long as that of the stocky type (Swaim, Bryant and Bean). In the former there is more possibility for change of position in faulty body mechanics, and therefore downward displacement has its chief effect through pull on the mesentery. Such a pull, although frequently compensated by gradual development, may affect the mesenteric blood vessels and the sympathetic nerves, which control the secretions and the innervation of, and the absorption from, the small intestine. Much of the malnutrition of the slender asthenic type can be ascribed to overstimulation of peristalsis in the short small intestine, to chronic passive congestion from venous stasis and to lack of absorption. Because of these disturbances, much of the food is not assimilated properly in the small intestine, thus making possible increased putrefaction and fermentation in the large intestine.

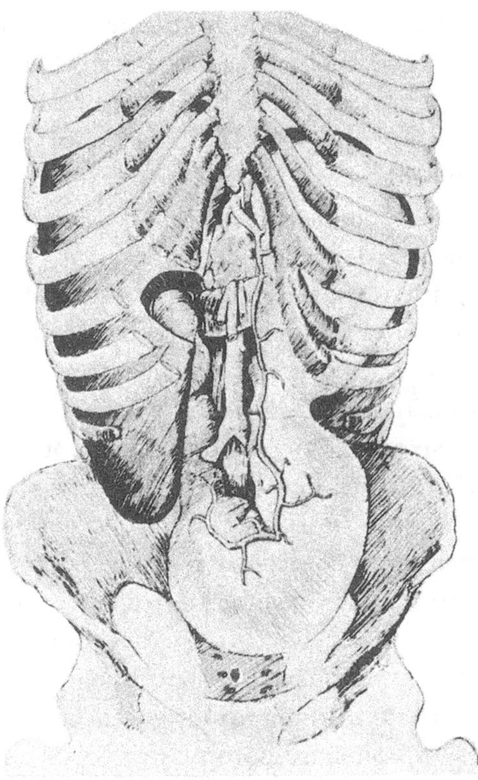

FIG. 68. Diagrammatic view of the organs of the upper abdomen in faulty body mechanics. Note that with the narrowing of the ribs all the movable upper abdominal organs are displaced downward and therefore must produce more or less pressure on the retroperitoneal organs and blood vessels, such as the pancreas, the duodenum, the celiac axis and its arteries and the sympathetic nervous system. This sketch is based on the actual findings in a roentgenogram.

THE CECUM

The cecum in the slender type is always loosely attached and has wide variations in position unless held down by adhesions of pathologic origin. Its tip, dilated and atonic, often is found lying over the brim of the true pelvis out of reach of the palpating hand. A "puddle" of barium is frequently found here in roentgenograms. If dilatation of the cecum has progressed far enough, the ileocecal valve may become incompetent, resulting in symptoms of absorption from stasis. The positions of the cecum, the ascending colon and the hepatic flexure, which are attached loosely in the slender type, are dependent on two factors: (1) the downward pressure from above and (2), the removal of support through relaxation of the abdominal muscles. As the ensiform approaches the symphysis in the drooped posture, the tonus and the strength of all the abdominal muscles become lessened; the stomach, the small intestine and the transverse colon therefore tend to sag, often to the brim of the true pelvis. This is particularly the case in the slender type, where the colon is especially movable, since embryologically it is unattached to the posterior wall except in the splenic and the sigmoid regions. Dilatation of the cecum, with stasis, may give rise to symptoms resembling appendicitis. Stasis and spasticity of the transverse colon may result in symptoms of colitis. These are not uncommon in the slender, drooped person, and the symptoms often are relieved by correction of the posture and the visceroptosis. Poor body mechanics may give rise to functional disturbances of the colon, and to these have been attributed a long list of symptoms, ranging from indigestion to neurasthenia and from auto-intoxication to arthritis. The primary factors in the production of these symptoms are chronic passive congestion, stasis and disturbed innervation, which may be caused by the abnormal positions of the organs always found in faulty posture.

In the stocky type, the cecum usually is attached to the posterior abdominal wall, and the appendix may be small and, not infrequently, retrocecal; the hepatic flexure is higher and less movable than in the slender type. Flaccid constipation is often the only intestinal symptom in the acquired ptosis of this group; probably it is one of the factors in the production of hypertrophic arthritis through chronic auto-intoxication, acting as a chemical irritant to the joints.

The stocky type has a long small intestine—often from 25 to 39 feet. This length increases the absorptive surface and may account for the better nutrition. However, such small intestines weigh more. This weight is no inconsiderable factor in producing the acquired visceroptosis so often found in faulty body mechanics. When acquired ptosis is established, it may give rise to the same gastric symptoms and intestinal indigestion as are seen in the slender group.

THE KIDNEYS

The kidneys, which are the chief organs of excretion, are not attached by ligaments but are held in their retroperitoneal pockets by fat. A loose kidney is found almost always with faulty posture. The drooped thorax obliterates the forward thrust of the ribs and relaxes the diaphragm, thus pushing the liver downward on the kidney to the right. Because of this pressure the protecting fat is rapidly lost, and ptosis of the kidney follows. Chronic passive congestion, kinked ureter, hydronephrosis, orthostatic albuminuria, urinary stasis, stones and infection are possible outcomes, since the function of the kidneys is dependent on a full blood and nerve supply and on free drainage—all of which ptosis may disturb. The normal position of the kidneys can be restored, and the protecting fat replaced, by relieving the downward pressure of bad body mechanics.

THE PELVIS

It remains to speak of the pelvic cavity and the pelvic organs, as these are subject to the same possibilities of disturbance of function from faulty body mechanics as may occur in any other part of the body. In fact, since they are below the abdominal cavity, they are perhaps subject not only to the disturbances which may come from their own displacement but also to the pressure from displacement and downward pressure of the abdominal organs.

In good body mechanics, in which the chest is held up, and the diaphragm is high, and the abdominal wall is firm and flat below the umbilicus, the abdominal viscera exert little or no pressure on the pelvic organs (Fig.69A). In poor body mechanics, where the chest and the diaphragm are both low, and the lower abdominal wall—that below the umbilicus—is relaxed and protuberant, there must be a marked backward thrust of the lower abdominal viscera directly into the pelvic cavity (69B). Not only can this cause local pressure and possible congestion but it also must have an effect on the pelvic organs, since their only method of drainage is through the great abdominal veins.

With such a conception of the mechanical factors influencing the circulation of the pelvic organs, is it not possible that here is an explanation of the congestion of the bladder and the prostate so often found in older men, which may lead to prostatic hypertrophy and malignancy of the prostate? In the female pelvis, the malpositions of the uterus and the weakened pelvic floor so common after childbirth may become the cause of symptoms, when associated with body mechanics, when by themselves they would not. The symptoms of dysmenorrhea, menorrhagia and irregular menstruation, so common in young girls, often have disappeared entirely when the mechanics of the body were improved sufficiently to remove the pressure from above.

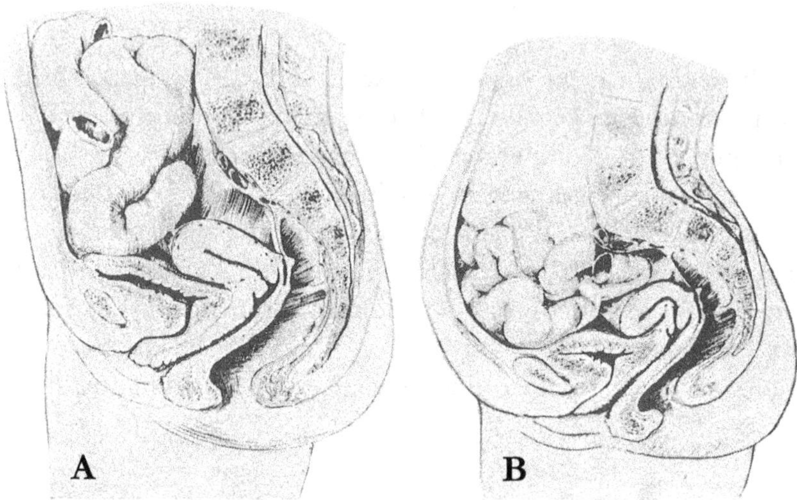

FIG. 69. Diagrammatic lateral view of the pelvis and the lower abdomen. (A) Good body mechanics. Note that the forward tilt of the pelvis (diagonal conjugate), combined with the flat lower abdominal wall, gives considerable support to the hollow viscera and that the axis of the urethra and the vagina approach the horizontal. (B) Faulty body mechanics. The increased forward tilt of the pelvis combined with the relaxed and protuberant abdominal wall gives no upward support to the intestines, permitting pressure on the pelvic organs. The increased forward tilt of the pelvis also tends to make the axis of the urethra and the vagina more nearly vertical, an important factor in pelvis prolapses.

Another condition which is very distressing and causes great disability and discomfort, and for which there is no cause given in the textbooks, is varicose veins. Faulty body mechanics, with the consequent congestion of the abdominal and the pelvic organs, and the pressure of these organs on the iliac veins and the arteries in the pelvis, as well as the diminished pumping action of the diaphragm on the abdominal and the pelvic veins, is a very important factor in the cause of varicose veins of the legs. It well may play a part in making the dilated veins associated with childbirth permanent varicosities.

CONCLUSIONS

An attempt has been made in this brief discussion to draw attention to the effect of bad body mechanics on the position of the abdominal organs and the possible disturbances which may take place in their normal functions and health. It has been shown that the main factors which determine the maintenance of the abdominal viscera in position are the diaphragm and the abdominal muscles, both of which are relaxed and cease to support in faulty posture. (Fig.66). The disturbances of circulation from a low diaphragm and ptosis may give rise to chronic passive congestion in one or all of the organs of the abdomen and the pelvis, since the local, as well as the general, venous drainage may be impeded by the failure of the diaphragmatic pump to do its full work in the drooped body. Furthermore, the drag of these congested organs on their nerve supply, as well as the pressure on the sympathetic ganglia and plexuses, probably causes many irregularities in their function, varying from partial paralysis to overstimulation. All these organs receive fibers from both the vagus and the sympathetic systems, either one of which may be disturbed. It is probable that one or all of these factors are active at various times in both the stocky and the slender anatomic types and are responsible for many functional digestive disturbances. These disturbances, if continued long enough, may lead to diseases in later life. Faulty body mechanics in early life, then, becomes a vital factor in the production of the vicious cycle of chronic disease and presents the chief point of attack in its prevention.

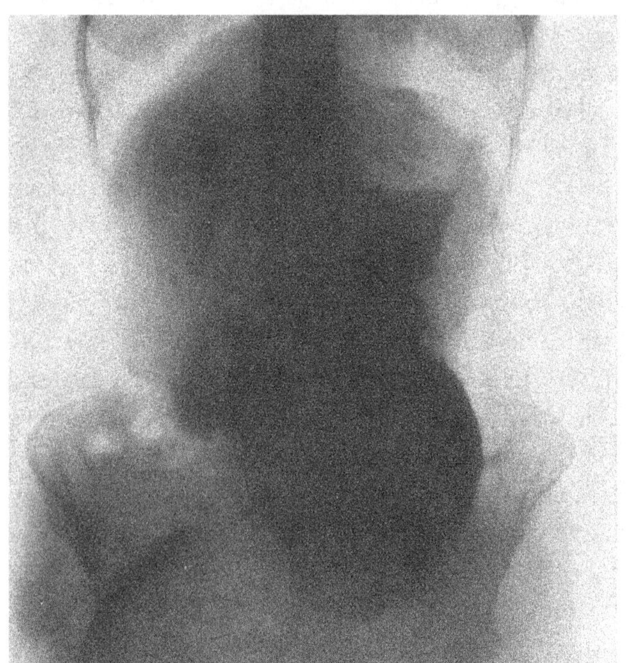 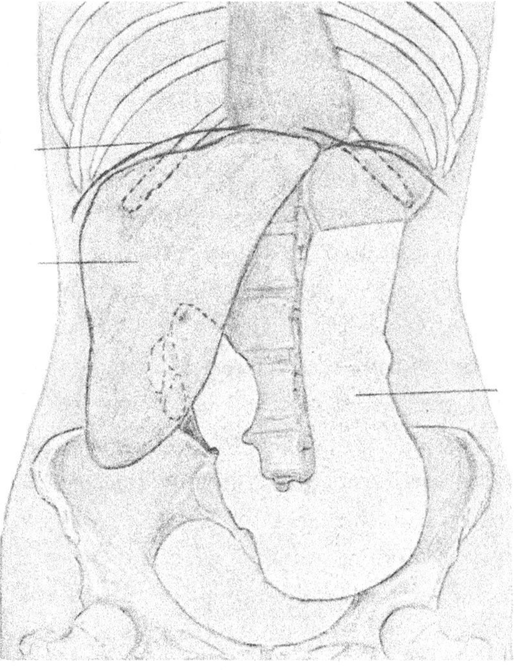

FIG.70

Roentgenogram and diagram showing that when there is downward displacement of the diaphragm, A, there must be also downward displacement of the other organs. The liver, B, is not only displaced downward but also is rotated to the right and is partially in the pelvis. Note that the axis of the liver is almost vertical instead of the usual horizontal axis. The stomach, C, is also in the pelvis. the kidneys, the spleen and the intestines must be displaced downward to a greater or a lesser degree, the exact amount varying with each individual.

9

Diseases of the Nervous System

Good body mechanics is essential for the proper functioning of the nervous system. The effects of bad body mechanics upon this system are expressed indirectly, chiefly through the locomotor and the circulatory systems.

The nervous system should not be considered as a distinct entity apart from the other systems of the body, since it integrates and regulates them, and they in turn support and nourish it. It is composed of cells somewhat more specialized in function and differing more widely in structure than those in other parts of the body; but they are affected in much the same way as are those of other tissues in fatigue, in intoxication and in circulatory changes. There are many cases on record which suggest that they are more vulnerable than those of other tissues.

CHANGES IN STRUCTURE

Nerve tissue subjected to a sufficiently severe insult dies. Nerve cells-the neurons—and the supporting structure, or neuroglia, may be damaged by a large number of destructive agencies. A series of changes in structure occur, which may go on to destruction and necrosis. In the early stages these changes are confined to the finer histologic elements of the cell, and a return to normal appearance and normal function is usually possible. With more serious injury there is a swelling of the body of the nerve cell, with structural changes in the chromatin and the fibrillary elements, a wandering of the nucleus to the periphery of the cell, vacuolation of the cell body and granular degeneration of the fibrils. Complete structural and functional recovery is rare. The next step is a decrease in size, and finally, a disappearance of the cell nucleus. At the same time the nerve fibers peripheral to the point of injury undergo degeneration, with progressive disappearance of the myelin sheaths.

Holmes has shown that fatigue alone may lead to a disappearance of the chromophilic substance in the nerve cell. Such variation in structure, he believes, under ordinary physiologic conditions does not produce permanent changes in the cell, but in so far as it lowers resistance and vitality, it may be a factor in bringing on pathologic changes primarily due to other causes. Nerve cells have a somewhat limited power of recovery from injury. So far as we know, when they die they are not replaced. The dead cells are destroyed by phagocytic cells, and their place is taken by neuroglia, producing scar nerve tissue. The peripheral fibers of nerve cells do repair and may resume their usual functions. Occasionally, the function of destroyed nerve cells is taken over by other nerve cells or pathways.

130

CIRCULATORY DISTURBANCE

It is believed commonly that no other tissue in the body is so dependent on a constant and efficient supply of blood as that of the nervous system. Even a temporary anemia may produce demonstrable changes in nerve cells, with serious temporary derangement in function, such as loss of consciousness, paralysis or anesthesia. The arteries of the brain and the cord are numerous and delicate and are supported somewhat poorly by the neuroglia and the membranes. These factors make even slight circulatory disturbances extremely serious. Moreover, the excessive vascularity of nervous tissue renders it particularly liable to the action of circulating toxins. It has been demonstrated that extreme cerebral congestion may produce violent pain and even convulsions. On the other hand, Leri has shown that continued cerebral anemia may produce cavitation, scarring and perivascular softening. Small repeated hemorrhages may produce similar changes in cerebral tissues. This may be seen particularly well in the brains of aged people. The part played by disturbances in the lymphatic circulation is more obscure, although edematous infiltrations have been produced by lymphatic blockage.

While the pathologic changes may be traced step by step in the nerve tissue, we have a much less clear conception of the disturbed physiology that is present in the nerve cells before irreparable damage has occurred. Our usual neurologic tests are not sufficiently acute to demonstrate these early changes, and the sufferer commonly does not consider a slight derangement of function to be of sufficient importance to make him consult his physician. Such changes often do not point to the nervous system primarily and are dismissed commonly as "nerves" or debility. The abnormalities that may be found, if carefully looked for, are increased irritability, decreased alertness, decrease in the rapidity and the skill with which volitional acts are performed, decreased activity of sensation, abnormal flushing and blanching of parts and increased sensibility to changes in temperature. These may suggest beginning inability of the nervous system to cope with injuries which it is receiving.

The nervous system is protected peculiarly by a bony covering against trauma from without, but is unprotected against mechanical trauma from within. While the circulation and the fluid exchange are regulated marvelously in health, their normal variation in nervous tissue is sharply limited (Fig. 71). This is true whether we consider the brain, the cord, the sympathetic ganglia or the peripheral nerves. In the brain in health, the vasomotor center in the floor of the fourth ventricle ensures an adequate blood supply, but severe trauma or disease, by markedly decreasing or increasing the peripheral resistance of the circulation or disturbing endocrine function, may and often does produce conditions with which the vasomotor center is unable to cope. The more severe grades of such circulatory disturbances and their effects on the nervous system have been studied carefully by physiologists and pathologists, but the milder forms and the effects of slight, long-continued derangement have not been recorded (Fig. 72).

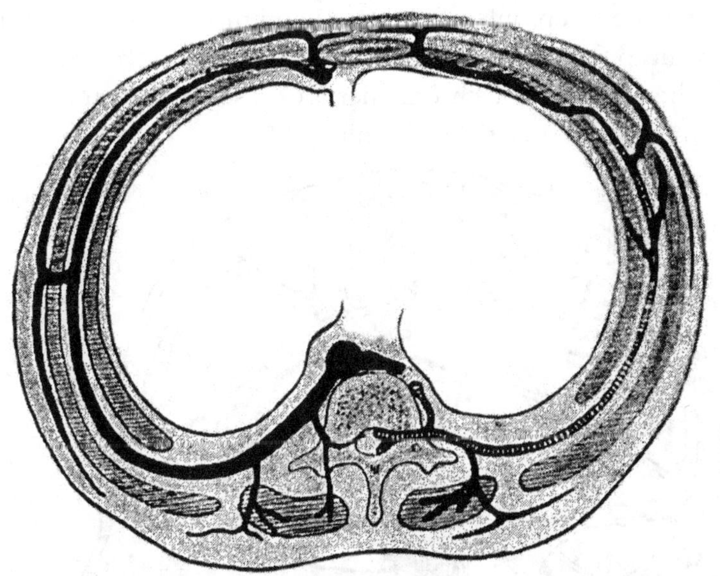

FIG. 71. Diagram of the arterial and the nerve supply in a single vertebra. Through each intervertebral foramen pass the arteries, two veins, the anterior and the posterior nerve roots and the branch of the sympathetic. All these, with the fat and other supporting tissues, occupy each intervertebral foramen, one side of which is formed by the tissues of the joint of the spinal articular facets.

VENOUS DRAINAGE

In the preceding chapters it was shown that slowing of the return flow of blood and serious congestion of various tissues could be produced from the constant assumption of faulty body mechanics, primarily through decreased function of the diaphragm. With visceroptosis and splanchnic congestion this may lead to anoxemia of certain organs, as reported by Sanders. In addition, stretching of vessels as they enter the spinal canal and pressure on nerves or ganglia may produce disturbances in function. In a series of experiments, Batson has shown that the venous return from the lower part of the body and the vertebrae follows three pathways: the vena cava, the splanchnic and the portal system, and the vertebral system. Normally not much blood is carried through the vertebral veins, but with abdominal or interference through the vena cava or the iliac veins, a much greater portion is found therein. Through mechanisms of this nature, damage to the spinal cord can occur because of faulty body mechanics.

In this short discussion no attempt has been made to review all the diseases of the nervous system. A discussion will be given only of the more common ones which can be related both in cause and in treatment to faulty body mechanics. Emphasis is given to certain factors which are of importance in the evolution of chronic nervous diseases and are concerned also in the development of a number of associated deformities.

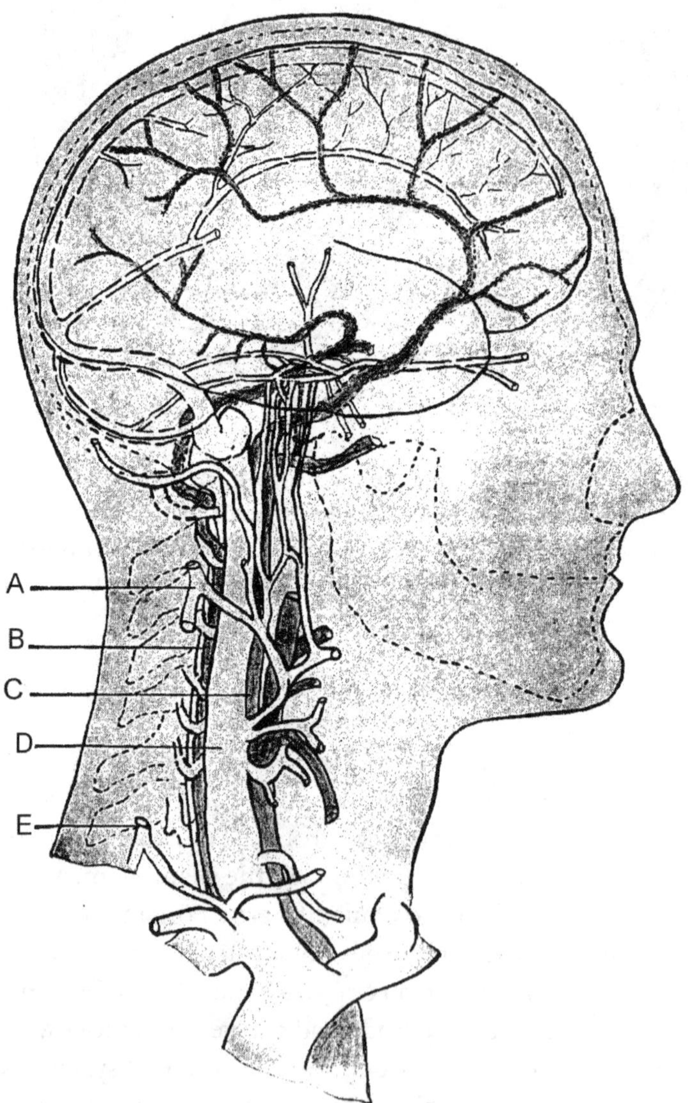

FIG. 72. Diagram of the cerebral circulation. Note how close the arteries and the veins are about the cervical spine. Stretching and kinking can occur readily with habitual faulty positions of the head. (A) Vertebral vein. (B) Vertebral artery. (C) Internal carotid artery. (D) Internal jugular vein. (E) External jugular vein.

DIVISIONS OF THE NERVOUS SYSTEM

For convenience, the nervous system may be divided into the vegetative nervous system, the sensorimotor system and the psychic apparatus. The vegetative system has for its function the maintenance of the metabolic processes of life. It regulates the glandular, the gastro-intestinal, the genito-urinary, the vascular, the respiratory, the muscular, the cutaneous and the osseous structures. The sensorimotor portion, through its sensory and motor nerves, regulates the balance and the interrelation of the various motor organs of the body. It ensures that the various parts of the body shall work harmoniously. The third and highest division, the psychological, is the most complex. Of the processes of thought, memory, reason and choice we know little. Only the outward expressions of these processes are apparent, but that they may be disturbed in physical disabilities is evident daily.

VEGETATIVE NERVOUS SYSTEM

It is impossible to describe all the disturbances which may occur in the vegetative nervous system. Its relation with all parts of the body, and particularly with the endocrine glands and the cardiovascular system, makes its alterations in functional activity of peculiar importance. **Disturbances.** The vegetative nervous system supplies all the smooth muscles and the secretory glands of the body. It controls functions which are absolutely essential to life. Disturbances of this system may result from stimuli of various kinds: in emotional response, as shown in palpitation of the heart, anorexia, fainting, crying, dilatation of the pupils and diarrhea; in the reaction to infections and toxins, as shown in reddening, swelling, gooseflesh, tachycardia, and gastric and visceral crises. Constitutional defects of the vegetative nervous system have been suggested as being the cause of the changes seen in acromegaly, scleroderma, dwarfism and the myopathies. It is related so closely to the other portions of the nervous system that nervous diseases usually have some manifestations in its disturbed functions.

Impulses from the vegetative nervous system apparently are involved in all our movements through their automatic regulatory mechanism. Evidences of disturbance in it are common in habitual faulty body mechanics. Functional changes may be produced by circulatory disturbances. Changes in position or pressure by the surrounding structures also may cause disturbances of the functions of the sympathetic ganglia and their connecting fibers. Pressure about the cervical spine from faulty posture or from arthritis frequently leads to changes in the sympathetic nervous system. These may take the form of sympathetic reflexes, which manifest themselves in the skeletal structures as visceromotor reflexes, viscerosensory reflexes and viscerotrophic reflexes. A moment's consideration will suggest the innumerable changes that may take place in the functions of viscera and in sensations referred to the various portions of the anatomy, such as the radiation of pain in gallbladder and renal disease, as well as in angina pectoris. Disturbances which are ascribed commonly to malfunction of the glands of internal secretion cannot be separated wholly from those resulting from abnormal nervous control by the vegetative nervous system. The normal physiologic equilibrium of the body is maintained ultimately, it is believed, through the interaction of this system and the hormones of the glands of internal secretion.

SYMPATHETIC NERVOUS SYSTEM

The vegetative nervous system is divided sometimes for convenience into the sympathetic system and the parasympathetic system. The sympathetic nervous system consists chiefly of chains of ganglia lying on each side of the vertebral column with, as a rule, one ganglion for each spinal nerve root. The parasympathetic system has a somewhat similar arrangement in the cervical and the sacral regions. The superior cervical ganglion is one of the most important in the sympathetic system. It innervates the blood vessels of the head, the muscles of the hair bulbs, the sweat glands of the head, the dilator muscle fibers of the eye and the orbital muscles of Muller. It connects with the first four cervical nerves and the pharyngeal and pharyngeal and the superior cardiac nerves. Its usual location is opposite the second and the third cervical vertebrae. Anteriorly, it is in contact with the internal carotid artery and the internal jugular vein. The middle cervical ganglion is found opposite the sixth cervical vertebra. The inferior cervical ganglion is located at the base of the transverse process of the last cervical vertebra (Fig. 73)

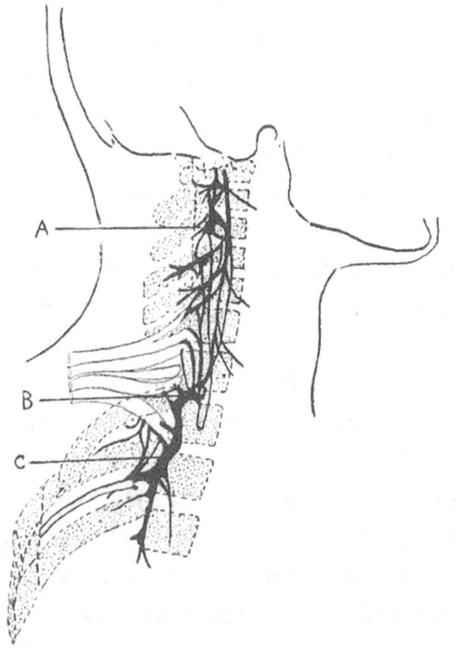

FIG. 73. Diagrammatic sketch of the cervical portion of the vegetative nervous system. Persistent changes in the position of the cervical vertebrae can produce functional disturbances in these ganglia. (A) Superior cervical ganglion. (B) Middle cervical ganglion. (C) Inferior cervical ganglion.

Disturbances in Sympathetic Ganglia. It can be seen readily that persistent changes in the position of the vertebrae, such as are found in faulty body mechanics, may produce disturbances in the sympathetic ganglia. With long-continued faulty body mechanics, actual pathologic changes are found in the cervical vertebrae, and symptoms referable to the cervical sympathetic nervous system are observed often.

The sympathetic ganglia connected with the dorsal nerve roots, so far as can be determined, are not as subject, as are the cervical ganglia, to mechanical trauma in faulty body mechanics. However, the position of the ganglia against the anterior surface of the heads of the ribs makes stretching of their afferent and efferent fibers no remote possibility. The cardiac plexus of the sympathetic system is situated at the base of the heart, one part lying in the concavity of the aortic arch, the other between the aortic arch and the trachea. While the functions of this plexus are not understood completely, it is known to send fibers to the muscles of the various cardiac chambers, and it has been suggested that it may play a role in the regulation of blood pressure. Marked sagging of the heart and the diaphragm (Fig. 74) must be considered as being a potential cause of disturbances of the normal function of this plexus.

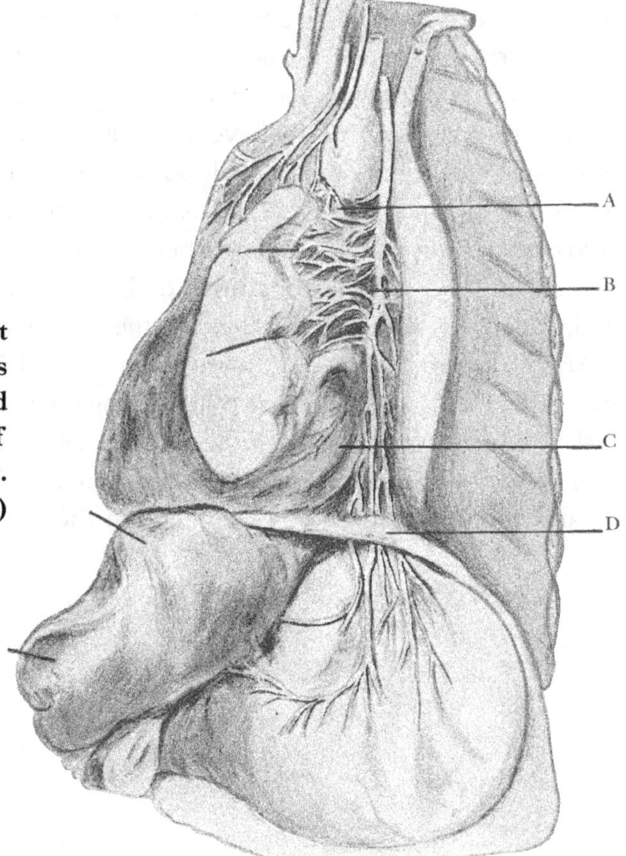

FIG. 74. Sympathetic plexuses about aorta and heart. Stretching of nerve fibers may occur readily from downward displacement of the heart. (A) Arch of aorta with plexus of sympathetic nerves. (B) Vagus nerve. (C) Base of heart. (D) Dome of diaphragm.

Probably the most important of the ganglia and the plexuses is the abdominal portion of the sympathetic nervous system. The celiac or solar plexus is the largest and is situated at the level of the upper portion of the first lumbar vertebra. It is intimately connected with a number of other plexuses supplying sympathetic fibers to the various abdominal and pelvic viscera. As has been shown, the greatest displacement of the viscera in faulty body mechanics occurs in the upper-abdominal region. Such displacement is seen commonly in patients with symptoms referable to the upper-abdominal region for which no cause can be found. Probably many of these are due, as Pottenger has suggested, to disturbances of the sympathetic nervous system which can be explained on a mechanical basis. We cannot evaluate satisfactorily the changes that result from disease or derangement in the vegetative nervous system because of their complexity, but no one will deny their importance (Fig. 75).

The autonomic (sympathetic) nervous system includes those efferent and afferent fibers which are concerned chiefly with the regulation of the internal processes of the body. Each efferent fiber has communication with one of the sympathetic ganglia. The afferent fibers serve many important reflex functions, as well as being the channels for the appreciation of visceral pain. The ganglia are chiefly distributing centers, although they serve also as local nerve centers for reflex action. To a certain extent, autonomic function is subject to control of the cerebral cortex. Without the autonomic nervous system, animals can live in a sheltered environment, but activity is lessened greatly because the stimulation and the activation of numerous reserve mechanisms have been lost. There is no longer heart acceleration, liberation of adrenalin, redistribution of the blood volume, dilation or constriction of the various smooth muscles. In the main, the two divisions of the autonomic system, the parasympathetic (craniosacral) portion and the sympathetic (thoracolumbar portion) are opposed to each other. Many organs have fibers from both divisions. Usually the sympathetic division helps the organism to maintain a constant environment for its cells or aids in calling out the reserves of the body in emergencies. The parasympathetic division has more conservative functions, slowing the heart, constricting the pupil, aiding digestion and elimination. Both are so integrated that they co-operate in maintaining a continued uniformity of the environment for all the tissues of the body. It is through this autonomic system that disturbances or improvements in visceral function are mediated by changes in the mechanics of the body.

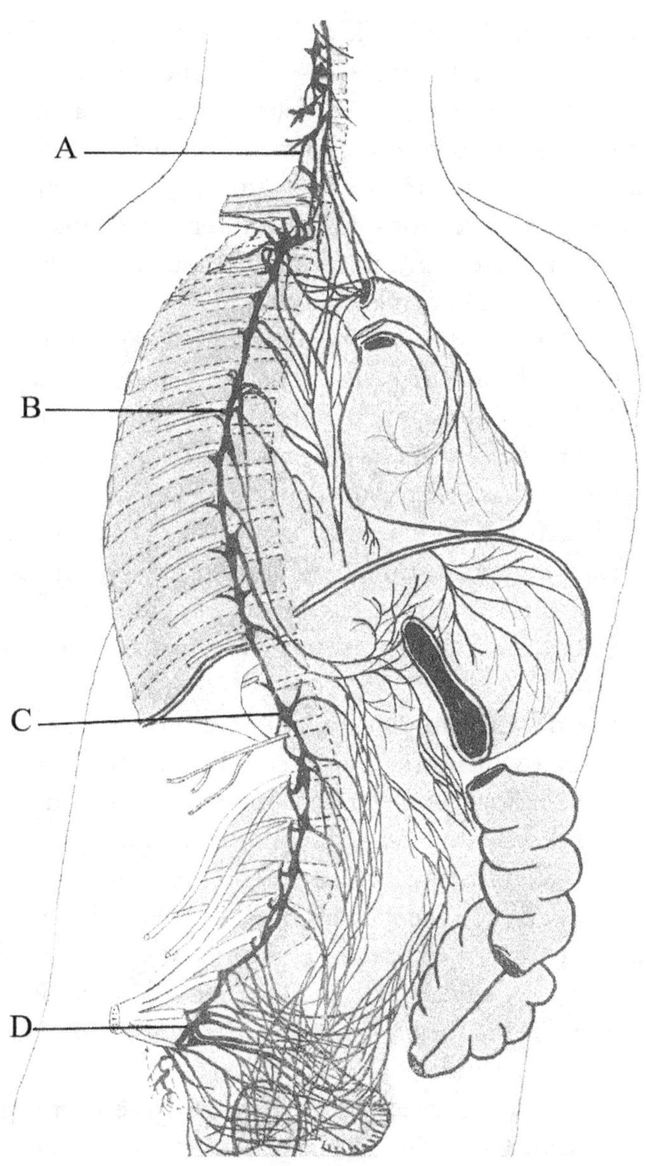

FIG. 75 diagrammatic sketch of the vegetative nervous system, from the right side. (A) Cervical sympathetic nervous system ganglia. (B) Thoracic portion of the sympathetic nervous system. (C) Celiac "solar" plexus. (D) Pelvic sympathetic ganglia.

Response to Sensory Stimuli. Most chronic diseases of the nervous system permit of proper evaluation of symptoms and definite diagnosis only at the sensorimotor level. Response to sensory stimuli in the voluntary system is immediate. In the vegetative system it is slower and less definite. These chronic diseases commonly manifest their development by disturbances either in the proper functioning of the motor apparatus or in sensation. It is believed generally that, except in occasional acute infections, the chronic nervous diseases do not appear in a normally functioning nervous system. A careful study of such cases shows a slow, progressive departure from what is considered normal function. Any study that does not take this into account does not progress very far either in the understanding or in the therapy of the disease

Progressive Involvement. Chronic disease in the nervous system, except where there is severe trauma or overwhelming infection or intoxication, progresses in the same manner as does chronic disease in any other tissues. It begins in a welter of vague symptoms which often do not in any way suggest involvement of the nervous system. The most common early ones are easy fatigability, lassitude, decreased stamina, loss of weight, irritability, purposelessness, overactivity, increased reaction time, disturbances in sleep, and change in appetite and in bowel function. If a cause is looked for, a number of departures from what is generally understood as good hygiene will be found. One of the most obvious of these will be the extremely faulty use of the body.

Root Pains with Symptoms. Probably the most common nervous disturbance directly due to bad body mechanics is that which finds expression in the various root pains without other symptoms. These have been variously called radiculitis, neuronitis and neuritis. They have been described fully where injury to one or more spinal or cranial nerve roots has been caused by toxic or irritative agents. Inflammation of these roots usually manifests itself in pain or disturbed sensation in the peripheral termination of the nerve in one or all of its portions. Motor disturbances have been recorded but are less common. Anything which causes increased pressure on the roots, such as coughing or stretching, increases the pain. Pathologically, there may be partial demyelinization of the nerve root, increase in the intrafascicular fibrous tissues, hemorrhage and lymphocytic infiltration.

Mechanical Irritation. However, there is another type of nerve-root irritation showing similar pathology and functional disturbance due to mechanical causes, usually the result of pressure or stretching of the nerve roots. The many joints and bony processes about the spine and the numerous ligaments and muscular attachments make the spinal nerve roots peculiarly liable to mechanical irritation. Examples of this have been found by many observers in radiating pains about the shoulder girdle and in the arm and in such pains as sciatica in the lower extremities. The same observers have noted the disappearance of the pain after the correction of the faulty body mechanics. Carnett and Gunther have described the frequent occurrence of symptoms which simulate visceral disease, particularly that of the gallbladder and the appendix. They disappeared with the removal of the mechanical irritation (Fig. 76).

Infantile Paralysis. In infantile paralysis, particularly during the early or acute stage, the application of the principles of good body mechanics has been found to be of value in conjunction with the usual types of therapy. The congestion and the edema which are all present in the central nervous system may be helped greatly by improving the diaphragmatic function and avoiding positions which interfere with the proper functioning of organs. In the convalescent and the chronic stages of the disease, the return of muscle function can be hastened and undue strain prevented by keeping the body mechanics as nearly normal as possible, without changing the use of splints to prevent deformities and without any modification of special treatment for muscle groups. In the so-called spastic paralyses much help also can be obtained, particularly in improving muscular control.

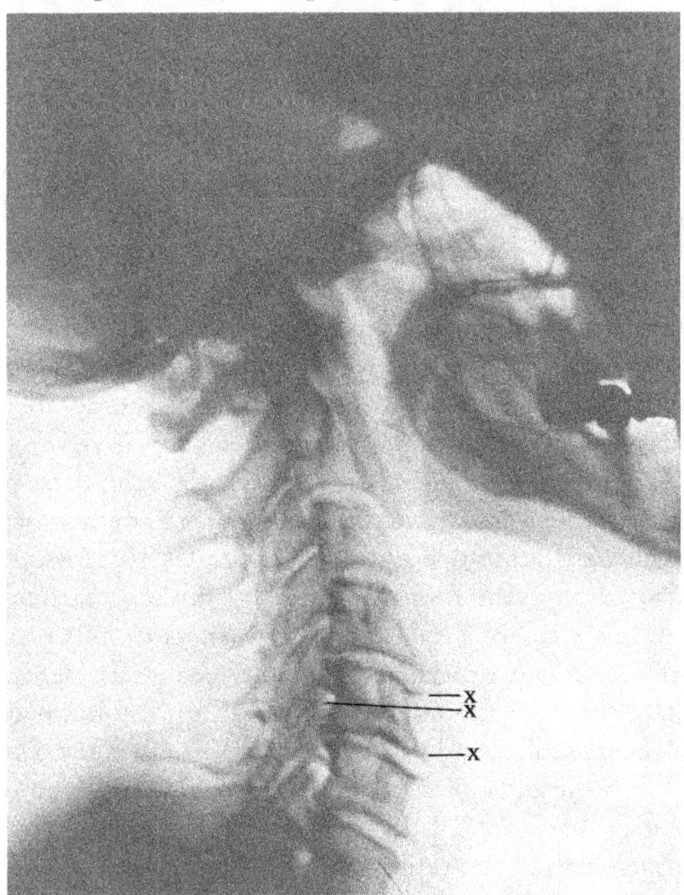

FIG. 76. Roentgenogram of cervical spine showing hypertrophic arthritis at X. Note the curvature of the spine and the faulty position of the head. This patient had pain along the fifth and the sixth cervical nerves. The hypertrophic spurs seen on the anterior and the posterior parts of these vertebrae in the roentgenograms are found, in anatomic specimens, to be on all sides of the vertebrae.

Multiple Sclerosis. One of the most serious of chronic diseases of the nervous system, and one which neurologists tell us is increasing, is multiple sclerosis, a chronic affection of the brain and the cord characterized by local lesions. The pathology of the disease has been described carefully. In recently invaded areas of the spinal cord there are infiltrations of lymphocytic cells and edema about the blood vessels. We know very little of the cause, but infection from a filtrable virus, a food deficiency and a lipolytic toxin have been suggested recently. What part strain and subsequent fatigue play in the development of these lesions, and to what extent the pathologic changes are induced or augmented by chronic circulatory stasis, we cannot determine. Both circulatory stasis and strain, with fatigue of muscle and nerve, as well as many other physiologic disturbances, are enhanced greatly by the increasing static deformities which always accompany this disease unless they are prevented. Much can be done to improve the general muscular control, lessen strain and fatigue and relieve circulatory disturbances by correcting the faulty body mechanics. If this correction can be accomplished in the early stages of the disease, its progression can be retarded, and in a number of cases improvement will result. Primary lateral sclerosis, which shows a somewhat similar pathologic picture, confined usually to the pyramidal tracts of the cord, has a similar relation to body mechanics in its cause and treatment.

Paralysis Agitans. Another severe chronic disease of the nervous system is paralysis agitans, characterized by disturbances of certain automatic and associated movements and tremors and rigidity. The pathology usually is confined to the globus-pallidus mechanism, the so called extrapyramidal tract. There may be atrophy and a decrease in the number of the large motor cells. In a number of cases mild symptoms of paralysis agitans have been observed in elderly persons. This has led to the suggestion that the disease, at least in these cases, may be due to senile degeneration and arteriosclerosis. We shall not discuss all the symptoms but shall merely call attention to the characteristic attitude and gait. The head is bent forward, the back is bowed and the gait is propulsive. A persistent forward position of the head, with the associated extreme cervical curve, may produce cerebral congestion. The effect of this on the progress of the disease must be harmful. In our experience not only have these deforming features been lessened, but a gradual improvement in the distressing symptoms has been observed also.

Muscular Atrophy. The muscular atrophies form a large group of the diseases of the nervous system of which we know little and for which medical knowledge can offer no satisfactory therapy. All are characterized by a gradual degeneration of the motor tracts. The nervous system shows atrophy of the large cells of the ventral horns in the spinal cord, a decrease in medullated fibers, a replacement of the degenerated cord tissue by neuroglia, a gradual atrophy of the muscles and occasional sclerosis of the ventrolateral tracts. We believe that faulty body mechanics, with its increased demands on the energy of the motor tracts, and with the accompanying congestion of the cord, may play a part in the onset and the development of these diseases.

Muscular Dystrophy. The muscular dystrophies form another group of chronic diseases of the nervous system the etiology of which is shrouded in mystery and for which medical science can supply no distinct therapy. These affections show muscular wasting, with or without an initial hypertrophy, beginning in various groups of muscles. Here degenerative changes are found in the muscles themselves, with hypertrophy of the fibers, increase in the nuclei and increase in the connective tissue. This is followed by atrophy of the fibers, the appearance of vacuoles and the deposition of fat. In muscular dystrophy and in muscular atrophy as well, re-education in the use of the muscles, prevention of deformities and improvement in all physiologic functions offer most for therapy. The application of the principles of body mechanics is of great value.

Mental States. The realm of the mind has for a long time been considered to be a thing apart. However, every day makes us realize more keenly the close association of the efficiency of the so called mental states with the state of health of the body. Moreover, fatigue and cerebral congestion, inevitable concomitants of faulty body mechanics, are frequently the cause of irritability, depression and faulty judgment in the chronically ill. The recent studies of Klein have shown the improvement in the school work of children following correction of body mechanics. In local sanatoriums the common association of poor body mechanics with psychoses and the improvement in the milder aberrations by its correction offered suggestive evidence of a causal relationship. William James has described the drooped position seen in failure and depression and the erect attitude in elation and optimism.

We do not wish to suggest that the correction of body mechanics will cure chronic nervous diseases However, we believe that whatever other measures are employed, it is necessary to apply these principles in order to secure the greatest functional recovery and to secure sufficiently normal physiology in the region of nerve tissue so that repair and return of function may take place.

ILLUSTRATIVE CASES

In order to show what has been accomplished by the correction of faulty body mechanics alone, a short summary is given of the histories of a few patients who were crippled by chronic nervous diseases. All these patients had one thing in common: extremely faulty body mechanics. Much that might have been of interest both in histories and in laboratory findings has been omitted purposely in order to present the results as simply as possible. One hesitates to speak of cure in chronic disease, but the improvement observed should demonstrate the value of treatment which attempts to correct the mechanics and to improve the function of the whole body.

Multiple sclerosis is a disease of the nervous system which leads to great crippling. The pathologic lesion is a degeneration of scattered areas throughout the spinal cord. Little is known of the cause, and the prognosis as commonly given is poor. Patients suffering from this disease usually are referred to the orthopedist when there is much disability. The treatment formerly given consisted of local exercises, and little if any improvement was observed. With a better understanding of the physiology of body mechanics, a very different expectation of improvement has come.

Case 1. Multiple Sclerosis with Extreme Disability. .A 49-year-old married woman was seen first in 1927, having been brought to the hospital from the Middle West in an unusually helpless condition. There was no control of the bladder or the bowel function, and practically every detail of care had to be given. The symptoms had begun 20 years before, including slight disturbance of sensation and of control of the leg muscles. These disabilities gradually increased, and there was also enhanced weakness of the arms and the hands. The patient was bedridden and for 10 years had received practically no special treatment, many remedies, among them the removal of the ovaries, having been tried previously.

The degree of helplessness and hopelessness was profound. A diagnosis of multiple sclerosis had been made by many physicians, and there was no reason for disagreement with it. After frank discussion of the condition with the patient and her husband, treatment for the correction of the bad body mechanics was undertaken. The special positions described later were begun, with special exercises, in an attempt to regain some of the lost control of the muscles. Hot fomentations were applied to the spine twice daily to stimulate the circulation of the skin; since the blood vessels of the spinal cord are branches of those which supply the spinal muscles and the skin, it was expected that, if the circulation of the skin was stimulated, that of the spinal cord would be also.

The contractures which had developed at the knees and the ankles were overcome chiefly by the repeated use of plaster-of-paris casts. These were applied with as much dorsiflexion at the ankle and as much extension at the knee as was possible without undue tension on the muscles. With the casts so applied (Fig. 77), the gradual relaxation of the muscles made it possible to gain further correction by the application of new casts. This was repeated with little or no pain until the deformities were corrected fully. While this treatment was in progress, everything possible was done to improve the general condition. At first the temperature remained one and a half degrees below normal; the blood pressure was very low, and the basal metabolism was subnormal.

Improvement came gradually. The muscles were controlled better. The patient was able to move herself and to do certain things with her hands. Little by little, control of the bladder and the bowels returned. This improvement continued, and spinal supports then were planned; when muscular strength became adequate, sitting was allowed. Soon thereafter, the use of a loom for weaving was permitted. This helped greatly, since the control of the foot pedals as

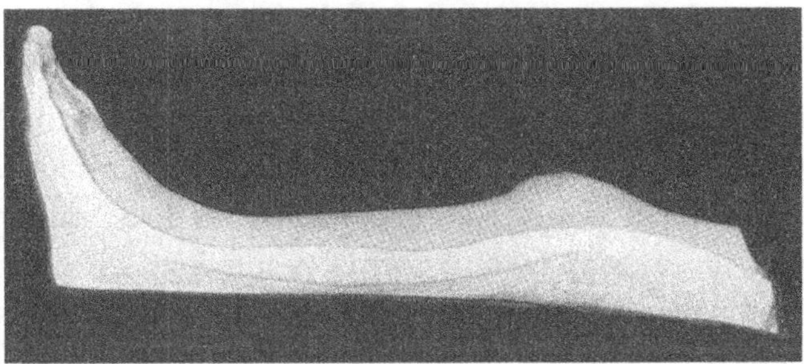

FIG. 77. Plaster shell used in correction of flexion deformities of the lower extremity. An attempt is made to bring the knee into full extension as nearly as possible, and the foot into a good weight-bearing position.

well as of the shuttle and the beater, involve training in the use of muscles of all the extremities; also, since all four extremities must be used independently, the loom is helpful in breaking up the common cross-stimulation of the muscles, the idle arm or leg not moving when its fellow is used. The muscular control improved until the function of the arms was but little impaired. The legs improved sufficiently to permit the patient to stand with caliper splints and to walk with assistance. The control of the bladder and the bowels became nearly normal.

To accomplish this result the patient was kept in the hospital for about a year. Within that time the general health improved markedly, with a return of normal temperature, normal blood pressure and a normal basal metabolism. The muscles of the extremities were still weak but were under voluntary control. It was finally possible for the patient to rise from a chair with but slight assistance, and by holding on to pieces of furniture, to walk about the room. From a condition of entire helplessness she recovered so that she was able to care for herself in part and to take her place at the head of her household.

In this case complete recovery was not expected, since there was undoubtedly some permanent damage to the nerve cells. However, if great improvement was possible in a patient so seemingly helpless as this, more could be expected if the proper methods were applied in the early stages of the disease. A spirit of hopefulness and infinite patience are necessary. Muscular training, the correction of faulty visceral positions and the adjustments of suitable apparatus in proper sequence can be expected to accomplish much. Since occasional periods of remission of symptoms are common in multiple sclerosis, it is of interest to report that the improvement which occurred in this patient under treatment has been maintained for a period of 10 years.

Case 2. Multiple Sclerosis with Diplopia; Very Faulty Mechanics. A married woman, 26 years of age, was seen first in January, 1928. Her symptoms were of 6 years duration, with gradual loss of vision in the left eye. The vision in the left eye improved, but this was followed by complete loss of vision in the right eye. There was double vision much of the time. Weakness of the back and the legs developed so that a wheel-chair was required. Later the arms became

144

involved, and the control of the bowels was partially lost. The patient had treatment at many clinics without benefit. The diagnosis given was multiple sclerosis.

At the time of the patient's arrival her general condition was poor. The body mechanics were extremely bad, with marked forward tip of the pelvis and with a low position of the ribs and the diaphragm. The reflexes were much exaggerated and the pulse was rapid. The basal metabolism was irregular, at times above the normal reading, at other times below it. The eyes showed no permanent impairment in vision, but the muscular co-ordination was imperfect, with double vision much of the time.

The patient was taken to the hospital, where treatment was begun for the correction of the faulty body mechanics, and other measures were used as described in Chapter 11. The marked contraction of the feet-with the foot-drop deformity was corrected by the use of plaster-of-paris casts, as described in the previous case.

The improvement was fairly rapid, and in a short time the patient was transferred to the convalescent hospital, where weaving with a loom was added to her activities. There was gradual, steady gain. She was able to return to her home in the Middle West in 4 and a half months after the beginning of the treatment. The control of the eyes was practically normal. The function in the hands had so improved that she was able to play difficult piano music again. The control of the bladder and the bowels became nearly normal, while that of the legs improved enough so that walking was possible with but little assistance.

The patient has been seen since at infrequent intervals, with occasional reports by letter. The gain made in the beginning has been maintained. She has given birth to a healthy child, the care of it, as well as many household duties, devolving upon her. Many of the muscles have remained weak, but there has been no further muscular involvement, and the improvement has persisted.

The diagnosis of such conditions in the beginning is often difficult because the symptoms are irregular and inconstant. We have seen complete recovery in patients who presented as chief symptoms weakness of the eyes, with double vision, disturbed sensation of the arms and the legs, weakness of the muscles and abnormal reflexes, all of gradual development. In the early stages, naturally, long confinement in the hospital is not necessary, but training in good body mechanics is essential, with the temporary use of a support. It is also necessary to see that the general activities are regulated to give more time for resting until the general health has improved greatly. If severe disability in chronic nervous disease can be benefited by carefully planned treatment having for its aim the development of the best possible function of all parts of the body, one can reasonably expect that if such a regime were started in the early stage of the disease, before permanent damage to the nerve cells had occurred, complete recovery would result.

Case 3. Multiple Sclerosis and Faulty Body Mechanics with Slowly Increasing Disability. A 46-year-old woman was seen first in April, 1927, when she complained of

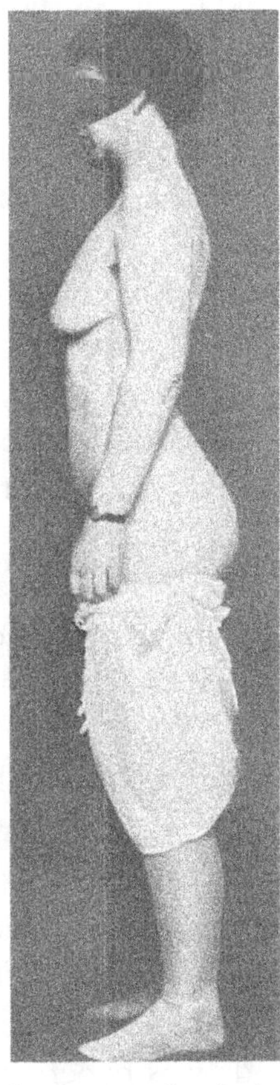

FIG. 78. Multiple sclerosis with slowly developing disability. The patient is not in her habitual relaxed position, as she is attempting to correct her body mechanics. Sag of the diaphragm is suggested by the hollows under the ribs in the epigastric region. The forward tilt of the pelvis accentuates the extreme lumbar curve.

difficulty in the control of the arms and the legs of 8 years' duration. There was also some disturbance of sensation in both arms and legs. The control of the bladder was normal, and there was only slight disturbance of bowel function. Examination showed marked exaggeration of the reflexes in arms and legs and considerable spasm of the muscles of the trunk. The body mechanics was poor, with lumbar spine used in the position of extreme extension and with hyperextension of the cervical spine (Fig.78). The diaphragm as shown by roentgenograms was in a low position. There had been no disagreement on the part of the many physicians who had seen the patient as to the diagnosis of multiple sclerosis.

The patient was admitted to the hospital, and treatment was begun for the correction of the faulty mechanics, in the hope that, with the improvement in the general circulation, there would be improvement in that of the spinal cord. With this treatment, with special positions and with muscular training in other ways, the general health was improved as much as possible.

Progress was fairly rapid. At the end of a month the patient had been fitted to a body brace and a special corset and was beginning to walk about. She was transferred to the convalescent hospital, where she remained for 3 weeks.

During this time the improvement continued. She then returned to her home in New York State to carry on the treatment there. She is now able to walk from her room to her place of business, a distance of almost a mile, without undue fatigue and with little peculiarity in gait. The recovery was much more rapid and more nearly complete than in Cases 1 and 2 because the trouble had been present a shorter time, and less damage to the nervous system had occurred.

One of the conditions found in any clinic which treats chronic and crippling conditions is progressive muscular atrophy, characterized by gradually increasing weakness of muscular groups and marked atrophy of the muscles. The textbooks give no definite cause for the trouble, nor is any hope of improvement offered following treatment. The expected result is increasing helplessness and death. The following case shows that a very different prognosis is possible.

Case 4. Muscular Atrophy. A man 33 years of age from one of the southern states was seen first in 1915. There was great weakness of all the muscles, with much atrophy and absence of the normal reflexes. The condition had begun 4 or 5 years before with slight weakness of the muscles of the legs. It had increased gradually so that walking was difficult, and if the balance was lost, there was no strength to prevent falling. Rising from a chair was impossible except by supporting the thighs with the hands and flexing the body at the hips. The weakness of the hands was so great that the patient was unable to fasten his buttons.

The body mechanics was extremely poor, the marked general muscular weakness leading to a much greater abdominal and diaphragmatic sag than is seen usually in chronically ill patients. Measures were taken at once to correct the faulty mechanics and the disturbed physiology. Since the ribs and the diaphragm were so low, the body was hyperextended at the mid-dorsal region and held in this position in a plaster-of-paris jacket; the ribs were held in the position of full inspiration. At first the patient was kept in bed, with the body horizontal. Special muscular training was begun, very gentle at first but gradually increasing in strenuousness as the strength returned. Further study showed a very low blood-sugar level and a low creatinine.

Clinical improvement began at the end of the first week, and after this general progress was rapid. At the end of 7 weeks the patient left the hospital, having been fitted to a brace to help support the body in the correct position. He remained in a near-by hotel for 2 weeks longer. During this time he was able to walk about and could step on and off curbstones, an act that was entirely impossible before. He returned home and continued the treatment. There was a gradual complete recovery of muscular strength, which has been maintained since.

While the exact cause of this condition is not understood perfectly, in many cases, when the faulty body mechanics with the associated physiologic disturbances are corrected, health is restored.

10

Chronic Arthritis

The group of symptoms called "arthritis" can be understood better when we look at them from the point of view of the student of body mechanics and realize the local and general functional disturbances which can be produced by habitual bad posture. Arthritis is not a disease of the joints alone but is a widespread disorder of the whole body, there being very few parts which are not damaged sooner or later. This is equally true of the more highly organized tissues.

Joints are highly specialized tissues developed for weight-bearing and motion alone and are therefore subjected to constant strain and trauma. Even in resting positions in bed strain is present, and irritation is exhibited by frequent changes in position and stiffness on rising from sleep.

The simplest classification of chronic diseases of the joints is that of the Empire Rheumatism Committee of the British Medical Society, which divides them into two groups: in the first the cause is known, the diseases including infectious, tuberculous, gonorrheal and syphilitic arthritis, gout, typhoid fever and hemophilic arthritis; in the second the cause is unknown, the diseases including atrophic (rheumatoid) and hypertrophic arthritis (osteo-arthritis).

Arthritis is inflammation of joints. There are many different forms of articular disease which are called arthritis. All of these may be acute or chronic. Most arthritis falls into five main groups: (1) arthritis due to infection (when a specific micro-organism is found); (2) atrophic (rheumatoid) arthritis of unproved etiology; (3) arthritis due to degeneration in tissues of which hypertrophic arthritis (osteo-arthritis) is the chief example; (4) arthritis which is the result of injury to joints; (5) metabolic arthritis, including gout. This classification, which includes over 95 per cent of inflammations in joints, leaves out neurogenic arthritis, new growths in joints and arthritis which is the occasional accompaniment of various system diseases. While correction of the alignment of the articular surfaces and the correction of the body mechanics is of value in all types of arthritis, it is an essential part of the treatment in atrophic (rheumatoid) and in hypertrophic arthritis (osteo-arthritis).

CAUSES

The two chief causes of articular injury are acute strain and chronic trauma and the irritating effects of injurious chemical substances carried to the joints by the circulation. Good circulation, as in other structures, controls the nutrition of the joints. One of the earliest signs of joint disease, whether from trauma or from poisons, is chronic passive congestion of the soft tissues about the joints, producing a swelling which, by its pressure on the lymph channels or the blood vessels, may impair the normal nutrition of a joint. Thus, mechanical and chemical irritations play a large part in the production of chronic arthritis.

There are unquestionably many cases where either the bacteria or their toxins produce the immediate picture of arthritis and the changes found therein. These changes are the reaction of the tissues to the foreign irritation and may be mild or severe, depending on the virulence of infection, the general vitality and resistance of the patient to infection, and the local health and resistance of the joint itself. There are also many cases, the result of chemical poisons from disturbed intestinal digestion or faulty metabolism, which give a similar appearance clinically to the changes brought about by bacterial products but which respond only to revised diet, intestinal care and correction of metabolic errors.

General resistance can be lowered by weak, irregular and abnormal functioning of the organs of the thoracic and the abdominal cavities, as shown in the previous chapters. Since general vitality depends upon the correct working of these organs, poor health is frequently the result of the handicap following the effects of bad posture. The lack of natural resistance so produced allows the infection to get a foothold and to spread. The converse is true also: not infrequently the spread of infection, and even the focus itself, can be influenced markedly by the increased resistance and the improved health resulting from the correction of a faulty posture and the restoration of normal functioning of the viscera.

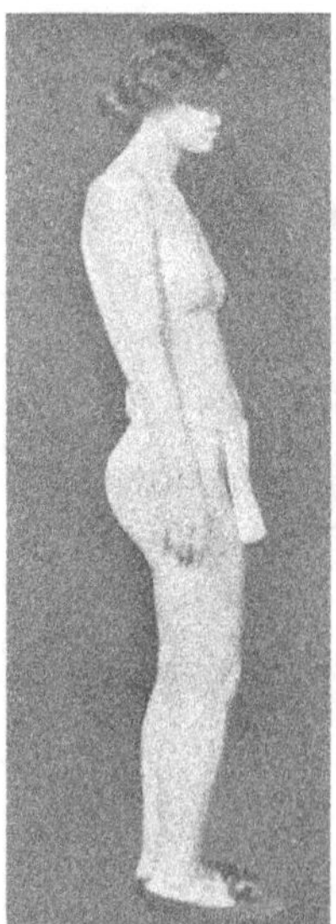

The local resistance not infrequently is dependent on the chronic strain to which the joint is subject in use. Habitual faulty use of the body produces such strain in most of the spinal and the joints of extremities, such as the shoulders, the knees, the ankles, and the feet.

Chronic arthritis may well be the result of the effects of bacterial or chemical poisons in a person whose physical vitality is low, who lacks local resistance in one or many joints because of the poor circulation and the trauma from faulty mechanical use of the body. Once joint injury has taken place, it is apt to be self-perpetuating. The wrong use of a joint through the strain of faulty posture will continue to produce the symptoms of arthritis even after the irritant no longer is present or the infection has died out (Fig. 79).

FIG. 79. Patient with atrophic arthritis.
Note the extremely faulty body mechanics,
with congestion of the hands and the legs.

THE ADRENAL CORTEX AND ARTHRITIS

Glandular disturbances for a long time have been considered to be a factor in the development of chronic arthritis. Chance observations have shown various glandular dysfunctions accompanying atrophic (rheumatoid) arthritis particularly, and an improvement or a disappearance of the arthritis with the correction of the glandular dysfunction. Hench and his associates have found that improvement occurred in almost all patients with arthritis during pregnancy, the studies of Selye have demonstrated that failure of adaptation of the organism was due to fatigue or failure of the adrenal cortex. More recently, an adrenal-cortical hormone, cortisone (Compound E) has been found to cause a temporary suppression of arthritis and other inflammatory symptoms. Adrenocorticotrophic hormone (ACTH), obtained from the anterior pituitary gland of hogs, has been found to stimulate the production or the appearance in the blood stream of cortisone and in this way has shown a reaction in the patient with arthritis similar to that observed with cortisone. Both of these substances have now been used for two years. In most patients with active atrophic (rheumatoid) arthritis the use of these symptoms has led to a temporary subsidence of pain and swelling. The pain and swelling have recurred in most instances 2 or 3 weeks after the use of cortisone or ACTH was discontinued. A prolongation of the action of the drug has been attempted by giving smaller maintenance doses for long periods of time. Useful as this type of therapy has been, it has wrought no lasting change in the body. Faults in the body mechanics, with their accompanying physiologic disturbances, remain; unchanged. Deformities in and about the joint are not influenced by these drugs.

TREATMENT

The removal of the focus of infection may give temporary relief in rare instances, but if the joint continues to be habitually strained through incorrect posture, no permanent recovery can be expected. After the arthritis has occurred all causative factors must be removed, and the general body condition brought to as near normal as possible before the reaction in the joints can be expected to disappear, and repair can be expected to take place (see Fig. 80). Therefore the joints must be protected constantly from all further insult. This can be done only by so rebalancing the body as a whole that local strain ceases, and the visceral functions are permitted to proceed normally. Old, quiescent arthritic joints are particularly susceptible to change of posture or fresh poisons and must be protected constantly from them. Often there may be no outward signs or symptoms demonstrable by roentgenogram or physical test. Still, changes are unquestionably present, usually to a greater extent than we suspect. This is the reason that it is so vital for the patient suffering from chronic arthritis to learn to use his body with the least possible strain to the joints and thus to keep them from deformity at all times.

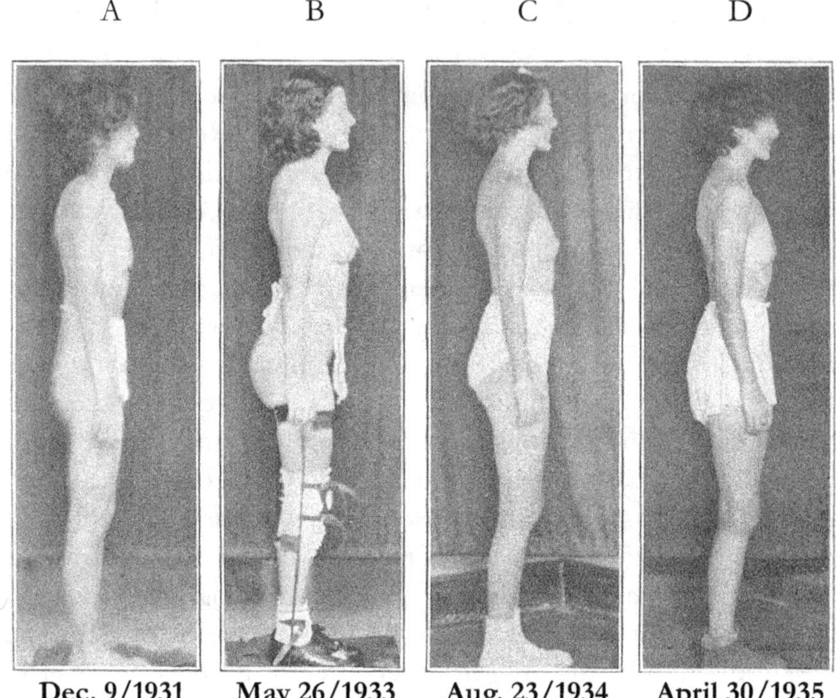

FIG. 80. Atrophic arthritis of 6 years' duration. There is some wasting of the tissues, A, but good nutrition of the body is shown in subsequent pictures, with steady improvement in posture. Note the good condition in B after a year of-bed rest, with special positions and exercises, in spite of a recrudescence of the arthritis between A and B. This patient has remained well, as in D, for 5 years. Compare Figure 84.

ATROPHIC (RHEUMATOID, PROLIFERATIVE) ARTHRITIS

Atrophic (rheumatoid, proliferative) arthritis is a chronic constitutional disease causing an atrophy of bone, muscle, skin, nails and most of the structures of the body. One of the first signs found by roentgenogram is bone atrophy, even before the joints (Figs. 82 and 83) show any destruction, or the symptoms of pain, swelling or tenderness appear. Muscular wasting with loss of weight and fatigue is also an early sign (Fig. 84). Young women are more subject to the atrophic form of this disease than are young men, but the spinal type of atrophic arthritis (ankylosing spondylitis or Strumpell-Marie arthritis) is more common in young men. Both diseases occur between the ages of 20 and 40 and almost always in the slender anatomic type (Fig. 85 and 86) (see slender type, Chapter 2).

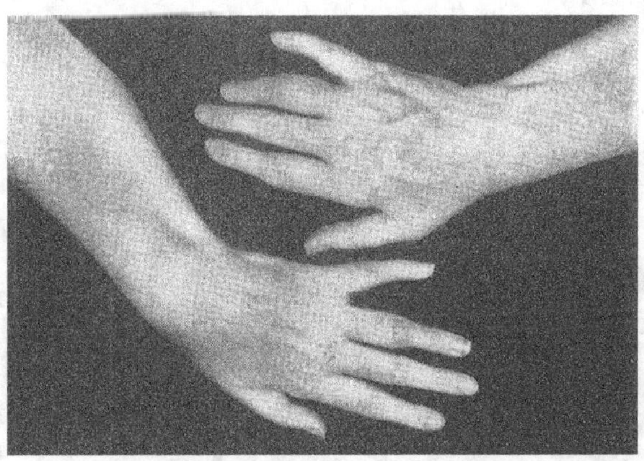

FIG. 81. Hands in early atrophic arthritis. Note the swelling about the metacarpophalangeal and the phalangeal joints. The skin and the nails show very little change.

Almost all the data relating to atrophic arthritis point toward a profound failure of the body to do its work. This failure is shown by subnormal temperature (Fig. 87), low blood pressure, low metabolism, diminished circulation in the extremities (cold hands and feet), secondary anemia, lack of appetite, malnutrition, loss of from 10 to 70 pounds in some cases, avitaminosis in vitamins A, B, C and D, muscular atrophy, decalcification of the bone, with abnormal calcification of the cartilages, and sometimes achlorhydria, with symptoms of excessive fatigue, nervousness, weakness and joint soreness. The picture is one of derangement of many functions of the body, all of which disturbances together produce the varied but constant signs of failure. With these conditions present infection can take place easily, but it seems improbable that it alone can produce the entire disease. The background of inherited anatomic structure, to which is added 20 or more years of visceroptotic existence with its weakness and faulty posture (this present in over 90 per cent of all atrophic cases), results in the increasing malfunctioning of the diaphragm, the heart the lungs and misplaced abdominal organs (Fig. 88). Thus, the whole vitality is diminished, and the physical signs of impending failure of the body functions appear.

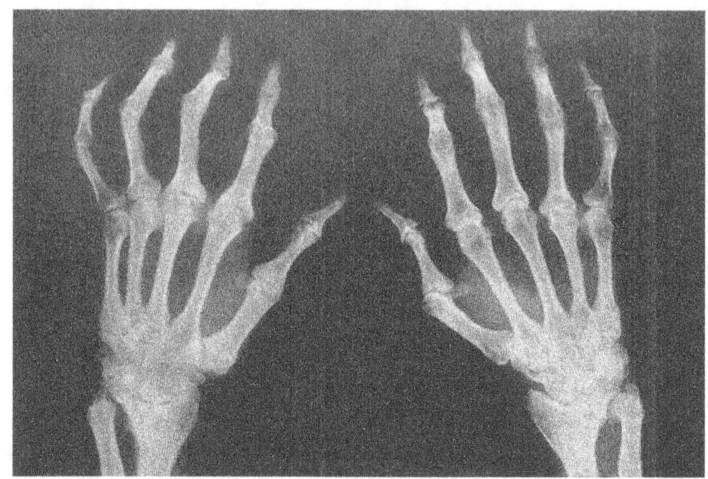

FIG. 82. Roentgenograms of hands in early atrophic arthritis. There is a moderate amount of osseous atrophy, most marked about the joints. Some soft tissue swelling is evident also.

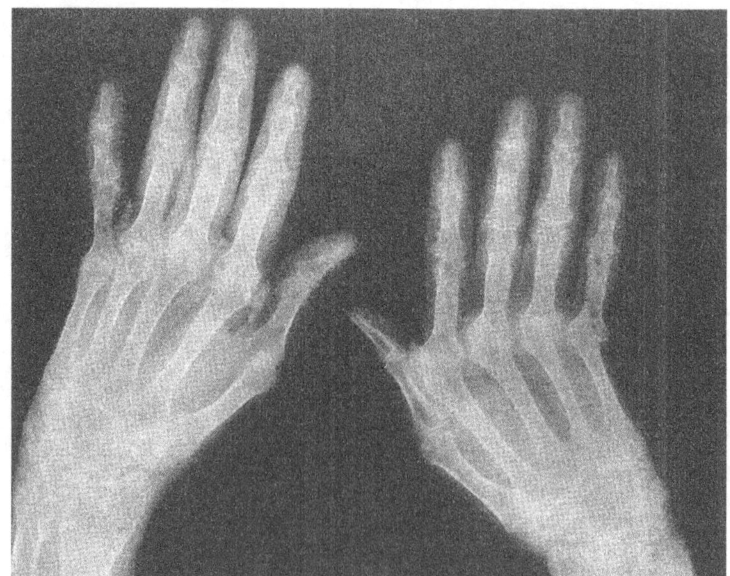

FIG. 83. Roentgenograms of hands showing advanced atrophic arthritis. There is extreme atrophy of the bones and destruction of the joints, with deformity of the fingers and subluxation of the thumbs at the metacarpophalangeal joints

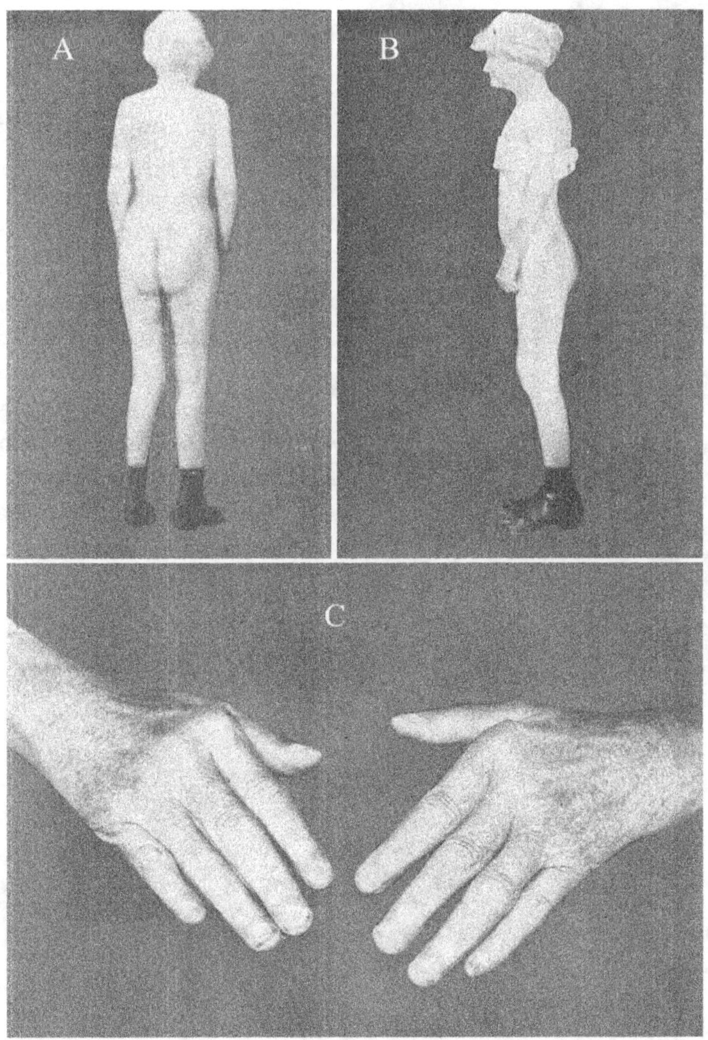

FIG. 84 Patient with advanced atrophic arthritis of many years duration. A and B show faulty body mechanics and residual deformities. There is atrophy of the muscles of the arms and the legs. (C) Hands of patient shown in A and B. There is marked atrophy of the skin of the hands and deformity of the nails. The joints of the fingers show no swelling at this time.

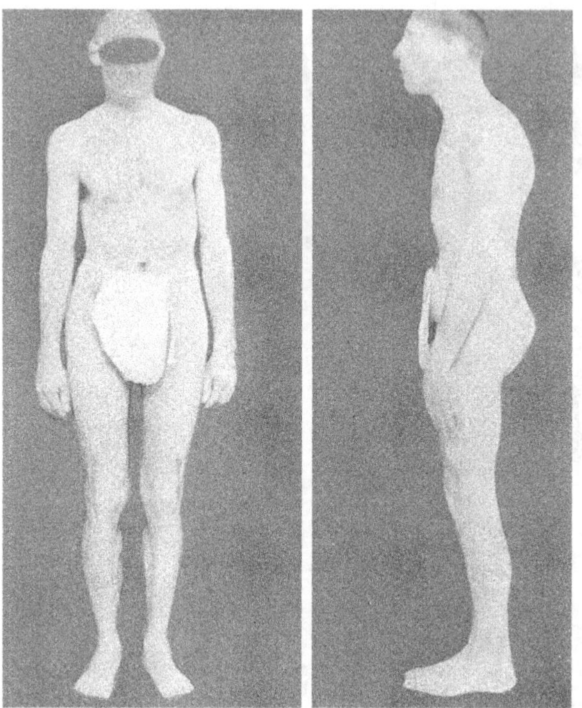

FIG. 85. (A and B) Atrophic arthritis of the spine, ankylosing spondylitis, Strumpell-Marie type, of 9 years' duration after 6 months of treatment based on correction of the faulty body mechanics. At the beginning of treatment the patient showed general atrophy and wasting of the body, with stiffness and deformity of the spine and the chest. There is now relatively good nutrition and improved body mechanics. All the symptoms except the stiffness of the spine have disappeared. The chest expansion has increased 2 inches.

FIG.86. (C and D) Roentgenograms of spine of the patient shown in Figure 85 (A and B). There is marked atrophy of the bones, with ossification of the spinal ligaments and fusion of the sacro-iliac joints.

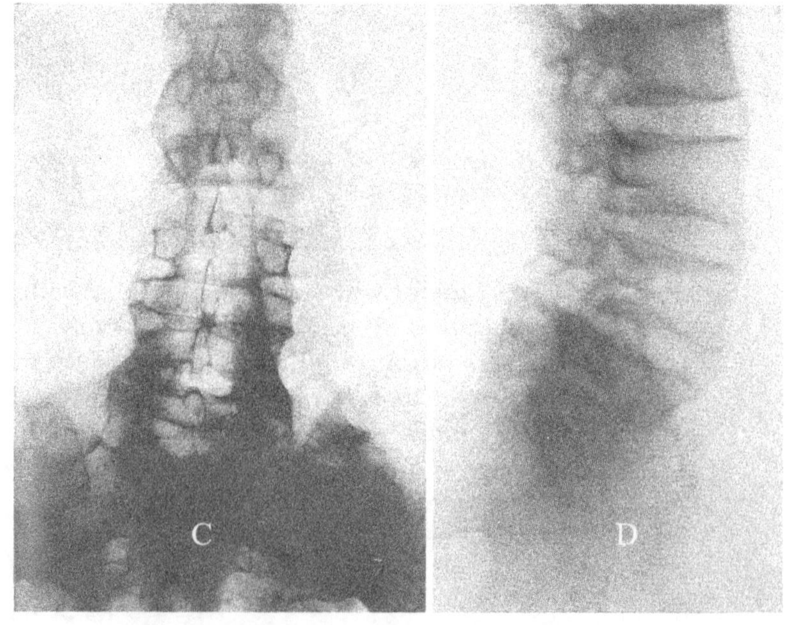

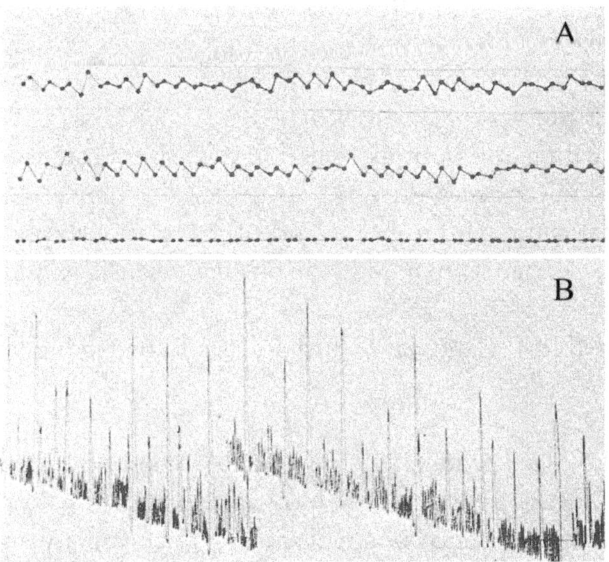

FIG. 87. Temperature chart and metabolism graph of patient with atrophic arthritis. (A) A persistent subnormal temperature varying from 95.5° F. a.m., to 97.8° F. p.m. This means profound fatigue and an inability to carry on the normal functions of the body. Subnormal temperature usually appears after the patient has been in bed several days. An approach to normal temperature usually means an improvement in the general physiology. (B) A very irregular metabolism graph. The computed test shows a rate of -17 and -18 per cent. This marked irregularity means a very unstable physiologic condition. The frequent long excursions on the graph denote air-hunger and occur frequently when the diaphragm is habitually low. This graph will become more nearly regular with improvement in the body mechanics.

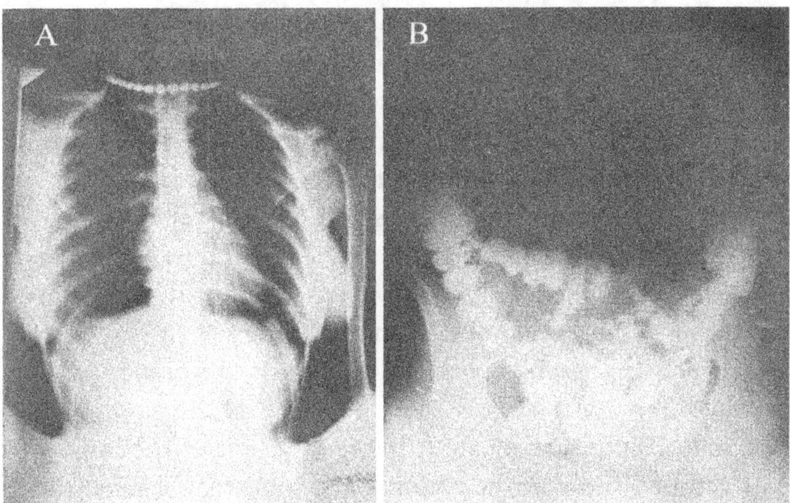

FIG. 88. (A) Roentgenogram of the thoracic cavity of a patient with atrophic arthritis, taken in the standing position. The domes of the diaphragm are flat and on the same level. The domes of the diaphragm are lower than the spinal attachments and are at the level of the twelfth rib instead of being between the eighth and the ninth ribs. The heart is sagged; the pleural cavity is very long. (B) Roentgenograms of the abdominal cavity. Both small and large intestines have sagged markedly; most of the viscera are in the pelvic cavity. These findings mean impaired function of both thoracic and abdominal viscera.

Some of the predisposing causes of atrophic arthritis may be listed as follows:

1. Weakness of the inherited type of anatomy.
2. Chronic handicap from faulty posture over the period of growth.
3. Imperfect metabolism plus bad habits of eating and poor assimilation of what is eaten.
4. Overwork, with its resulting fatigue in a handicapped body.
5. The nervous strain of modern life, especially in regard to home and office relationships, and frequent fears, insecurities and drift (the slender type of individual is hypersensitive and introspective).
6. Chance infections, accidents, strain of childbirth, glandular disturbances and bad living conditions.

The changes called atrophic arthritis take place gradually in all parts of the body, often insidiously but persistently, until the disease is clearly evident. If we look upon atrophic arthritis in this light, recognizing its multiple causes, its incidence in age and sex, its chronicity and resistance to treatment, occurrences with physical and nervous strain, after pregnancy and with exacerbation at menstruation, the general physical failure and the pathologic changes are understood more easily. The gradual undermining of the none-too-good vitality of the slender type, associated with habitual faulty mechanical use, requires only a little extra poisoning from food, fatigue, nervous strain, infection and bad living conditions to disturb seriously the balance of physiology. The longer the imbalance is allowed to go on, the greater is the permanent damage done, and the greater the susceptibility to additional burdens from without or within. If allowed to take its course, atrophic arthritis produces great crippling, with emaciation, weakness and degeneration of practically all the tissues of the body, such as kidneys, arteries, muscles, bones, eyes and hair. The effect on the joints is only part of the general disease.

The degenerative changes are preventable, and the progress of the disease can be stopped if taken in hand early and approached with the previously mentioned etiologic points clearly in view. The body mechanics must be corrected in order that the diaphragm, the great venous pump of the body, may function adequately; that the heart and the lungs may have their full capacity to work effectively; and that the abdominal organs may resume their full, unimpeded function. What use is it to feed a corrected diet to a handicapped body if we have not first put it in good working order, thereby improving the circulation and relieving chronic passive congestion? These changes cannot be accomplished without correcting the body posture to allow every organ to do its work to its full capacity and in perfect harmony. After this, diet, warmth, physical therapy, removal of infection, regulation of fatigue and a more normal attitude toward life can be instituted, with some degree of expectation of stopping the disease changes. This seems fundamental in the handling of all cases of atrophic arthritis, 9 out of 10 of which fail to improve permanently unless all the primary factors of physical strength are restored through correct use of the body, correct feeding and a knowledge of correct living, mental and physical. Nothing short of complete treatment will prevent a recurrence of chronic arthritis, no matter whether the focus of infection is removed, or a vaccine given or a temporary burden lifted. Recurrence will take place unless the body as a whole is functioning at its full capacity, and the mind is at peace. The changes of chronic illness may be fast or slow, but they are inevitable with the continued misuse of the body, bad living habits and poor diet in the hereditarily predisposed slender person.

The functional disturbances resulting from poor posture, as explained in the previous chapters, therefore make the symptoms found in atrophic arthritis understandable. The disease then becomes one of imbalance with biologic failure. Disease of the joints is merely the result of inevitable tissue changes, occurring observably there, but invisible in other organs, such as the intestines, the liver, the kidneys and the blood vessels.

HYPERTROPHIC ARTHRITIS

Hypertrophic (osteo-degenerative) arthritis has fewer constitutional signs than has atrophic arthritis. It is found commonly in men beyond the age of 40 years and in those who have worked at hard labor. It always is found at points of chronic strain, such as the spine, the neck, the fingers, the toes, the knees and the hips. These joints, with the exception of the fingers, are all subject to the strain of weight-bearing, and frequently this strain is increased markedly by faulty weight-bearing. Hypertrophic arthritis is most marked at points of the body where postural strain can be demonstrated as abnormal (Fig. 89). The changes seen in hypertrophic arthritis cannot be ascribed to infection alone; the slight traumas to the structure of the joints of an individual with a background of poor body chemistry due to age, fatigue and acquired visceroptosis, with an accompanying constipation, appear to be more important.

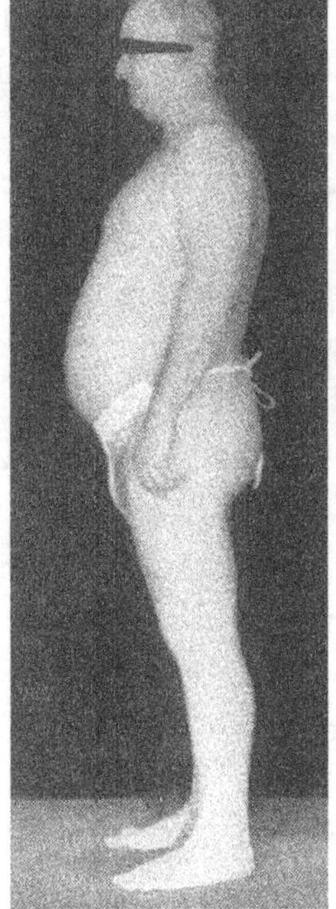

FIG. 89. Hypertrophic arthritis of the spine. Stocky type with prominent abdomen. There is strain on the cervical, the dorsal and the lumbar regions, with strain on the hips and the knees.

Retarded functional capacity and gradual degenerative processes are expected after the age of 45 years, but much of the spurring, the lipping and the eburnation of the bones, with degeneration of the cartilages, seems unnecessary, as it is the result of the unnecessary strain to which the joints have been subjected. Disability in this condition is due chiefly to pain, as is shown by the relief obtained through rest, correction of posture and weight-bearing lines and support of the strained parts of the body (Figs. 90 and 91).

Thus posture, or body mechanics, plays a leading role in the production, and in the successful treatment of chronic arthritis. Inflammation in a joint cannot heal as long as the joint is irritated by sprains associated with poor body mechanics. In hypertrophic arthritis also, bony overgrowth about the joint will continue as long as these sprains occur.

ILLUSTRATIVE CASES

In the above discussion it was stated that a large number of patients who have had chronic arthritis recover with little if any treatment. Such cases at least partially increase the percentage of so-called cures in every vaunted treatment for chronic arthritis. However, a large number of patients do not recover spontaneously, and usually little if any improvement is observed following the ordinary medical procedures. The cases reported here were of long duration, and all the patients had received many forms of treatment, all of which failed to influence the course of the disease and to prevent crippling.

Case 1. Atrophic Arthritis. A 22-year-old unmarried woman-was seen first in October, 1914. There had been pain and stiffness in the joints of 6 years' duration. The joints of the extremities were chiefly involved. The spine, except for the neck, was quite free, but the temporomandibular joints were involved, making chewing difficult. The disability occurred chiefly in the flexed knees and in the feet, which were stiff in valgus. The finger joints were involved, all showing the typical spindle-shaped swelling.

The body mechanics were poor, with a marked droop of the head and the shoulders, and with a low position of the ribs and the diaphragm (Fig. 92). There was marked prominence of the lower abdomen, with little space in the upper abdomen for the viscera, and with practically no retroperitoneal fat. The subcostal angle was narrow. There was marked osseous atrophy, as well as atrophy of the muscles. The digestion was poor, and there was constipation.

The patient entered the hospital, and reconstructive measures were begun to improve the improper functioning of the whole body. Special positions and exercises were given. Plaster-of-paris jackets were applied first in order to raise the ribs and the diaphragm and to make room in the upper abdomen for the abdominal viscera. Casts and exercises were used to improve the position of the flexed knees and the feet, and everything possible was done to improve the general health.

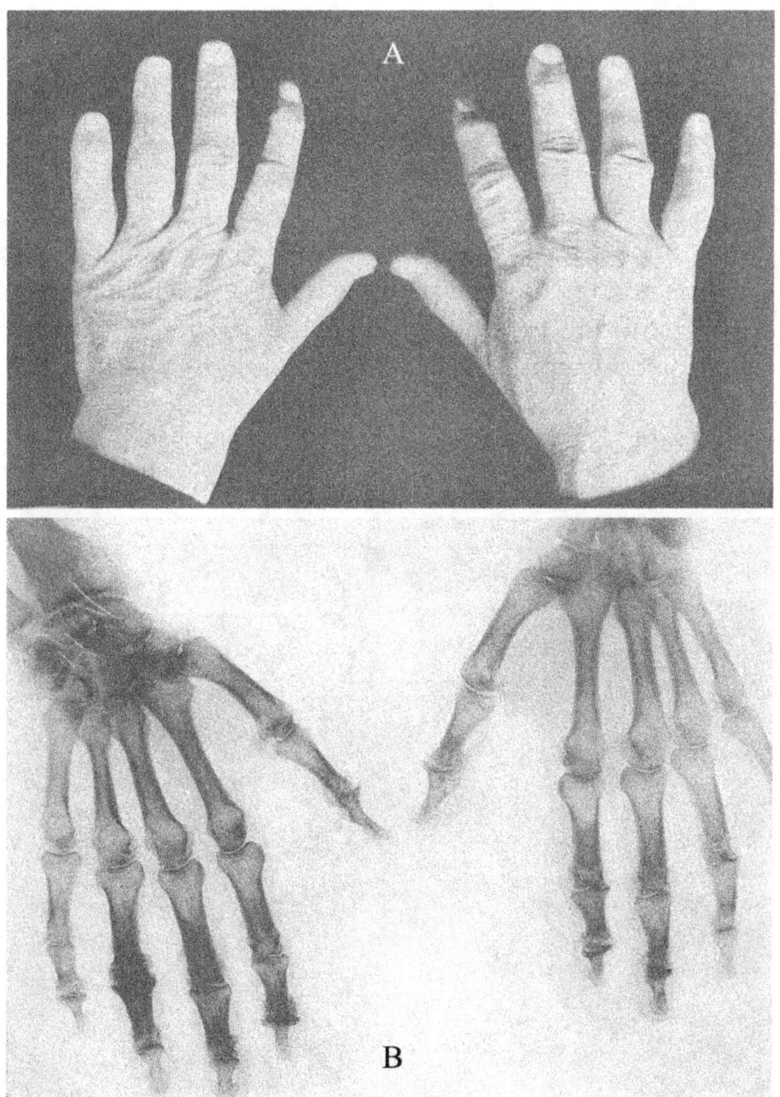

FIG. 90. (A) Hands of patient with hypertrophic arthritis. There is no atrophy of the skin or the nails; Heberden's nodes are shown at the terminal phalangeal joints. (B) Roentgenogram of hands showing hypertrophic arthritis. The bones are dense, there is no osseous atrophy; bony proliferation and spur formation are present at the terminal phalangeal joints and about the thumbs. Compare with atrophic arthritis. Figure 82.

After a considerable gain while the patient was in bed, caliper splints were fitted to support the knees, a body support was fitted, and she was permitted to be up for short periods. She returned to her home after 8 months with little evidence of active disease. With the body support, the special exercises and an adequate diet, all continued at home, she gained steadily. However, stiffness of the knees persisted and caused much limitation in her activities.

The disease being quiescent, an operation was performed on the right knee in 1919-a partial synovectomy, separation of adhesions, and removal of bony spurs. (No operation should be performed on joints when the disease is active.) The result of the operation was so satisfactory that a similar one was performed on the left knee 2 years later. Ninety degrees of motion resulted in both knees. Since that time the patient has continued to do well. She has been able to go about freely and to lead a reasonably normal life. Naturally, the knees and the hands do not have full motion, but the limitations in function are slight. She does her own housework, going up and down stairs easily.

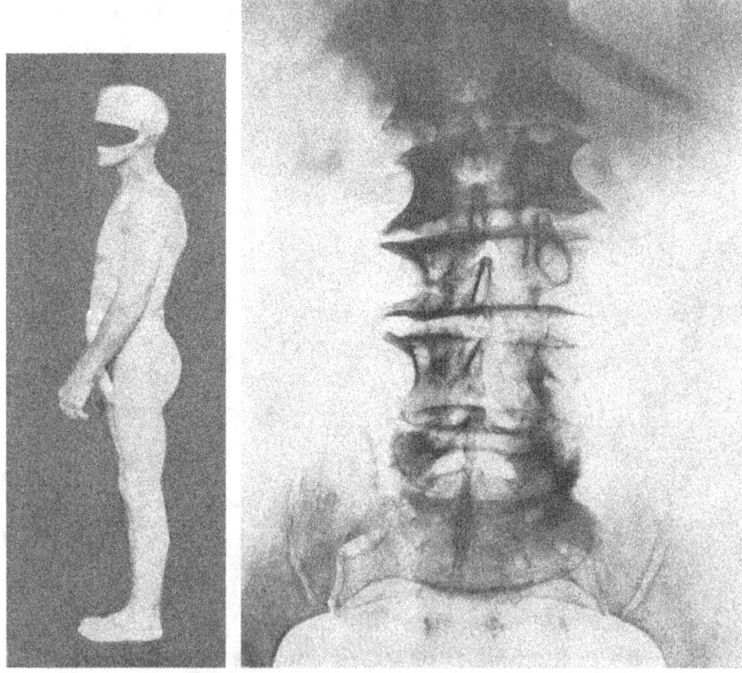

FIG. 91. (Left). Patient with hypertrophic arthritis involving all the joints, but with symptoms referred to the low back. After treatment and complete relief of symptoms the body mechanics, although improved, are not very good but there is no longer sufficient strain on the spine to cause symptoms. (Right) Roentgenogram of spine of this patient. The vertebrae are of the stocky type; there is marked lipping of the bodies, but no ankylosis.

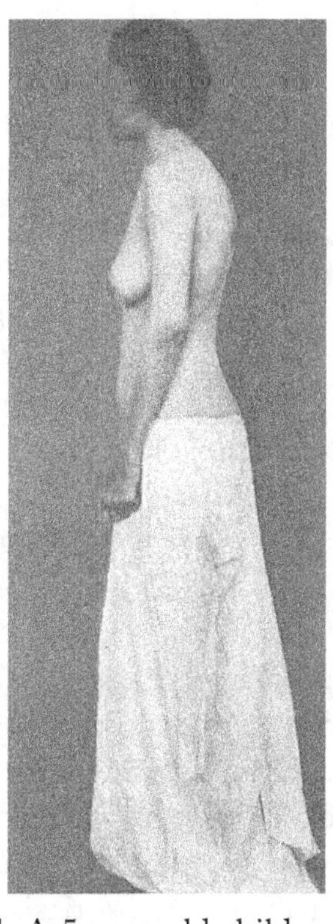

FIG.92 Case 1. **Slight deformity of upper extremities, flexion deformity of fingers; flexed knees are concealed by garment. The body mechanics are very faulty; the chest and the spine have sagged as much as is possible with this patient's type of anatomic structure.**

Case 2. Still's Disease. Atrophic Arthritis in Childhood. A 5-year-old child was seen first in August, 1931, because of trouble with the joints of several months' duration. The patient was of slender build and was in poor general condition. The color was poor, and there was a slight fever, ranging around 100° F. The sag of the abdomen was marked, and the whole body was much drooped. The knees were swollen and flexed, with outward rotation of the tibia. There was arthritis in both elbows, the wrists, the right hip, the feet and the ankles. The diagnosis was severe atrophic arthritis (Still's disease). There had been much treatment, including the removal of the tonsils and the use of special vaccines, without modifying the progress of the disease.

The patient was taken to the hospital, and medico-orthopedic measures were begun to improve the poor body mechanics and to assist in the imperfect function of the organs. The bowel function had been considered normal, but with the free use of castor oil a large amount of very old and offensive material was evacuated. Plaster-of-paris casts were applied to the lower extremities for the gradual correction of the flexion of the knee and the outward rotation of the tibia. As correction was obtained in both the knee and foot, new casts were applied. Correction occurred very slowly, and manipulation was necessary, particularly to correct the rotation of the lower leg. This naturally was not undertaken until the active symptoms of the disease had passed. The flexion deformity of the wrists which was present on admission was corrected by the use of cock-up splints and special exercises.

At first the child remained in bed for 2 weeks. During this time the special positions and exercises were given. As the condition improved with better development of the upper abdomen, a body brace was fitted, as well as caliper splints, and the child was allowed to be up for short periods. At first the improvement was very slow but later it became more rapid. Evidence of active disease disappeared with good development of the upper abdomen, with the diaphragm high and the abdominal organs in place. The damaged joints recovered so that the child returned to school and got about freely, the knees did not become entirely normal, being limited slightly in extension, but the improvement continued, and the deformity which was present did not interfere with his activities. The child returned to the hospital for manipulation of the joints, but most of the treatment was carried on at home, with the child returning to the office only for further supervision.

It required two years to bring the disease completely under control and to secure good function in the disabled joints. But when one considers that the treatment also involved the careful guidance of the growth of the child, with remodelling of the body so that the organs could have proper space in which to function, this has not been a long time. With these patients it is unreasonable to expect rapid cures.

Case 3. Atrophic Arthritis with Psoriasis. A physician, 50 years old, was first seen 20 years ago because of a progressive disease of the joints with increasing disability. He was trying to carry on his practice but with much effort and with much suffering. For many years he had had an unusually severe psoriasis; the arthritis had been present for only 4 or 5 years. He was of a mixed anatomic type, being partly slender and partly intermediate. There was a generalised involvement of the joints of the extremities mostly in the knees and the hands. The general condition was poor with poor body mechanics. The abdomen was large and much sagged with displacement of the abdominal organs and dilatation and poor muscular tone in the colon. The psoriasis was quite marked. On the anterior side of body there was a solid confluent mass of scales from the pelvis to the neck and the skull was completely psoriatic.

The patient was taken to the hospital, and measures were begun to improve the faulty mechanics and to make possible better function of the organs. At first the patient was kept horizontal in bed with special positions and exercises and fomentations to the spine. Because of the marked distention of the colon, irrigations of the bowel were used as well as regular cathartics. The patient remained at the hospital for about 2 months. The improvement in the joints was steady, so that after 4 weeks a body brace was fitted, and the patient was permitted to be up for short periods. Exercises were given at first, with the body horizontal, but with the improvement they were increased in number and were given largely with the patient standing. The skin became better, and in a few months the psoriasis had practically disappeared. It recurred on one occasion a few years later but was relieved quickly by further improvement in the body mechanics. The patient returned home and was able to continue with his work as a general practitioner. A modified routine was continued until all symptoms of both the psoriasis and the arthritis had disappeared. There was no return of either the arthritis or the psoriasis.

Case 4. Atrophic Arthritis with Subcoracoid Bursitis. A man, 34 years old, a rural free delivery mail-carrier in northern Vermont, was seen first in 1932 for pain in the arms that had been called neuritis. He had had much treatment, including the removal of several teeth and the tonsils, and had been on a special diet, none of which had changed the course of the disease. At the time of the examination he was much disabled, with limited motion in both shoulders, rotation being particularly painful. There was pain down the arm, worse at night. The elbows, the hands, the knees and the feet were involved also.

The mechanics of the body were extremely poor in both the sitting and the standing position. The ribs were low, and the body was sagged. In the sitting position in which the patient drove his car the arms and the shoulders were far forward, and the body was much drooped. The sag of the abdominal viscera was marked; the diaphragm was low with a limited excursion. There was very little retroperitoneal fat in the upper abdomen. The condition represented a typical atrophic arthritis with a subcoracoid bursitis of both shoulders (Fig. 93).

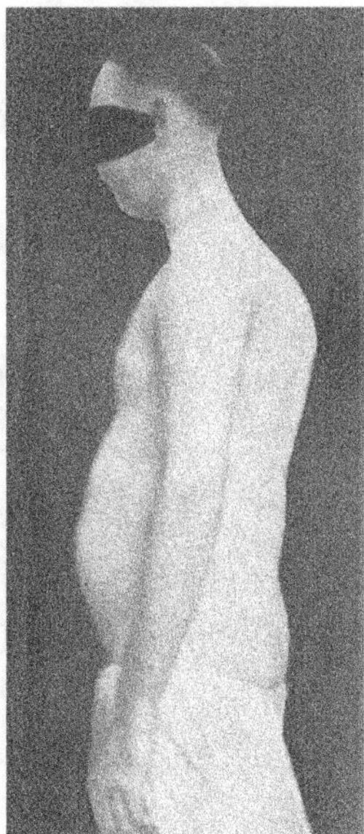

FIG. 93. Case 4. Atrophic arthritis with subcoracoid bursitis; extremely faulty body mechanics. The shoulders are low and forward, with an increased dorsal curve of the spine, flat chest and prominent abdomen. This position of the shoulders allows the humerus to pull away from the glenoid cavity and leads to strain of all the structures about the shoulder joint.

The patient was taken to the hospital, and positions and exercises to correct the poor body mechanics were begun. He was kept on his back most of the time, with the shoulders held in abduction, and with external rotation with pillows under the elbow and the forearm to relieve pain. The acute pain in the arms at night was due chiefly to rotation in the relaxation of sleep. Exercises were begun also for the better control of the muscles of the shoulders, with the patient lying supine, since in this position the head of the humerus fell away from the coracoid process, thus lessening the pressure on the bursa. Only active exercises which could be controlled and limited by the patient's sensation of pain and spasm were given; no passive exercises were permitted. The patient remained at the hospital for only 8 days; during this time he was learning the routine to be carried out at home.

A short back brace with an attached elastic shoulder brace was fitted, and foot plates were supplied also because of the weakness and deformity of the feet. A wholesome diet was planned, with much fruit and vegetables.

The patient gradually improved; he made 4 subsequent visits to the hospital, and plaster casts were applied, with caliper splints later, for the correction of the deformities at the knees. Treatment was planned each time to secure the best possible mechanics of the body, as well as to improve the function of the joints.

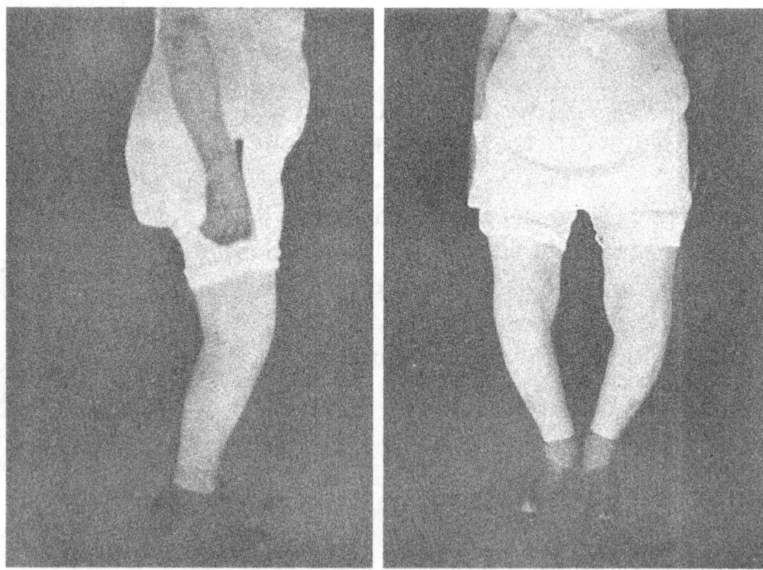

FIG. 94. Case 5. Hypertrophic arthritis of spine, hips and knees with marked visceroptosis. The faulty body mechanics are shown in both the lateral and the anteroposterior views, particularly in the lower extremities. There is a forward tilt of the pelvis which, in the stocky type of individual such as this patient, strains the hip and the knee joints and is an important factor in the development of the hypertrophic arthritis. The flexed knees also are sources of strain.

The patient has remained free from the pain in the arms since his first visit to the hospital. He returned to his work after 6 months. In driving his car he has improved his faulty sitting position, so that the tendency to bursitis and the disturbance in function in the organs are no longer present.

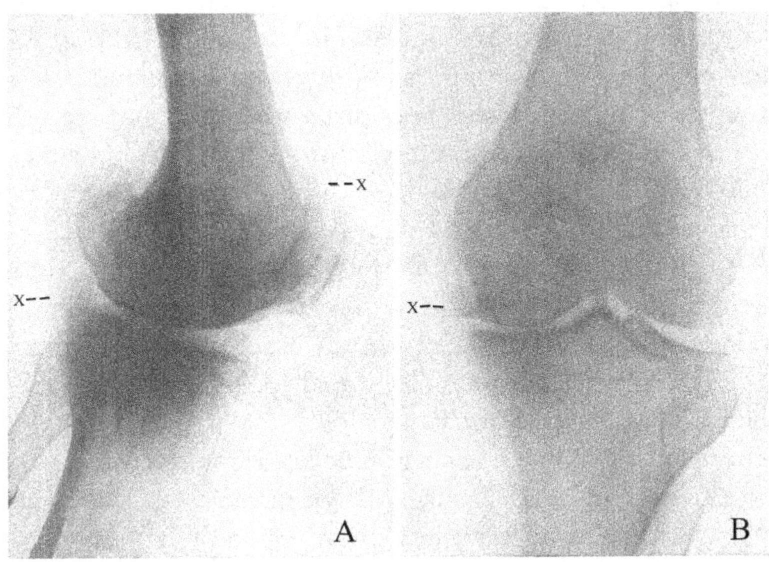

FIG. 95. Roentgenograms of knees. (A) Lateral view, hypertrophic arthritis. The bones are dense; there is bony overgrowth about the margins of the joint and at the edge of the patella. (B) Anteroposterior view of knee showing hypertrophic arthritis.

Case 5. Hypertrophic Arthritis of Spine, Hips and Knees, with Visceroptosis. A 64-year-old woman was seen first in 1926 for pain in the knees of 4 years' duration; there was also pain in the low back. The patient was of the stocky type. She stood with the knees bent, the legs rotated outward at the hips, and the pelvis tipped forward, with extension of the dorsolumbar spine and marked sagging of the abdomen (Fig. 94). Walking or prolonged standing was difficult and caused increasing pain. The knees showed a flexion deformity of 15° and they could be flexed only to a right angle (Fig. 95). There was limitation in abduction and rotation in both hips, the result of deformity of the femoral heads, which were mushroom in shape, with nodes about the margins of the cartilage. The increase in the outward rotation of the legs was the result of the forward tip of the broad pelvis, with flaring ilia, which not only forced the legs apart but caused the weight to be thrown on the posterior part of the acetabulum. (In the slender type, with a narrower pelvis and a longer femoral neck, a forward tip of the pelvis does not lead to outward rotation of the legs.)

For treatment, a short back brace was used, with a special corset, the purpose being to flatten the lumbar spine and to correct the forward tip of the pelvis. This relieved the strain on the knees by making the weight-bearing lines better. The apparatus also decreased the marked abdominal sag and improved the function in the abdominal organs. Elastic supports reinforced with felt were applied to the knees to protect the joints and to lessen the irritation. These did not prevent motion at the knees. Foot plates were used to correct the weight-bearing lines of the feet. Special exercises were given to improve the faulty body mechanics.

The patient did well from the beginning, and pain soon disappeared entirely with improvement in the mechanics of the body. She was able to do her own housework and to lead an active life, in spite of slight permanent limitation in the affected joints. No medical treatment was given except such remedies as would favor free elimination of the body wastes through the bowels and the kidneys. The result was exactly as was expected once the faulty mechanics were corrected, and better-physiology made possible. There has been no extension of the disease, and pain has ceased entirely.

Of the different forms of arthritis, hypertrophic arthritis is the simplest to control, and if the patient is seen early before much damage has occurred to the joints, the control of the disease should be so complete as to leave little if any limitation of function.

Osteitis Deformans (Paget's Disease). Among the progressive crippling conditions affecting the bones and the joints osteitis deformans has a definite place, and while few cases go on to the extreme deformity shown in Sir James Paget's original article, there are a great many patients in whom a less general manifestation of the disease exists. It is not uncommon for one or two bones to show it without other evidence in the skeleton than a generalized atrophy, apparently the first stage of the disease (Fig. 96), the condition, with the general weakness of the muscles, resembling atrophic arthritis. Apparently the weakening of the shafts of the long bones is greater in atrophic arthritis and not infrequently leads to bowing. The increased density of the bones seen in the later stages of the disease is apparently Nature's attempt to repair or support the weakened parts (Fig. 97).

The similarity of this disease to atrophic arthritis is suggested further by the frequent presence of lesions in the joints. One may expect to arrest and improve this condition in much the same way as in atrophic arthritis. In the light of our experience it seems reasonable to give a favorable prognosis in osteitis deformans, except in the cases in the healed or "dense-bone" stage of the disease.

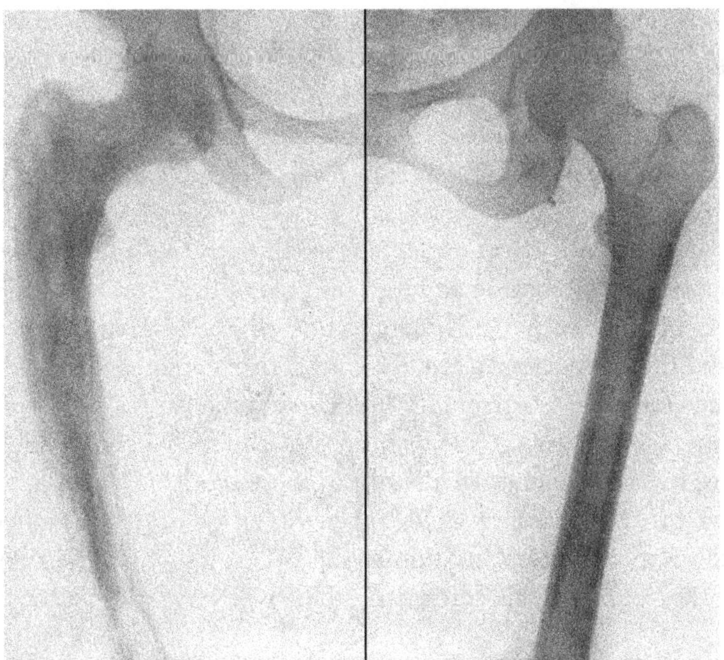

FIG. 96 Osteitis deformans (Paget's disease). The disease is shown in the right femur, with bowing and increased calcium deposit in the upper part of the femur. The disease is beginning in the left femur, where there is slight generalized atrophy.

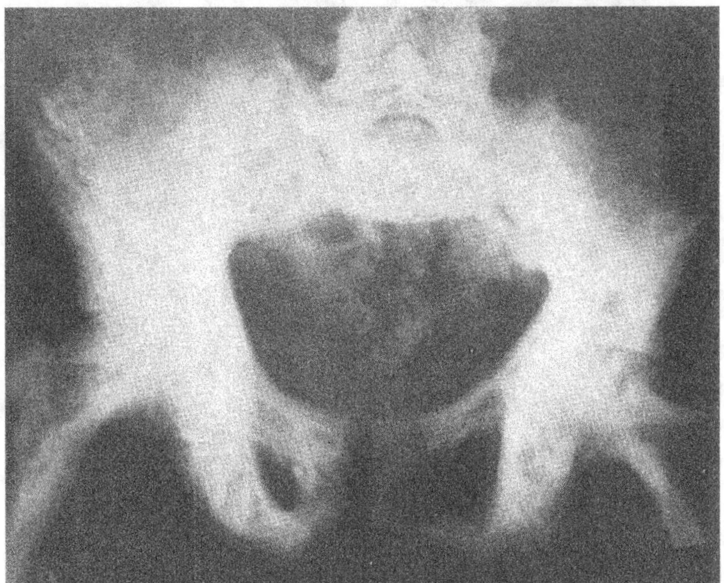

FIG.97 There are areas of thickening and areas of atrophy in the pelvic bones. The femora also are involved.

Case 6. Osteitis Deformans. A school-teacher, 61 years of age, was seen first in 1931 for pain in the right leg. She had fallen 3 years before, striking the upper part of the lower leg. There was rapid recovery, with no recurrence of the difficulty until 1 year later, when she began to have pain which extended up and down the entire lower leg. The attack lasted only a short time but recurred in about a year, this time being worse. The attacks came on without apparent cause.

The patient was of the intermediate type. She stood with the body markedly relaxed, and the abdomen much sagged. The body had been supported by a corset, which did not correct the faulty mechanics. There was marked exaggeration of the lumbar curve of the spine, the knees were flexed, and the legs were rotated outward. The right knee was held in slight flexion, but motion at the knee joint was normal. Hip motion was free, as was also motion at the ankle and the foot. The general muscular tonus was poor. Abdominal palpation showed the acquired type of visceroptosis, but no evidence of disease in the viscera.

X-ray study showed marked atrophy of the skeleton as a whole, with a beginning atrophic arthritis in the joints of the low back and in the sacro-iliac joints. In the right tibia there was the characteristic appearance of osteitis deformans; there was very little involvement of the fibula.

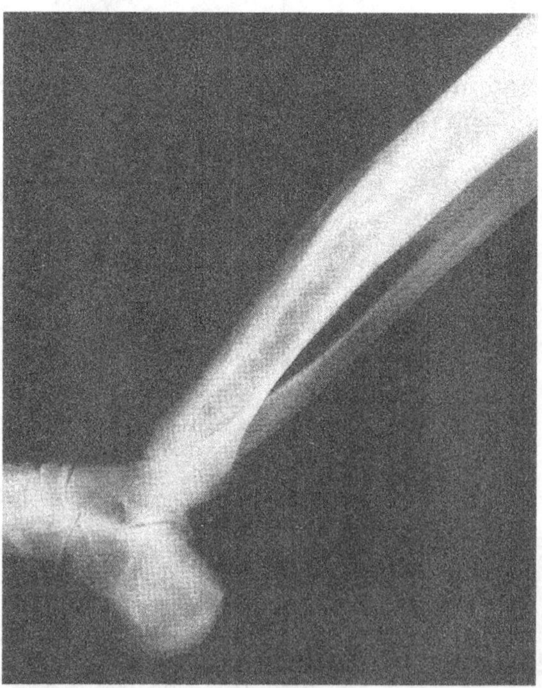

FIG. 98. Osteitis deformans (Paget's disease). There is atrophy in the pelvic bones. The femora are involved also.

The left os calcis showed the same disease but no local symptoms. X-ray examination of the entire skeleton showed no evidence of osteitis deformans other than the marked atrophy of the bones.

Correction of the faulty mechanics of the body was begun at once. A support was fitted to the body to correct the increased lumbar curvature, to support the markedly relaxed abdomen and to tip the pelvis downward at the back, thus balancing the body and bringing the weight properly on the legs. Medication was planned to improve the general condition. Special exercises were begun, and special positions were prescribed for short periods several times during the day. The patient was followed at intervals in the office, with gradual improvement in the condition, and marked general improvement. The patient is able to do her work with no inconvenience; the slight flexion of the knee that was present in the beginning has been overcome, and the disease in the left os calcis has remained inactive.

With the improvement in the general condition, there has been some improvement in the generalized skeletal atrophy, although the bones do not show as much density as would be considered normal in an individual of this type.

From the results obtained it seems proper to expect an improvement and gradual arrest of the condition which otherwise would go on to serious crippling. In this case the result was secured chiefly by improving the functional mechanics of the whole body.

11

TREATMENT

GENERAL CONSIDERATIONS

Once the foregoing conception of health and disease is grasped, the treatment for the individual case naturally consists, first of all, in correcting the faulty mechanics so that the different structures may be able to work as nearly normally as possible. This is fundamental and should be begun before other special forms of treatment which may be indicated for the special type of disease are used.

First, one must put the machine in order so that all the parts can work. Whether the primary symptoms represent a static strain, an arthritis, a progressive paralysis, a visceral disturbance, varicose veins or some other chronic condition, the different parts should function so that general good health is reasonable to expect; after that, such special treatment as may be indicated may be employed. To resort to special diets, physiotherapy, apparatus, medicine or operation without first correcting the faulty mechanical relationships must produce unsatisfactory results, since the basic features of the physiology have not been appreciated or correct function made possible. These features should be corrected first, after which special diets, or medicines, or operations or anything else that may be necessary to relieve the patient may be added.

At times, as the result of disease, injury or congenital defect, the parts may be so damaged that the ideal normal is not possible, but under such conditions the faulty mechanics should be corrected so far as possible, so that there may be the smallest amount of remaining handicap from the incorrectible features.

The special treatment required to bring about correct body mechanics must depend on the degree of the faulty features and whether or not actual disease already has resulted. Many times the disturbance is relatively slight and shows itself as static strain of the back, the feet or the knees, as mild digestive disorders or as prominence of the veins of the legs, without evidence of serious derangement. Under such conditions it is usually possible to accomplish the desired end without serious interruption of the normal activities of the patient.

Co-operation of Patient. In all cases, irrespective of the severity of the condition or the disease, the nature of the problem and the general plan of treatment first of all should be explained to the patient in simple terms. This genuine understanding and co-operation are absolutely necessary if the results are to be satisfactory. The physician can indicate the line of work, but the carrying out of the details must rest with the patient, and this co-operation is hardly to be expected unless the nature of the problem is understood fully. To make this clear, anatomic charts, silhouette photographs and roentgenograms are usually helpful, and for such presentation the physician himself must understand clearly the nature of the problem and be able to demonstrate on himself much that is expected of the patient.

Education of Patient. The next step is so to educate the patient, both mentally and physically, that the normal reflex muscular control will be developed. For this purpose special exercises are used, as well as special positions in which the body is placed for varying periods.

It should be explained that these are given with the sole aim of improving the general balance or position of the whole body. It should be understood clearly that these exercises are planned, not to make stronger or larger muscles but so that the muscles may be controlled properly, and so that the balance of the body ultimately may be such that the muscle action will be instinctively correct.

In learning to play golf, much time is spent in practicing the correct standing position or stance, as well as the proper use of the arms and the legs in making the strokes. None of this is done to make large muscles but simply to get the existing muscles under such control that unconsciously they will be used rightly. The perfect player gives little thought to form, since that has been assured by early practice. The same is true of the exercises and the positions used to correct faulty body mechanics. The aim is a well-poised body, with muscles under proper control and able to perform their proper function without conscious effort.

Planned Exercises. Frequent assumption of the correct position is the most important step. The simple doing of exercises will accomplish little unless they are planned properly. The aim is to obtain the correct poise of the body, with all the muscles in balance, and to this end exercise of the right type is of great help. The same is true of braces or mechanical supports, which are needed frequently in the treatment. The braces are intended simply to help in obtaining body poise and to obtain more rapidly the proper muscular reactions by relieving some of the temporary strain.

In mild degrees of faulty body mechanics there need be little change from the regular routine of life. The special muscle training, as mentioned above, should be carried out with the exercises performed two or three times daily. Frequent checking of the position of the body as the patient goes about or sits or stands should be practiced, and whenever possible he should lie flat on his back for 5 or 10 minutes without pillows under the head, but with the hands clasped under the head or the neck. A longer time in bed at night than usual, 9 hours at least, to lessen the downward drag of the structures in the upright position, should be encouraged, and the regular general physical activities should be kept well under the fatigue limit.

When the conditions are more extreme, or when actual disease is present, it is necessary to have the body recumbent for varying periods while the faulty mechanical features are being overcome. The ideal method is to have the patient in a properly equipped hospital where the special staff is trained to care for such cases. The ordinary hospital for acute diseases is of little benefit, since acute ailments receive most of the attention, while the chronic type of case, partly because but little understood, receives slight care. In chronic cases the most rapid progress can be gained by beginning the treatment in the recumbent position. In this position the force of gravity, which increases the sag of the organs and the strain on the body as a whole in the upright position, is removed to a large degree, and the bed itself can be used as a splint to help the patient acquire the correct position.

With the horizontal position the first aim is to flatten the lumbar spine, to tip the pelvis backward and to elevate the ribs, thus raising the diaphragm and the organs attached thereto (Fig. 99). In the horizontal position, since most severe cases are of the slender anatomic type, the lower ribs drop backward as well as downward with the general droop of the body, thus deepening the lateral spinal spaces. This allows the organs to drop backward more than is normal, and therefore they must drag or press on the structures which lie in front of the spine in the upper abdomen; these structures, which include the veins and the arteries, are interfered with under such conditions.

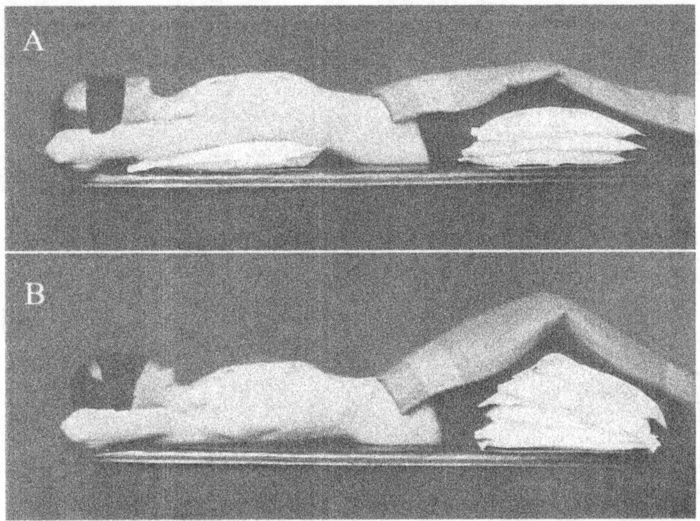

FIG.99. (A) Hyperextension position, with the body in a horizontal position with pillows under the knees. The arms extended over the head help to raise the ribs still farther and to flatten the dorsal spine. The pillows under the knees remove the strain from the lumbar spine. Note how the thorax is raised to what is practically the position of full inspiration. With such a position of the thorax the excursion of the diaphragm must be as free and as great as possible. Compare this figure with Figure 39, which has been modified for strain of the back. At times the patient must begin treatment without any pillow under the chest, as in B, going on to the position at A as soon as it can be taken without too great discomfort.

There is also the possibility of draw and pressure on the pancreas, the duodenum or the bile ducts, or interference with the sympathetic ganglia, which are so numerous in this region. The possibility of such disturbance is avoided unconsciously in the slender type, since it is a well-recognized fact that such persons rarely sleep on the back but are more comfortable on the face or the side..

Use of Pads. While the back position is important in order to flatten the low back and to raise the ribs with the diaphragm, yet, with these features in mind, it is often well to place pads under the loin at the sides so that the sag of the lower ribs is prevented or lessened. Often this can be accomplished by using carefully selected small pillows or soft sandbags, or, what is many times best of all, a plaster-of-paris shell that is molded to the back when the patient is lying on his stomach (Fig. 100). During the molding the ribs are raised as much as possible, and the soft parts below them are pushed up or forward. After hardening, such a shell can be used for the patient to lie in for certain periods during the day, thus obtaining the benefit of the back position without the harm of the marked backward visceral sag.

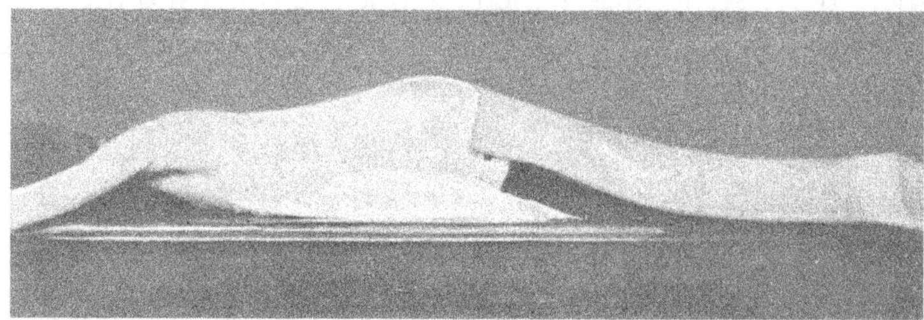

FIG. 100. "Face-prone" position. The patient lying prone, with pillows under the abdomen. Note the flatness of the back and the fullness of the chest. In this position the organs fall away from the structures at the back of the upper abdomen.

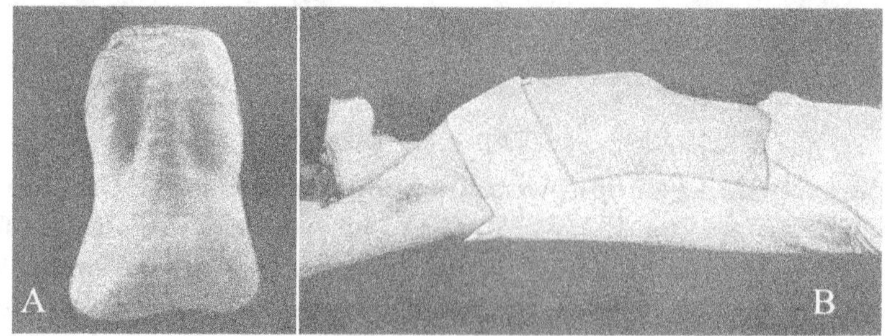

FIG. 101. (A) Plaster shell. Note the molded depressions which raise the lower ribs. (B) Patient in shell, showing the elevation of the lower ribs.

In spite of such measures, since there will be some backward drag or pressure on the nerves and the vessels at the back of the upper abdomen, after periods of not more than a half hour on the back, the "face-prone" position, with the body rolled over on the abdomen (Fig. 100), should be taken. In this position the organs fall away from the structures at the back of the upper abdomen, and any discomfort that might come from long continuation of the first position is avoided. The occasional marked changes in the pulse rate which occur as these positions are taken suggest strongly the extreme delicacy of the adjustments of the body mechanics.

With the beginning of the treatment, not only are the positions in which the body is placed carefully planned, but exercises are begun at once with the idea of developing gradually a proper control of the muscles on which the ultimate proper use of the body must depend. The first essential is to control the abdominal muscles. The average person has little if any ability to control or even contract intelligently these muscles and this is brought about often only after teaching. With this, similar control of the muscles of the buttocks must be taught also, so that the usual forward tip of the pelvis can be corrected. At the same time an attempt is made to widen the usually narrow angle formed by the ribs as, through the costal cartilages, they join the sternum at the subcostal angle. Following this comes a regular progression of exercises, as shown later in this chapter, taking in the neck, the chest, the arms and the legs.

Development of Muscle Control. As stated above, in developing muscle co-ordination the intent is not to build strong muscles but to secure normal control of the important groups of muscles on which so much of the proper use of the body depends. When it is thought that the correction of the faulty mechanical features has been accomplished as much as is possible with the body horizontal and that the muscular control is reasonably satisfactory, the use of the body in the upright position is begun.

Resumption of Active Work. To determine when the patient is ready for active work, not only is the ability to control the important muscle groups checked, but the different physiologic tests which have been made during the time of recumbency are studied. The temperature and the pulse are taken daily (Fig. 102). In the beginning the temperature is usually low or, if nearly normal, it drops, in the first few days of relaxation, 2° or occasionally 3°, below normal. The pulse is usually rapid and irregular; with relaxation and the use of special positions to improve the action of the diaphragm, it should become slow and more regular. The blood pressure, which is generally low, the systolic pressure being often 100 or less, should gradually approach the normal for the individual. Before much freedom of activity is allowed, the pressure should be taken during rest and then after a brisk walk; with normal physiology there should be little difference between these two. In estimating the blood pressure and in studying the basal metabolism or the temperature, the anatomic type of the patient should be considered.

The slender type should have a blood pressure from 10 to 15 points below the so-called normal, while in the stocky type it should be that much above normal. The temperature also is usually lower in the slender type. The basal metabolism in this type should be +10 or 15, while in the stocky type it should be about the same amount minus. The basal metabolism test is employed to indicate the condition of the general physiology, and in interpreting these tests the graph is depended on more than the computed figure. At the beginning of treatment the metabolism may be high, suggesting a hyperactive thyroid gland, while the graph may be so unstable as to suggest that this activity was simply a reflex struggle in an effort to preserve the physiologic balance. With rest and with special exercises to improve the general circulation, the metabolism is usually minus. Moderate doses of thyroid extract generally hasten recovery, suggesting that the reactions as seen are largely those of fatigue.

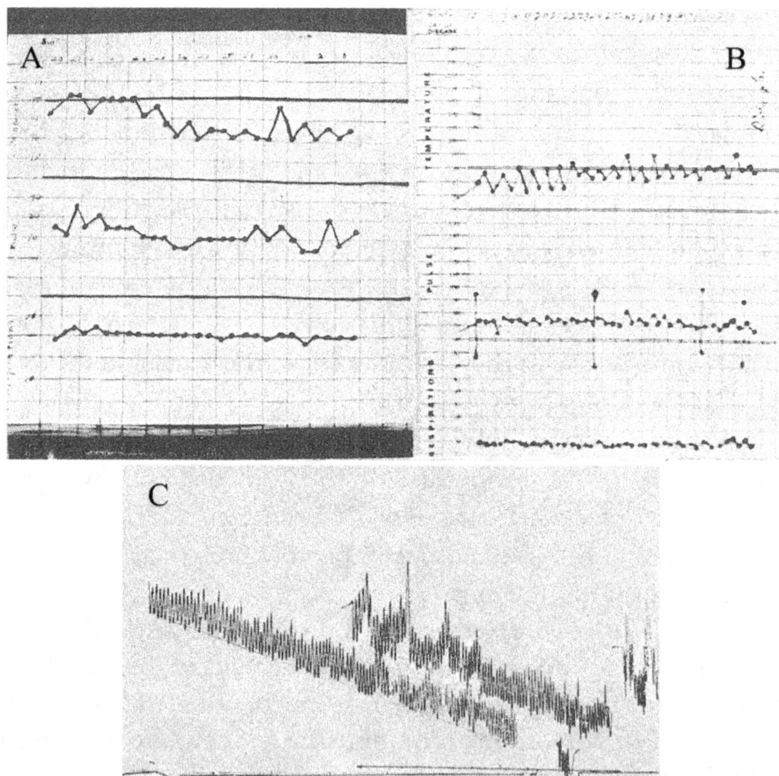

FIG. 102. (A) Temperature chart showing drop in temperature after patient has been recumbent several days. (B) Approach to normal. (C) Irregular tracing in basal metabolism at beginning of treatment. (A) The temperature chart shows that the patient, even after two weeks in the hospital largely at rest in bed, with the special positions and exercises, is still physiologically unstable and is not ready for too active work. Note the nearly normal temperature for the first few days, and the marked drop not only in the A.M. but also the P.M. The pulse showed a similar variation. The irregularity in temperature and pulse in the last 4 days was caused by the patient's beginning to get up and around. (B) Approach to normal temperature after fatigue has disappeared. (C) The basal metabolism graph shows marked irregularity of breathing. Although the computed rates are only plus 9 and plus 14, the character of the graph represents marked physiologic instability and a labored breathing. This graph indicates that the patient needs much more rest and treatment before he can be considered well, even though at the moment he may be free of symptoms.

Another finding is that in the beginning practically all the cases of any type show very little retroperitoneal fat, as can be demonstrated by palpation through the loin from the back to the front, the fingers usually touching except for the layers of skin. This factor, with its correction, is of the utmost importance for health and should be watched very carefully.

When it is time for the patient to be allowed to be up, all the foregoing factors should be checked. The temperature should be normal and regular; the pulse should be of normal rate and steady; the blood pressure should show little variation at rest or activity; the basal metabolism test should show a reasonably regular graph and computed figure, and the fat pads in the back of the upper abdomen should be palpable, with good tone in the abdominal muscles (Fig. 104).

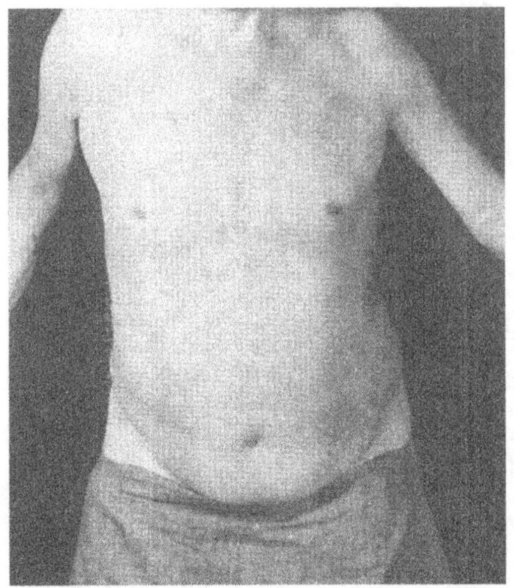

FIG. 103. Faulty mechanics with poor muscular tone in the abdominal muscles.

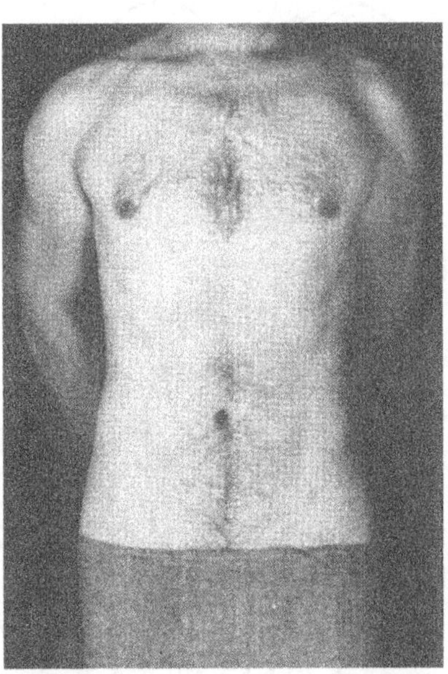

FIG. 104 Good body mechanics with good muscular tone in the abdominal muscles.

SUPPORTS AND BRACES

When these features have improved sufficiently, and when the patient has learned the principles of good body mechanics, supports are used to assist in maintaining the correct position of the body until enough time has elapsed for normal tone to develop. This is because the muscles are not yet fully developed, and the ligaments have not yet adjusted themselves to the new positions.

Temporary Use. Supports or braces should be understood to be temporary means to an end, not for permanent use. As commonly planned, they assist chiefly in maintaining the correct position of the pelvis, the structural base of the body. They also help to prevent the usual sag of the body backward from the hips by pushing forward on the dorsal spine and helping to elevate the ribs. Since, with the usual long use of the body in the incorrect position, the joints of the pelvis have become strained, and those of the low lumbar region weakened, the apparatus is employed to give support about the pelvis, as well as to protect the joints of the low back.

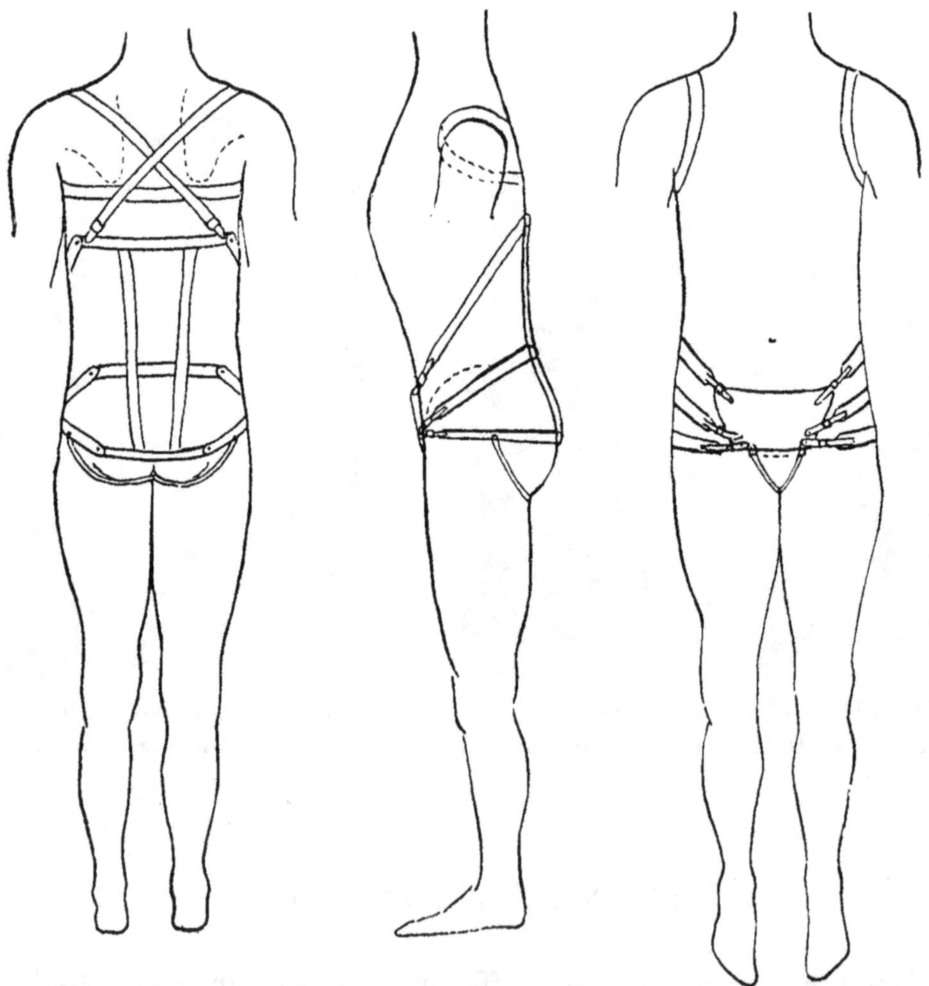

FIG. 105. Back brace commonly used when the patient is first permitted to be in the upright position. The upper crossbar is made as wide as the thorax. In this way the upper straps attached to the crossbar do not pull the lower ribs downward and inward.

We recommend no one brace or appliance, since the chief aim is to accomplish the results described above. How this is done is of little matter, and rarely are the tools used by different individuals the same. However, since it may be of some interest to others or suggestive of the principles of treatment, the type of brace most commonly used by us in this stage of the treatment is shown here (Fig. 105). The uprights are of flexible steel, tempered hard enough to hold their shape in ordinary use but soft enough to be reshaped with a wrench as the body changes with the improving conditions. There are two crossbars at the bottom, so placed that they can be molded to fit the shape of the posterior part of the pelvis. Both these straps encircle the body below the crests of the ilia and above the top of the trochanters, thus giving the needed support to the pelvic joints.

The lower part of the brace should extend down to the level of the tip of the coccyx; the upper part should reach to the ninth dorsal vertebra. When fitted, the brace should exert pressure at the top and the bottom but should not touch in the midlumbar region, in the expectation that the body will be gradually drawn back to the brace at this level. The upper crossbar should be long enough to extend around from the back of the body slightly to the sides. It should also be long enough so that the straps to be fastened to it and to the anterior pad will not exert lateral pressure on the lower ribs and thus interfere with the action of the diaphragm.

The anterior part of the brace is a reinforced leather pad to which the straps can be attached. The two lower straps are fastened close together at the bottom of the pad so that their pressure is entirely about the pelvic girdle. When they are fastened the lower part of the pad should be drawn in, thus forming a support for the commonly sagging abdomen. The top strap is attached to the upper part of the anterior pad and serves to hold the upper part of the brace against the back, as well as to draw the abdomen into place. The pad must be wide enough to ensure freedom of the lower ribs.

Elastic Shoulder Strap. With such a support, if the shoulder position is poor, and if the patient has a marked tendency to droop forward in the standing and the sitting positions, thus compressing the chest and crowding all the organs in the epigastric region, an elastic shoulder strap can be added. A rigid shoulder brace is not used, since this sacrifices the support at the bottom, which is by far the more important. Such a support can be worn under a specially fitted corset or canvas belt if it is deemed necessary to have more support or, for esthetic reasons, to hide the brace.

With this brace, the normal motions of the body can be made by bending from the hips in stooping, by sideward bending at the waistline or by the usual twisting if the body is used correctly. Drooping or buckling at the waistline is made difficult, and activities, such as golf, become easily possible.

The purpose of the brace is to assist the patient, through his muscles, ligaments and especially his brain and nerve cells, to gain the right or best use of his body. It should be used, as crutches are used after a broken leg, until the parts are strong. The brace is only a means to an end; it is intended to assist in maintaining good alignment of the body until the muscles can keep this alignment constantly without fatigue. As muscular strength and co-ordination approach the normal, the brace is gradually discarded.

Other Supports. At times, other supports are required, usually as a temporary measure, rarely as a permanent aid. In women, when the weakness is chiefly in the muscles of the lower abdomen, a firm corset often will keep the body in improved alignment until the body becomes stronger. This corset should be sufficiently firm to pull the abdomen in and up. The corset should lace in the back, since in this way better support will be given to the back, and the abdomen will be held firmly (Fig. 134). When there is arthritis or a severe deformity a brace, such as is shown in Figure 135, may be required also. This usually is covered by a corset in women because the clothing fits over it better, and because firmer support is given in this way. When there is very severe or fixed deformity of the spine a well-molded jacket of leather or plaster is required sometimes. Such jackets are applied with the patient lying on a metal frame (Goldthwait frame). The low back is flat, and the dorsal spine is in extension. The jacket is well-molded over the anterior superior spines and in the loins. This jacket usually is cut in front to permit removal for other treatments and for bathing. Jackets of this type often relieve symptoms by holding the body passively in an improved mechanical position. It aids little in the active correction of the body. Except in the presence of severe fixed deformity of the spine, a jacket should be used only temporarily for the relief of symptoms.

Such should be our aim, but it must be understood that where serious disease exists, and the ideal result is unattainable, the nearer to it we can come, the less will be the ultimate handicap. If Nature is given only a slight chance, it is surprising how much she is able to do in restoring function in what seems to be a badly damaged or helpless body.

MUSCLE RE-EDUCATION

The technic and the reasons for the exercises which have been found to be helpful in acquiring and maintaining good body mechanics are explained in the following pages. Extensive surveys reported at the White House Conference for Child Health and Hygiene showed that 80 per cent or more of the children of this country exhibit bad body mechanics. This indicates that the so-called systems of exercises, games, rhythmic dancing and sports in any plan of physical education have not produced good body mechanics in either children or adults. This is an educational problem; the fundamental principles must be taught first, and once these have been acquired, the more elaborate forms or systems of exercises, supplemented by games, rhythmic dancing, sports, and so forth, may be adopted.

The aim of postural exercises is to secure the poise of the body in the proper balanced line, without muscle tension or rigidity (Fig. 102 C). A well-poised body means better health through improved organic function, better work, both physical and mental, and greater strength and endurance, through a lessening of skeletal muscle tension and its resultant fatigue.

Good body mechanics mean the use of the body as a whole in proper poise. The following five requirements, which have been accepted by the American Academy of Orthopaedic Surgery, give a standard of measurement which can be applied easily and can be used in conjunction with other more complicated methods if so desired. They are as follows:

The first requirement is that the curves of the spine from the sacrum to the occiput shall not be exaggerated. For example, in the habitual standing or sitting position the lumbar curve, particularly at the lumbosacral junction, must have further motion in extension as well as in flexion. In the common faulty standing position, with the pelvis in a forward position, and the lower abdomen prominent, the lumbosacral joints are used in the position of complete extension. This applies to the other parts of the spine as well.

The second requirement is that the subcostal angle of the ribs shall be at least a right angle. If it is less than this, a disalignment of the costovertebral and the costotransverse joints results.

The third requirement is that the circumference of the chest at the xiphoid in the habitual or natural standing position shall be approximately halfway between the girth at full inspiration and that at full expiration. If the second and the third requirements are met, the costovertebral and the costotransverse joints are of necessity mechanically in a position where there is the least in congruence.

The fourth requirement, which can be recognized by observation and palpation of the patient or in a photograph, concerns the development and the prominence of the upper abdomen in the region of the lower ribs and the loins; palpation from back to front should show firm, resistant structures. In long-continued poor body mechanics such palpation shows little more than the two layers of skin. The upper abdomen should be larger and bigger around than the lower abdomen, or that part below the umbilicus. If this development is not present, even though the rest of the body is in excellent position, and the first four requirements are fulfilled, the examiner knows that the patient's posture or body mechanics is habitually poor, because such mechanics in any structural type tend to cause pressure or constriction in this region, with consequent sagging of the abdominal organs.

The fifth requirement relates to the position in which the feet are used habitually in relation to the patella. In good mechanics the line drawn through the patella and the middle of the ankle should strike the base of the second or the third toe. In poor mechanics, with the pronated foot, this line will fall inside the great toe (see Fig.127).

The ability to use the body rightly should be taught in the lying (Figs. 99, 109 and 110), sitting (Figs. 107, 116) and standing positions (Figs. 106, 108 and 117), as well as in the change from one position to another, such as rising from a chair or stooping. The teaching of proper body mechanics does not involve the development of great muscular strength in any one muscle group; it concentrates on the ability to utilize the muscles that are present, letting the normal use in daily life develop muscular strength according to its needs.

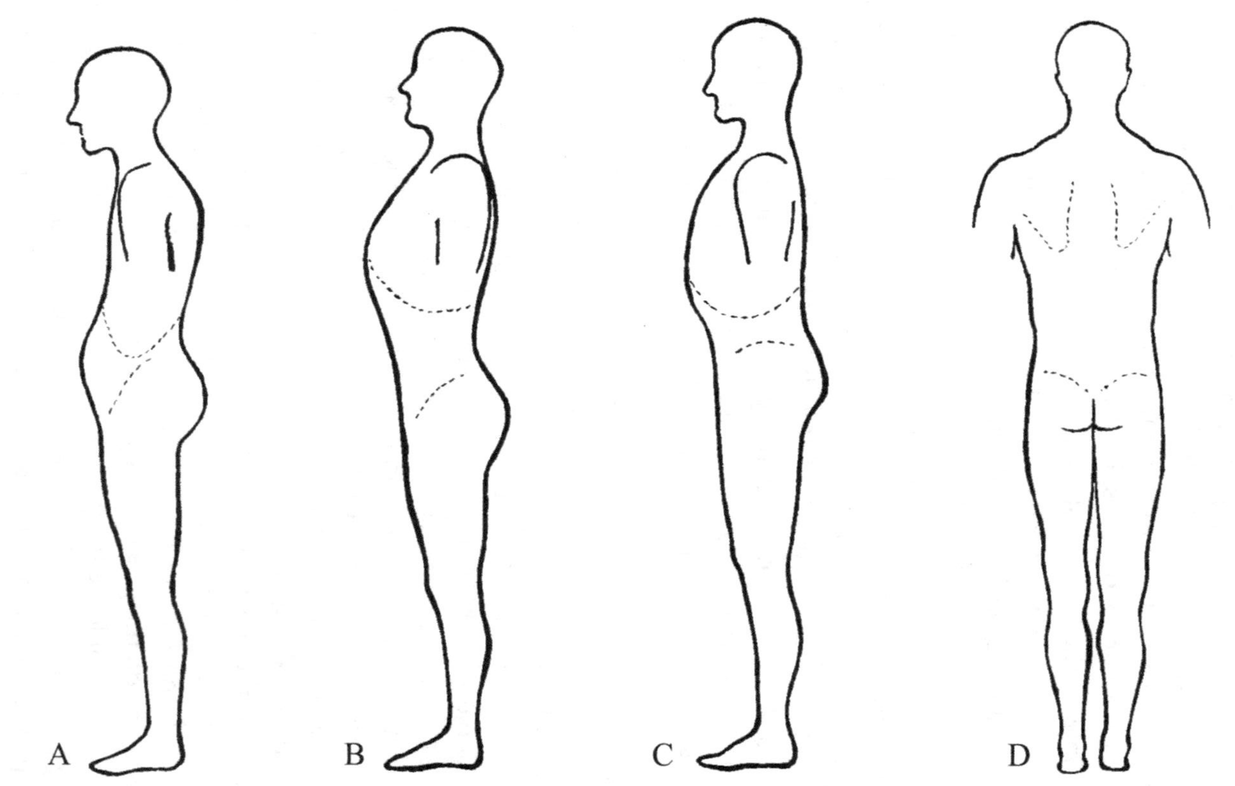

FIG.106. (A) Lateral view showing poor body mechanics and faulty muscular tone. (B) Lateral view of same individual , showing attempted correction. Note the rigidity and the posterior tilting of the thorax. The forward inclination of the pelvis is unchanged. (C) Lateral view of the same individual, showing good body mechanics. (D) Posterior view showing good body mechanics.
The upper dotted line in A, B and C shows the position of the lower ribs. The lower dotted line shows the slant of the iliac crest.

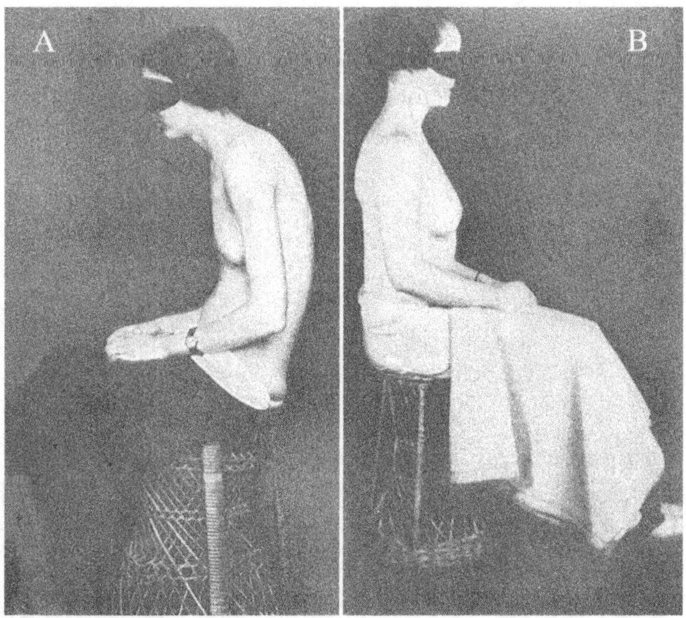

FIG. I07. Incorrect sitting position, A. Compare with diagram, Figure 112. Note the extreme narrowing in the region of the epigastrium. There are many ways of sitting incorrectly, each one being dependent on the anatomic structure of the individual. There is likewise no one way of sitting correctly, B, the correct one being that in which the organs are not crowded, as has been explained in previous chapters.

Balance. The aim of exercises in the development of correct sitting and standing is good balance of the body. Through co-ordination of the pull of opposing groups of muscles, the head is balanced over the torso, and the trunk is balanced over the pelvis. This co-ordinated contraction of gravity and antigravity groups of muscles is tedious at first and difficult to maintain. With practice, it soon becomes habitual and almost effortless, the various portions of the body being held with minimal muscular effort over the center of gravity. Eventually, the patient develops an awareness of the manner in which the body is held, a posture sense. When this is acquired the patient instinctively pulls the body back into good balance because the position of bad body mechanics, or slump, has become uncomfortable.

Incorrect Standing Position. The commonly exaggerated standing position, with the shoulders back and the chest high, and the accompanying hollow back and pronated feet, is not one of good mechanics (Fig. 106 B); continued and abnormal muscular effort are required to maintain it, and so fatigue is induced. This position is as incorrect as the extreme slumped position, which is marked by a prominent abdomen, round shoulders, hollow chest, and a forward inclination of the head and the neck (Fig. 106 A).

In either of these positions the body is out of balance, and muscular and nervous energy are wasted. The degree of faulty posture in either case varies according to the anatomic type and the age and the occupation of the individual, but it always indicates unnecessary fatigue which, sooner or later, will cause untoward results.

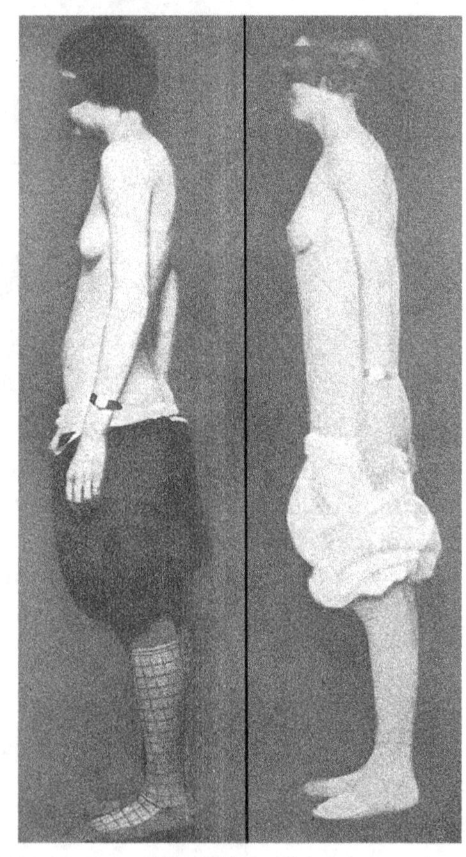

FIG. 108. (Left) Incorrect standing position. Compare with diagram, Figure 106. (Right) The same patient 5 years later. The upper abdomen is not full and rounded. The body still is not balanced efficiently. While this degree of correction is usually enough to relieve the symptoms, it should not be considered as good correction. Further training is necessary.

Trunk Alignment. If the body is to be used properly, the trunk alignment should be correct. This means that the weight must be well forward and on the outer borders of the feet, the lower abdomen pulled in and up, the back flat, the head up and the chin in. The body should be stretched tall, without being rigid; then the shoulders and the chest will fall into their own balanced line (Fig. 106 C).

The old method of throwing out the chest and pulling the shoulders back was faulty in that it disregarded the keynote of practically all posture correction-the ability to use the lower-abdominal muscles. When a person is told to lift his chest and pull his shoulders back, he almost invariably assumes a position of extreme lordosis (Fig. 67 B). He has thus diverged greatly from the correct weight-bearing lines, and when he relaxes, has every prospect of settling back to his original faulty posture. He has not learned how to develop a firm, flat, lower abdomen, which is the foundation of good body mechanics. Therefore, he should be taught a position which not only throws the weight well forward on the feet but also emphasizes the inward and upward contraction of the lower abdominal muscles. To accomplish the latter, he should be taught to get the feeling of pulling the abdomen in so hard that it pushes the head up, with the chin in. This pull should not interfere with normal breathing, for the contraction should be only from the lower attachments of the abdominal muscles. The upper abdomen should be broad, and the rib angle should be wide. If the chest is forcibly raised, as mentioned above, there is a consequent flattening of the abdominal wall which takes place without any actual effort on the part of the abdominal muscles and therefore is of no value because, when the chest relaxes, the abdomen sags to its original position.

In the upright position, as one becomes older, the tendency is for the abdomen to relax and to sag more and more, allowing a ptotic condition of the abdominal and the pelvic organs unless the supporting lower abdominal muscles are taught to contract properly. As the abdomen relaxes, there is a great tendency toward a drooped chest, with a narrowed rib angle, forward shoulders, prominent shoulder blades, a forward position of the head and probably, pronated feet. When the human machine is out of balance, physiologic function cannot be perfect; muscles and ligaments are in an abnormal state of tension and strain. A well-poised body means a machine working perfectly, with the least amount of muscular effort, and therefore better health and strength for daily life.

The Habit of Proper Use. The value of the exercises listed later in this chapter lies, not in the amount of motion or muscular work obtained, but in the way in which the exercises are done; the amount of motion increases with the ability to use the muscles, and the strength of the muscles comes with proper use. Fifteen minutes of intelligent exercise twice a day is of more value than extended periods of hard-driving exercises. It is of value to the patient to attempt to stand tall a number of times during the day, flattening the low back by contracting the abdominal and the gluteal muscles in co-ordination. In this way an awareness is obtained of the way in which the body is carried, sometimes called a posture sense. When the patient acquires this posture sense, he begins to find the slumped position uncomfortable and instinctively brings the body into better mechanical alignment.

Trunk-muscle Groups. The development of the various trunk-muscle groups is of the greatest importance and of real corrective worth. Exercises of the legs and the arms are mainly of circulatory value unless they are particularly indicated for some corrective measure.

The first exercises should be taken in a recumbent position, preferably on a hard surface. This position is most favorable for good mechanical alignment and muscular relaxation and allows the exercises to be performed and controlled easily.

Breathing exercises generally begin the list and may be worked in with others as time goes on. The two most essential points in these exercises are the forward and upward chest elevation and the lateral spread of the mid or lower-rib region. True diaphragmatic breathing should be used always. This means elevating the chest during inhalation, holding it in that position, and exhaling by an inward and upward pull of the lower abdominal muscles. This may allow only a partial exhalation of the amount of air drawn into the lungs. The same conditions hold true of the lower-rib region; here the expansion is lateral, and the rib spread is held during exhalation. Elevating and expanding the chest allows for the greatest possible excursion of the diaphragm.

It will be noted that nothing has been said so far about the correct diaphragmatic breathing; this is not important. A chest that is held habitually in a correct mechanical position and has a relatively small amount of expansion will have, in the ordinary respiration, better diaphragmatic action than one with a large expansion which is held habitually in a poor mechanical position. The drooped chest of faulty body mechanics brings the origin and the insertion of the diaphragm so close together that correct action is difficult.

Abdominal Group. The most important muscles in the teaching of good body mechanics are the abdominal group. It should be noted that these muscles have two separate nerve supplies. The muscles below the umbilicus therefore can be contracted independently of those above it; the patient must be taught to use them properly, that is, from the lower attachment upward. The control of the abdominal muscles and the ability to use them, whether lying, sitting or standing, are the foundation of this work.

A patient should be confined to a number of exercises to be done lying down until he has learned how to employ the abdominal muscles. The aim is to teach good habits for daily use, not hard muscular effort.

The following exercises need no apparatus or machines. They can be done on a table, a firm couch or bed, or the floor.

EXERCISES

Lying on the Back

Exercise 1 (Figs. 109, 110 and 111). Lie flat, with hands at back of neck or on top of head, knees flexed and lumbar spine flat. Breathe deeply, raising chest, but do not allow lower abdomen to bulge or protrude forward, or lumbar spine to lift. Hold chest upward and exhale by drawing lower abdomen inward and upward. Take the next breath with chest still lifted; exhale as before without allowing chest to drop or lower abdomen to bulge. (The amount of breath that passes does not matter; the essential points are the constantly lifted chest, which is pushed higher with each breath, keeping the lumbar spine flat during inspiration, and exhalation by the inward and upward contraction of the lower abdomen).

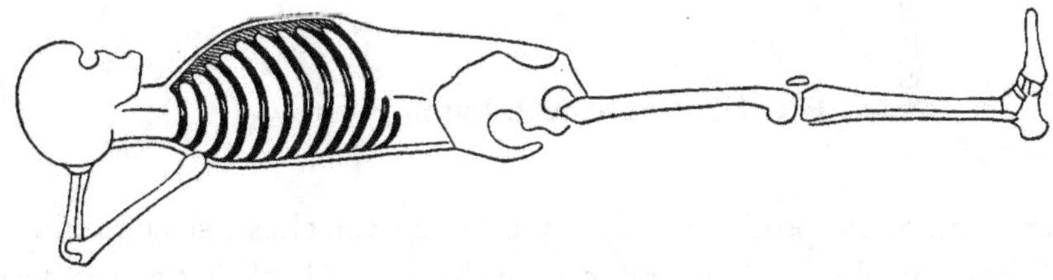

FIG.109 Correct lying position. Chin in; chest up; normal cervical, dorsal, and lumbar curves of spine with normal angles of the ribs and the pelvis.

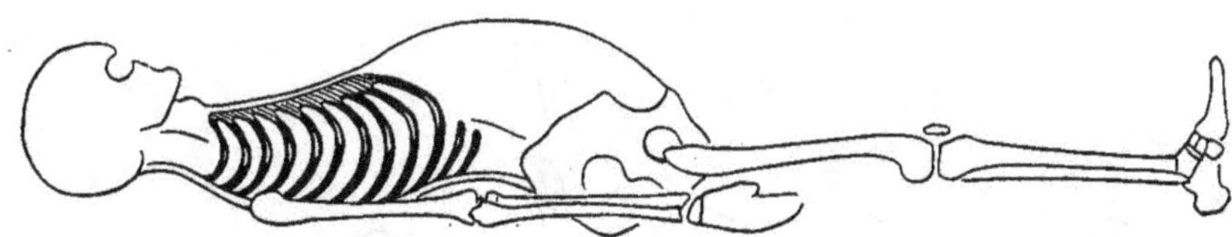

FIG.110. Incorrect lying position. Chin out; chest down, with increased cervical, dorsal and lumbar curves of the spine; ribs lowered; pelvis tipped forward.

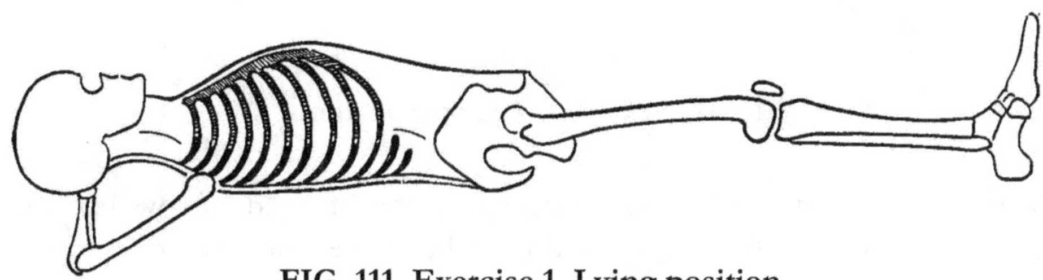

FIG. 111. Exercise 1. Lying position.

Exercise 2 (Fig. 112). Same position, with chin in. Contract lower-abdominal muscles with inward and upward pull; relax and repeat.

Exercise 3. Same position. Contract the lower abdominal muscles with inward and upward pull; relax and repeat. Tighten and lift the buttock muscles slightly and thus flatten the whole back against the floor; relax and repeat. (This is not a breathing exercise, so that the chest must be held up and the chin in when the abdominal muscles are contracted. The muscular effort is entirely in the pelvic region and the low back.)

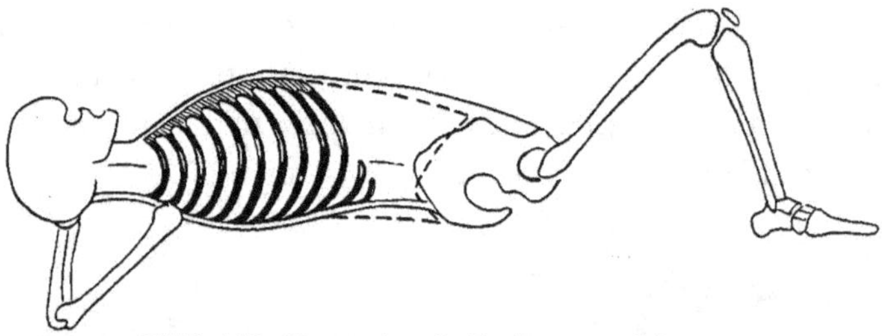

FIG.112. Exercise 2. Lying position.

Exercise 4 (Fig. 113). Same position. Bend one knee over chest, straighten leg and lower it slowly, holding chest up, chin and abdomen in and keeping back flat as leg descends. Repeat with other leg and alternate.

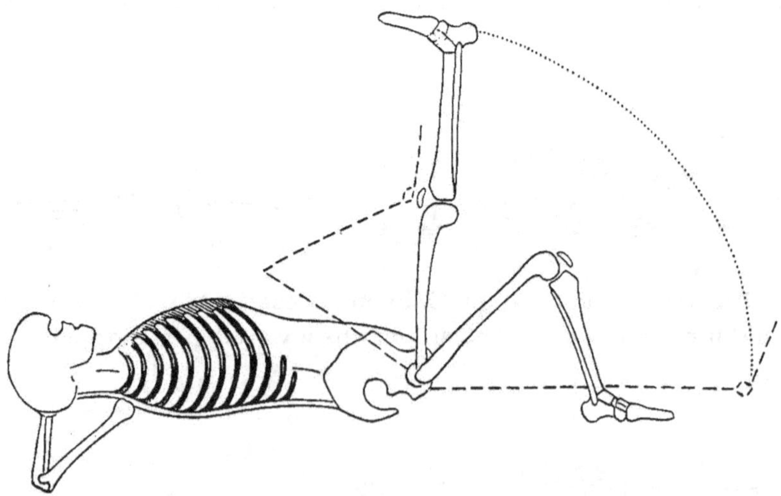

FIG.113. Exercise 4. Lying position.

Exercise 5 (Fig. 114). Lie flat, with hands clasped on top of head, elbows back, chin in and back flat. Stretch one side of the chest but do not bend the spine; see that a lateral upward spread of the ribs is felt; repeat with other side and alternate.

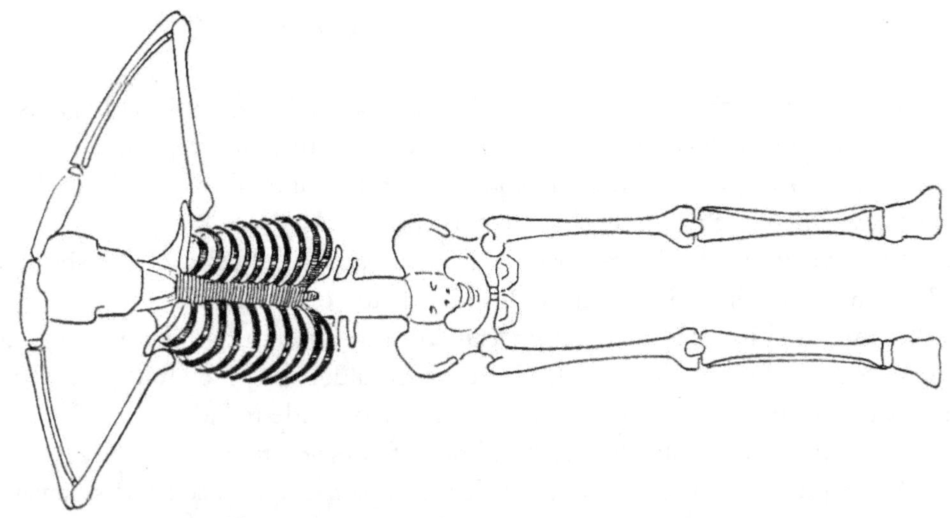

FIG. 114. Exercise 5. Lying position. Chest and ribs lifted while
in lying position. Ribs of one side separated by muscular pull.

Exercise 6 (Fig. 115). Lie flat, with chin in, chest up and back flat. Grasp ribs at costal margins firmly with both hands; breathe deeply, pulling ribs outward, but do not allow lower abdomen to bulge outward. Hold ribs out and exhale by drawing upper abdomen inward and upward. Hold lateral spread of ribs and inhale again, spreading ribs farther, but do not allow lower abdomen to bulge or protrude forward. Relax, but do not allow ribs to drop until 10 breaths have been taken. (The amount of air passing is not important: the lateral spread of the ribs and the increased motion of the diaphragm are the essential points in this exercise.)

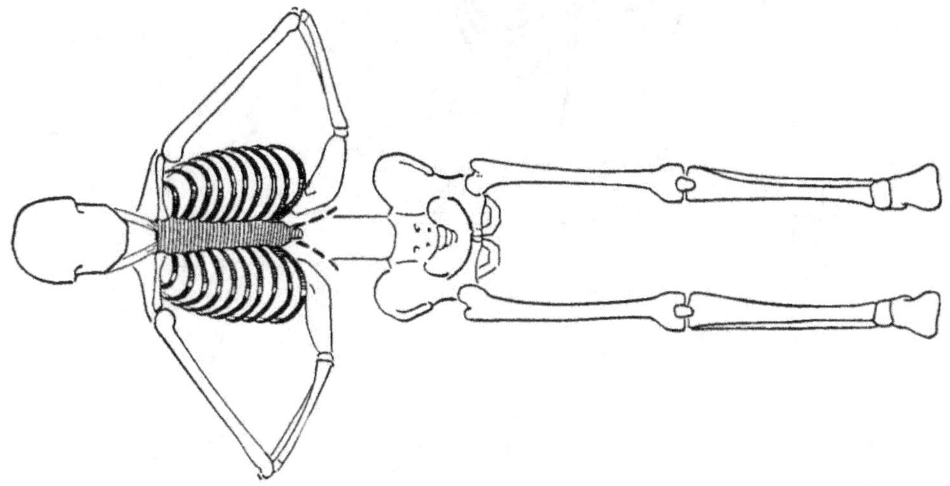

FIG. 115.Exercise 6. Lying position. Ribs and chest lifted
by lying position. Lateral spread of lower ribs at inhalation.

Exercise 1. Lie flat, with chin in, knees flexed, and elbows flexed and held against the ribs. Extend arms out to side at shoulder level, palms upward; return and repeat.

Exercise 2. Same position. Extend arms above head, keeping elbows on body level, palms facing upward, with arms at full extension; return and repeat.

Exercise 3. Same position. Hold arms extended sideways at shoulder level. Let shoulders relax. Let shoulders carry arms in order to allow rhomboids to contract.

Exercise 4. Same position, hands on hips. Pull chin in, stretching back of neck to flatten cervical spine; relax and repeat. Do not lift head or shoulders off the table or the floor.

Exercise 5. Same position. Hold chin in, rotate head from side to side.

Exercise 6. Same position. Hold chin in, bend head from side to side.

Exercise 7. Same position, arms straight at sides, and palms up. Raise arms sideways to back of head, keeping them on body level; stretch whole body upward. Keep chin in. Do not allow abdomen to bulge or protrude forward or lumbar spine to lift.

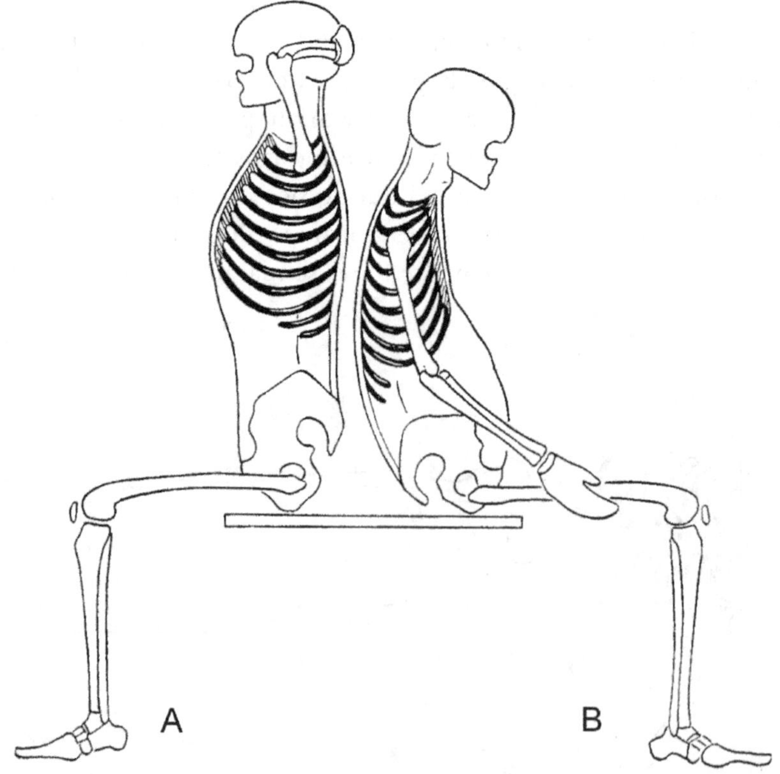

FIG.116. (A) Correct sitting position, chin in, ribs up, back flat, pelvis nearly horizontal. (B) Incorrect sitting position, chin out, ribs down, increased cervical, dorsal and lumbar curves. Pelvis tipped backward.

Exercise 1 (Fig. 116). Sit straight and tall, with abdomen in, back flat, head up, chin in and hands on hips. Breathe deeply, pulling chest upward and forward, but do not allow lower abdomen to bulge or protrude forward; hold chest up and exhale by drawing lower abdomen inward and upward; relax and repeat.

Exercise 2. Same position, hands clasped on top of head, elbows back, chin in, head up, and chest up and forward. Pull lower abdomen inward and upward and keep lower back flat. Repeat.

Exercise 3. Same position. Stretch one side, spreading ribs apart and pulling abdomen in, but do not bend spine laterally; repeat with other side and alternate.

Exercise 4. Same position. Bend upper part of trunk to side; alternate.

Exercise 5. Same position. Rotate upper part of trunk from side to side.

Exercise 6. Same position. Tighten buttock muscles; relax and repeat. Hold rest of body in good line. Stretch tall, with abdomen and chin in and back flat.

Exercise 7. Same position, with hands clasped on top of head, elbows back, head up, chin in and back flat. Breathe deeply, pulling chest upward, but do not allow lower abdomen to bulge or protrude forward; hold chest up and exhale by drawing lower abdomen in; relax and repeat.

Standing

Exercise 1 (Fig. 117). Stand tall against wall, with heels from 4 inches to 6 inches away from it, head, hips and shoulders against wall, and chin in. Stretch tall,
hands on hips. Breathe deeply, pulling chest upward. Hold chest up; exhale by drawing lower abdomen inward. Do not allow back to arch away from wall or lower abdomen to bulge.

Exercise 2. Same position, with abdomen in, back flat, head up, chest up and chin in. Pull lower abdomen inward; relax and repeat.

Exercise 3. Same position. Pull lower abdomen inward and upward; tighten and pull buttocks down to flatten back against wall; relax and repeat. Keep chest up and chin in; do not bend knees. (This is not a breathing exercise.)

Exercise 4. Same position. Hold abdomen in and chest up. Pull chin inward, stretching back of neck; relax and repeat. Do not lift shoulders or let head leave wall.

Exercise 5. Same position. Place hands on top of head and stretch elbows back. Stretch ribs upward; alternate; relax and repeat.

Exercise 6 (Fig. 118). Good standing position away from wall. Stretch tall, with feet apart, head up, chin in, abdomen in, back flat, chest forward, hands on top of head and elbows back. Bend upper part of trunk from side to side. Do not sway at hips or ankle joints.

Exercise 7. Same position. Rotate upper part of trunk from side to side. Do not let hips move.

Exercise 8 (Fig. 119). Same position. Bend one knee to right angles at hip and knee but do not move back; alternate. Keep tall, with head up, chin in, chest forward, abdomen in and back flat.

Exercise 9. Same position, hands on hips, weight well forward, head up, chin in. Stretch tall. Walk on straight line, make forward heel meet backward toe, toe in slightly.

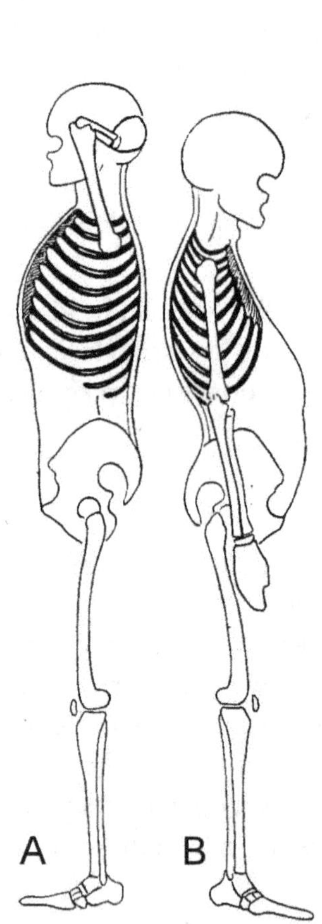

FIG.117(A) Correct standing position. Head up, chin in, ribs up, pelvis nearly horizontal, back almost flat. (B) Incorrect standing position. Chin out, ribs down, increased cervicodorsal and lumbar curves, pelvis tipped forward.

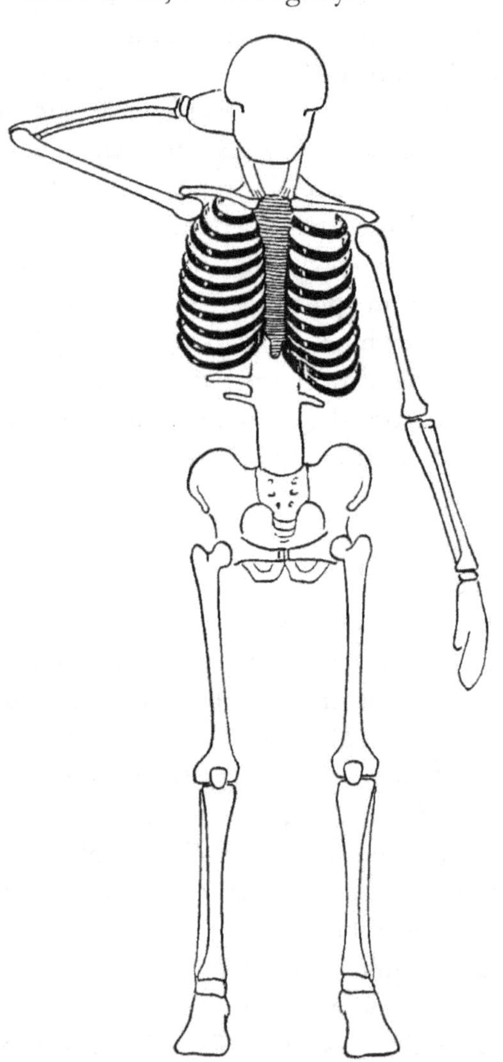

FIG.118. Exercise 6. Standing position. Lateral flexion of dorsal spine. Hips and pelvis fixed. Elbow and head back, chin in.

Exercise 10 (Fig. 120). Same position. Inhale. raising arms forward and upward, rise on toes, stretch tall. Let arms sink to side as heels sink; exhale by drawing lower abdomen in. Keep chest up and forward, and back flat.

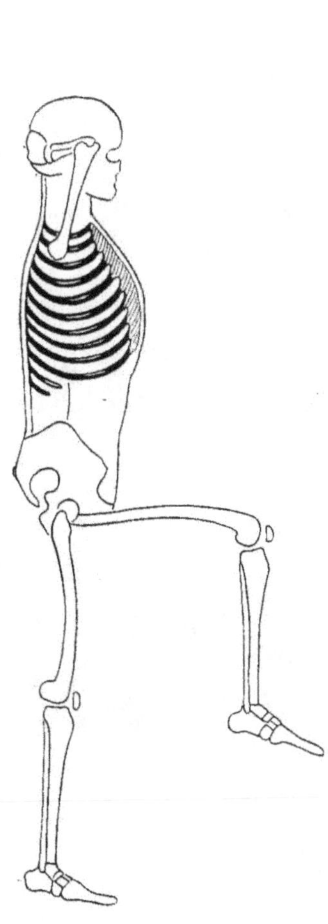

FIG. 119 Exercise 8. Standing position. Flexion of knee and hip. Ribs, chest and head up, back flat.

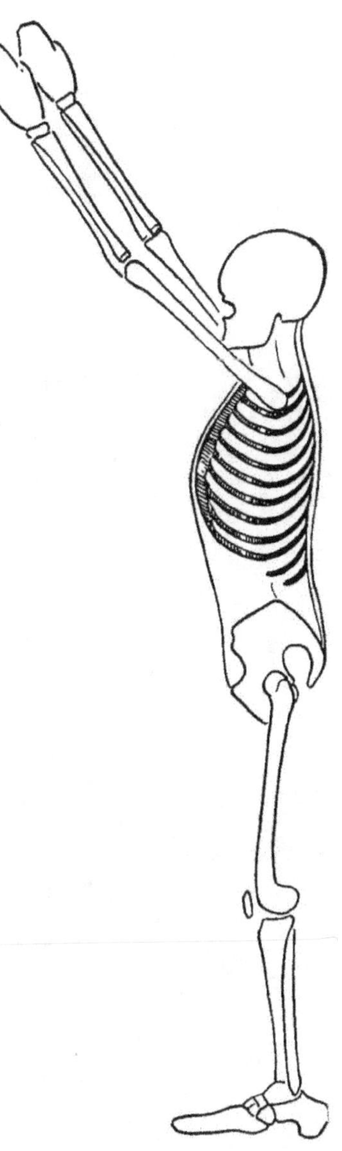

FIG. 120. Exercise 10. Standing position. Forward upward lift of arms, chest and ribs, back flat and head up, weight forward.

12

The Foot and Body Mechanics

INTRODUCTION

The foot plays an important part in the balance and the movement of the entire body. Disabilities of the foot should not be considered apart from the body as a whole. A disalignment or a disturbance in function in the remainder of the body is soon reflected by faults in walking and standing. Frequently, disabilities in the feet—most commonly muscular imbalance and valgus—accompany faulty body mechanics. Disturbances in the function of the foot are reflected by changes in the muscles and the joints above. With severe and prolonged disability in the foot, there may be pain in the muscles of the calf, in the thigh or even in the pelvis or the low back. Treating the foot alone, when it shows disability, usually will lead to only partial correction. Good body mechanics are essential for the proper distribution and carriage of body weight in the foot, for good function of the muscles in walking and for the best circulation of the blood in the extremities. In our experience it has been found to be most practical to train the individual in good body mechanics and then to proceed to special training and exercises for the feet. For this reason disabilities of the foot are taken up after consideration of the mechanics of the body as a whole.

Minor disabilities of the foot often get better by correcting the body mechanics, but the more serious disabilities of the foot require local treatment as well. In this way more effective and lasting relief is secured.

DEVELOPMENT AND ANATOMY

The human foot has passed through many changes in its development from the plantigrade (quadrupedal) to the orthograde (bipedal) type of walking. The changes have been described by Sir Arthur Keith and by Morton. There has been an increase in the number of bones, a gradual increase in the amount of weight borne on the heel, with an elongation of the heel bone (os calcis), a rearrangement of the weight thrust through the tibia, a more compact arrangement of the tarsal bones, a shortening of the metatarsal bones and the phalanges, and an adduction of the great toe to bring it in line with the other toes. Through this complicated process of evolution, which probably is not yet completed, various faults appear not infrequently in the feet and may lead to permanent weakness.

The normal foot consists of 26 bones: 7 tarsal bones, 5 metatarsal bones and 14 phalanges. These bones are held together by ligaments, and their balance and position are maintained by muscular pulls. The normal foot transmits the weight of the body through the os calcis and through the heads of the first and the fifth metatarsal bones. The other bones (with the head on the outer side. The transverse arch extends across the foot between and behind the heads of the first and the fifth metatarsal bones, extending back to the midtarsal bones. The metatarsal heads are all in contact with the weight-bearing surface, when standing, but, when the foot is at rest, are held in the form of a low arch by the transverse ligament and the intrinsic muscles of the foot. The toes are in contact with the floor in standing and walking. They serve a mild prehensile function but do not bear weight except in running or dancing. The flexor muscles of the toes aid in holding up the arches of the foot and in balancing the foot when weight is borne. exception of the heads of the second, the third and the fourth metatarsal bones) rarely transmit weight to the ground. There are two so called arches in the human foot, a longitudinal arch and a transverse arch (Fig. 121). These arch like arrangements of the bones of the foot lessen the jar of impact in walking and add to its resilience. The longitudinal arch extends from the os calcis to the first metatarsal head on the medial side and from the cuboid to the fifth metatarsal head on the outer side. The transverse arch extends across the foot between and behind the heads of the first and the fifth metatarsal bones, extending back to the midtarsal bones. The metatarsal heads are all in contact with the weight-bearing surface, when standing, but, when the foot is at rest, are held in the form of a low arch by the transverse ligament and the intrinsic muscles of the foot. The toes are in contact with the floor in standing and walking. They serve a mild prehensile function but do not bear weight except in running or dancing. The flexor muscles of the toes aid in holding up the arches of the foot and in balancing the foot when weight is borne.

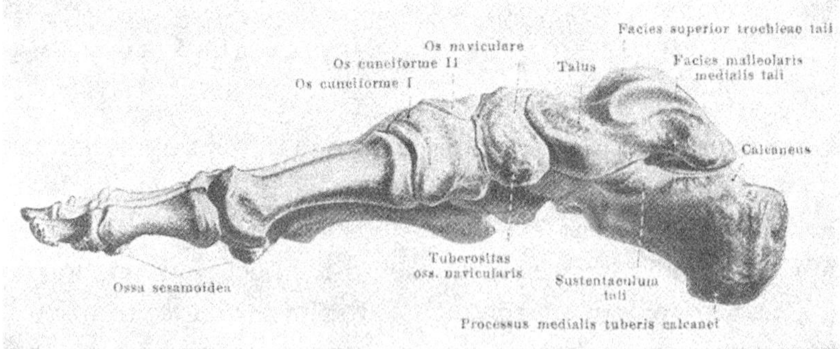

FIG.121. Inner side of the foot, showing the longitudinal and the transverse arches.

The leg is balanced over the astragalus and the os calcis by muscles which can be divided into two main groups (1) the inverters, which turn the foot inward, and (2) the everters, which turn the foot outward. In addition, the there are anterior muscles (dorsiflexors), which lift the foot up, and plantar flexors. These help to a certain extent to maintain balance and a good position for function. The inverters are the tibialis anterior, the tibialis posterior and to a lesser degree, the extensor hallucis longus. The chief everters are the peroneus longus and the peroneus brevis. Normally, the inverters should be a little stronger than the everters. Any weakness in the muscles which allows the ankle to roll inward leads soon to valgus of the foot (Fig. 122).

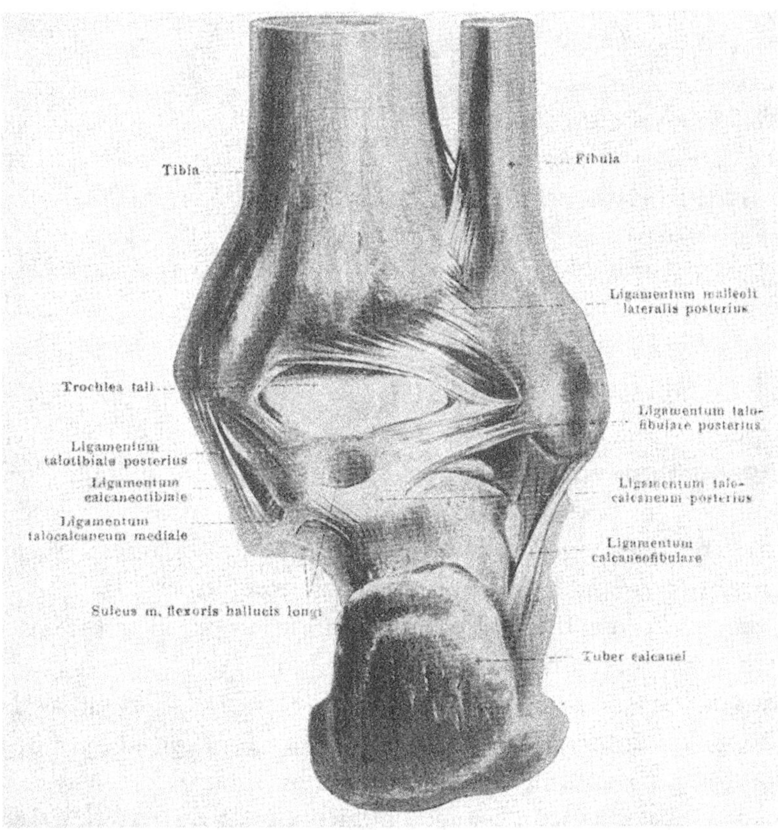

FIG. 122. Ankle joint, showing weight thrust and balance of the tibia upon the talus and the calcaneus.

TYPES OF DISABILITIES

The various kinds of disabilities of the foot can be grouped as follows:

1. Muscular and ligamentous sprains
   A. Acute
      1. Ligamentous tears
      2. Associated with fractures and other trauma
   B. Chronic
      1. Associated with muscular imbalance and deformity of foot
II. Fixed deformities
   A. Congenital
   B. Developmental
III. Infections
   A. In soft parts
   B. In bones and joints
IV. Circulatory disturbances
   A. Arterial
   B. Venous
V. Constitutional diseases affecting the foot

Not all of these conditions will be discussed. Only those that are related directly to body mechanics will be considered.

Muscular and ligamentous sprains may be the result of any acute injury which may involve the bones, the soft parts or both. Chronic sprains are seen more frequently than acute ones. They usually come after prolonged use of the feet in faulty alignment. Such chronic sprains may be found in any part of the foot, but occur most commonly about the longitudinal arch. Less commonly, they are seen in the forepart of the foot associated with spread of the forefoot and lowering of the transverse arch.

Fixed deformities of the foot may be divided into those which are congenital and those which are acquired. The most common congenital ones are Clubfoot and congenital flatfoot. In congenital flatfoot, seen commonly in small children, there is extensive relaxation of the supporting ligaments, with or without changes in the bones of the foot (Fig. 123); a long second metatarsal bone often accompanied by an excessively movable first metatarsal bone is relatively common. This type of deformity usually leads to sprain in the forepart of the foot. Among the acquired deformities, a contracture of the tendo achillis is the most common. While this deformity may be congenital, it is much more frequently acquired. It may result from injury or disease. It may follow the constant wearing of high-heeled shoes.

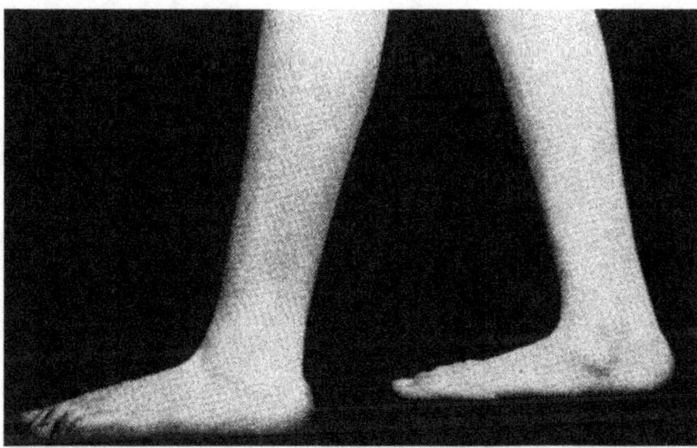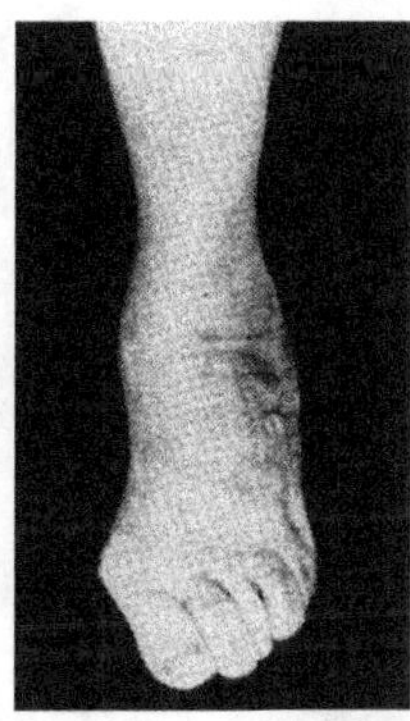

FIG. 123 (Left). Congenital flatfoot. There is ligamentous relaxation, with lowering of the longitudinal and the transverse arches. FIG. 124 (Right). Adult flatfoot, showing valgus, spread of the forefoot, with hallux valgus and hammer-toe deformity.

The next most common deformity is a fixation of the foot in valgus. Often this is associated with spasm in the peroneal muscles and sometimes is accompanied by arthritis in the intertarsal joints. In the forepart of the foot a turning outward of the great toe, usually called hallux valgus (Fig. 124), follows depression of the anterior arch and widening of the forepart of the foot. This is followed usually by a bursa or a bunion and by bony overgrowth about the first metatarsophalangeal joint. Hammer-toe deformity, an extension at the metatarsophalangeal joint, and a flexion of the proximal interphalangeal joint may be present also (Figs. 125 and 126).

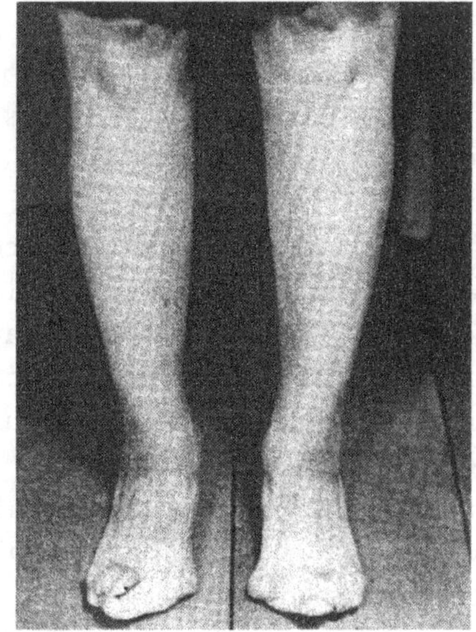

FIG. 125. Severe deformities of the feet associated with poor body mechanics. There is limitation of motion in the ankle. The foot is held in valgus. The fore foot has spread, with hallux valgus and hammer-toe deformity.

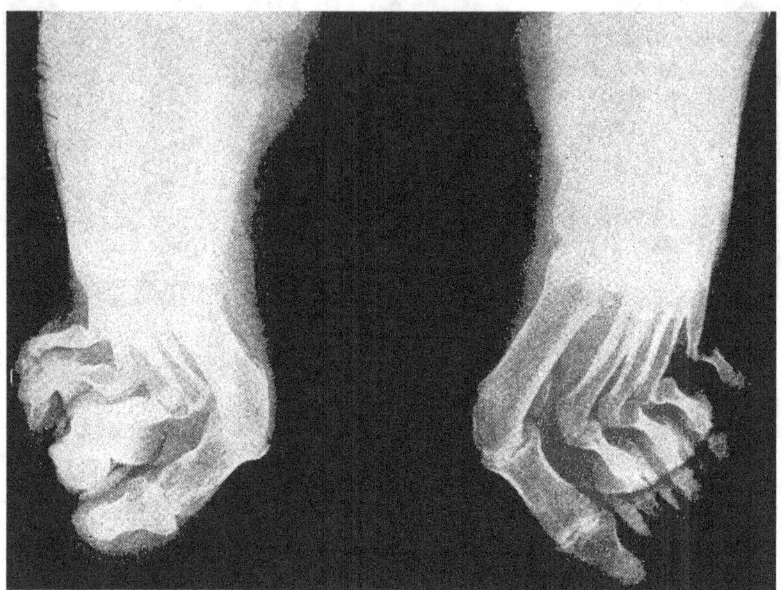

FIG. 126. Roentgenogram of the feet in Figure 125. There is subluxation of the proximal phalanges on the metatarsal bones. There are arthritic changes about the toe joints.

Infections about the foot are not related primarily to faulty body mechanics but frequently are the cause of much disability. Infections may involve the bones, the joints and the soft parts. Infection of the soft parts, a cellulitis, may follow a wound and not infrequently is seen after a blister on the foot or subsequent to "athlete's foot" infection. "Athlete's foot" infection, a fungus infection of the skin, is very common and at times can produce severe disability. **Circulatory disturbances** in the foot may be local in character or may be associated with a constitutional disease. Intermittent interference with the circulation follows the wearing of constricting clothing, such as circular garters. It may be observed as a general congestion of the lower extremities when faulty body mechanics is present. Spasm of the blood vessels may result from an excessive response to heat and cold or from Raynaud's disease. Constant interference in the circulation to the feet occurs from occlusion of a large vein or from a decrease in the size of the artery.

Constitutional diseases may affect the foot through weakness and in-co-ordination of the supporting muscles, through interference with the circulation, through the nerves, through the skin or through involvement of the bones and the joints.

The Normal Foot. The recognition of what is normal function is as important as the understanding of disabilities of the foot in an examination of the body mechanics. A normal foot should have a normal weight-bearing line (Fig. 127). This is a line projected from the anterior superior spine through the patella and over across the foot, with the patient standing. In normal weight-bearing this line should come over the mid-portion of the foot and through the first or the second toe. If the line falls to the inner or the outer side of the foot, the foot is being strained whether symptoms are present or not. There should be no obvious deformity of the foot; the foot should be balanced. There should be no varus or valgus of the foot, and no unusual spread of the forefoot. No corns or calluses should be present. There should be the usual range of motion in the ankle joint, in the posterior tarsal joints and at the toes. There should be no swelling about the ankle or over the dorsum of the foot. The foot should have the same warmth as the lower leg, and pulsation should be felt in the palpable arteries. The skin and the nails should show no abnormality.

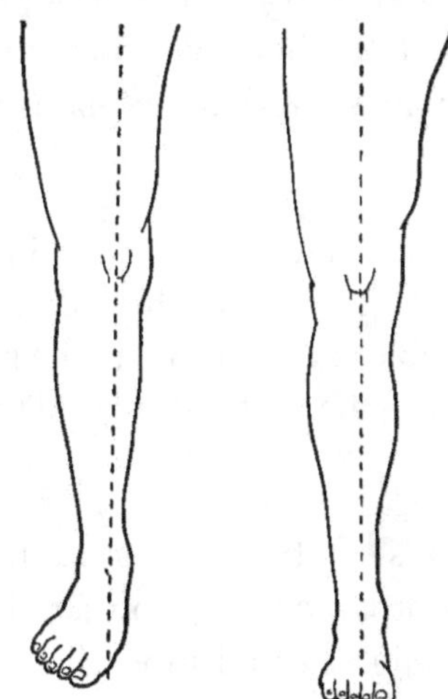

FIG.127. (Left) Poor weight bearing line. (Right) Good weight bearing line.

Tests for Disability. Although it may be symptom-less, the foot is functionally weak when it shows a marked deviation from the normal weight-bearing line. Helpful information can be obtained by observing the tilt of the back of the heel and the Achilles tendon and by seeing how far inward the midportion of the foot projects on weight-bearing. The height of the longitudinal arch is no indication of the strength or the weakness of the foot. It was stated in Chapter 2 that a low-arched foot was found usually in the stocky type of individual, and the narrow, high-arched foot in the slender type. In either type there should be only slight depression of the arch in weight-bearing. The symptoms found with sprain of the longitudinal arch are pain, tenderness on the inner side of the foot, sometimes along the outer side of the foot, swelling about the malleoli and pain in the muscles of the calf of the leg. Sprain in the forepart of the foot gives symptoms of pain under the metatarsal heads and cramp like pains radiating to the ends of the toes. The forefoot becomes wider. In about 10 per cent of the patients the second toe is longer than the first toe, indicating a long second metatarsal bone. Hallux valgus and hammer-toe deformity may be present. There may be calluses under the metatarsal heads. A contracture of the Achilles tendon is shown by an inability to bring the foot beyond a right angle when the knee is fully extended. With a short Achilles tendon there is often pain in the gastrocnemius muscle, or a sense of tightness about the heel. Circulation in the foot is tested commonly by feeling the warmth of the foot in relation to that of the leg. The finding of normal pulsation in the anterior tibial and in the posterior tibial arteries is suggestive of good circulation. If faulty circulation is present, a more exact determination of the type and the degree is obtained by x-ray of the vessels, the measurement of the temperature of the skin and by oscillometer tests.

Deformities Usually Seen with Faulty Body Mechanics. The most common deformity of the foot is found in children with poor posture. This is a pronation of the foot, a depression of the longitudinal arch and valgus of the heel. Various gradations of this deformity are seen in every child with faulty body mechanics. Graham explains the mechanics of such deformities as follows:

Associated with faulty body mechanics there is an increased forward inclination of the pelvis. This shifts the center of gravity forward a little. To support this shift in the weight of the trunk, the femoral columns rotate inward. Rotation is possible at the hip and at the posterior tarsal joints; it is not possible at the knee and ankle joints. Consequently, the foot is displaced inward at the ankle with pronation and valgus of the foot.

During adolescence further changes often are found in the foot. In addition to the pronation there is often a spread of the forefoot which is encouraged by soft, loose fitting shoes and by walking constantly on hard surfaces. High-heeled shoes, if worn for long periods, lead to serious changes in body mechanics and in the alignment of the foot. In the foot a shortening of the tendo achillis develops; there is thickening of the tissues about and above the ankle. Because the weight thrust comes upon the front part of the foot when high heels are worn, there is a tendency to spread the fore-foot. In adult life there is a slow increase of the deformities found in childhood and youth. In addition to pro-nation and valgus, contracture and spasm develop in the peroneal muscles. Arthritic changes (hypertrophic arthritis) begin to appear in the joints of the foot. To a spread of the forefoot is added a turning laterally of the great toe, called hallux valgus, with a bunion forming on the side of the first and of the fifth metatarsophalangeal joints. Hammer-toe deformity, an extension of the proximal phalanx with calluses over the proximal toe joint, is common. Calluses appear under the metatarsal heads. In this way severe deformities develop in the foot (Fig. 125).

TREATMENT

All disabilities of the foot disturb the balance and the movement of the body to a certain extent. But a discussion of the treatment of many of them-e.g., congenital deformities, infections and circulatory disturbances-is beyond the scope of a treatise on body mechanics. In treating disabilities of the foot, one must remember that the foot cannot be treated apart from the body. The interrelationship of the body and the foot in body mechanics has been most clearly described by Graham, who has shown that deformity in the foot rapidly follows the appearance of faulty body mechanics. With faulty body mechanics there is an increase in the anteroposterior curves of the spine and a greater forward inclination of the pelvis. This greater inclination of the pelvis forward causes a shift of the center of gravity more anteriorly. To meet this change in weight thrust, the femoral columns rotate internally as well as anteriorly. This rotation can take place only at the hip joint and the posterior tarsal joints (not at the knee or ankle joints (Fig.28). This internal rotation in the posterior tarsal joints is shown immediately by a faulty weight-bearing line and by pronation or valgus of the foot.

A change in the carriage of body weight is produced also by the constant wearing of high heels. Here, in addition to forward tilting of the pelvis and internal rotation of the leg, the weight of the body is carried for the most part on the front of the foot. This leads to sprain and spreading of the forefoot.

In the treatment of disabilities of the foot four things are usually essential:
1. A good shoe.
2. Training in good body mechanics.
3. Special exercises for proper co-ordination and balance of the foot.
4. Support to the foot until it regains normal function.

Foot disabilities cannot be corrected unless a proper shoe is worn. The best shoe for the foot is usually an oxford, since it gives more support to the longitudinal arch and to the sides of the foot than a pump or a strap fastening shoe. Since we spend more of our walking hours on hard surfaces, the sole of the shoe should be of relatively thick leather and the shank or midportion of the shoe should be fairly rigid. Flexible shoes should be used only on soft, yielding surfaces and with feet which are strong and used correctly. The inner side of the sole should be straight. There should be no sharp pointing at the toes as this cramps the foot and prevents the action of the muscles of the toes. There should be from ½ to 3/4 of an inch between the great toe and the front end of the shoe, since the foot becomes a little longer in weight-bearing. The shoe should fit snugly but should not be tight on the sides when weight is borne. The vertical depth of the shoe over the great toe joint should cause no compression on this joint. The heel should be low and fairly broad. It should not be higher than 1 and1/2 inches in women. For dress, when little or no walking will be done, a less well fitting shoe can be worn for short periods without harm. The counter should fit snugly about the foot just above the heel bone. It should be remembered that a good shoe alone will not correct disabilities of the foot. It simply provides the best environment in which the foot may function.

When there is evidence of acute sprain in the foot, with pain and muscular spasm, rest and heat, with the avoidance of weight-bearing, may be necessary until the acute symptoms subside. In the severe sprains the foot may require immobilization with a plaster cast or adhesive strapping. When the pain and other symptoms subside, exercises are begun, first without weight-bearing, and then exercises with weight-bearing are given. These are continued until the muscular balance and the co-ordination improve sufficiently to permit good function of the foot. The most important thing is to teach the patient how to keep the foot in correct weight-bearing lines when standing or walking.

Sometimes exercises alone are insufficient to secure the return of normal use in the foot. In such instances supports, usually plates or pads worn in the shoe, make it easier for the weakened muscles and ligaments to hold the foot in good balance. A milder form of aid to the weakened foot is a raise from 1/8 to 1/4 of an inch high on the front inner corner of the heel; this is usually called a Thomas heel. When lasting deformities have occurred in the foot it may be necessary for the patient to wear supports for the remainder of his life, in order to keep the feet in a good weight-bearing position. In a certain number of these feet, manipulation of the foot or an operation may secure better alignment and permit the discarding of support. In the milder deformities the wearing of a corrective plaster cast at night often improves the position of the foot.

EXERCISES

The exercises which are given to correct faulty body mechanics help greatly in obtaining better alignment of the legs and the feet. Exercises for the correction of the body mechanics come first and should be continued when special exercises are given for the feet. Special exercises for the feet are given to secure better co-ordination and improved strength in the muscles which support the ankle and the foot, to improve the circulation in the foot, to increase the range of motion in joints and to correct deforming positions in which the foot is used. Frequently these exercises are given at first without weight-bearing, and, as the patient develops facility in these, weight-bearing exercises are given. Many elaborate studies have been made, with motion pictures and with electrical apparatus, to determine the most efficient manner of standing and of walking. The position of the foot in standing and in walking is with the foot pointing directly forward, with the greater amount of weight on the outer side of the foot.
Exercise 1. Sit in a good position. Cross knees. Push foot downward, turn foot inward and then raise foot in dorsiflexion. In this way slowly make a circle with foot. The inward and upward pulls are the essential part of the exercises (Fig. 128).

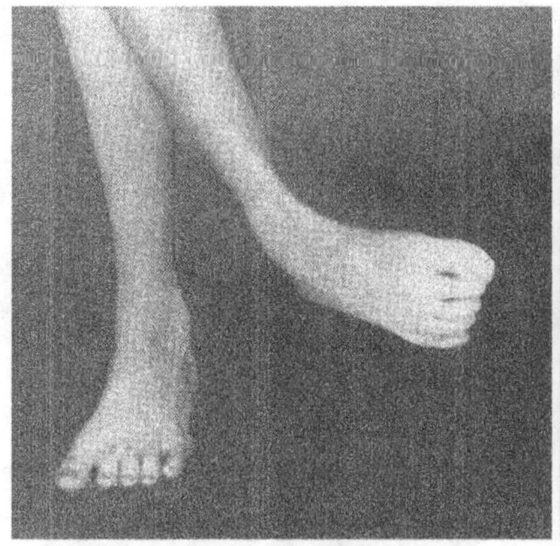 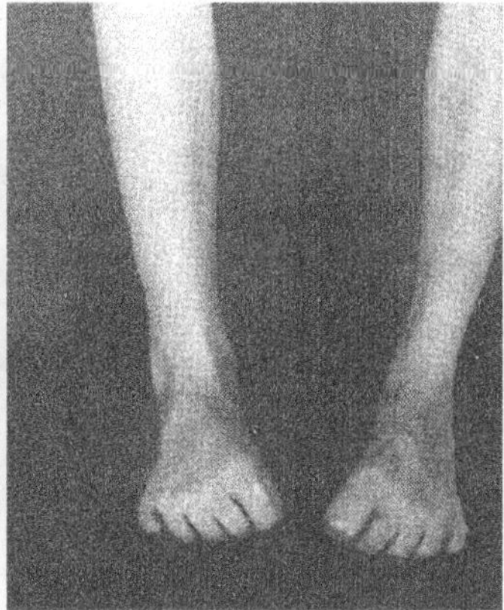

FIG.128 Exercise 1   **FIG.129 Exercise 3**

Exercise 2. Sit in the same position. Turn foot in slightly. Pull foot up and then push down slowly, using ankle joint.

Exercise 3. Sit with feet resting on floor. Curl toes under foot, pulling hard with flexor muscles. Then pull foot upward in dorsiflexion, with toes curled (Fig. 129).

Exercise 4. Sit with feet resting on floor. Curl toes under foot. Then roll foot inward so that soles of feet touch each other.

Exercise 5. Good sitting position. Pick up marbles with foot. Turn foot in varus so that marbles may be taken in hand.

Exercise 6. Good sitting position. Place a towel on floor. Using toes and outer border of foot, draw towel gradually toward you. Do not permit heel to rest on towel.

These are non-weight-bearing exercises. The first four exercises can be performed in the lying, as well as in the sitting position.

Exercise 7. Stand with body in good alignment, weight well forward on toes. Lift inner border of foot, bringing it into varus; relax partially and repeat.

Exercise 8. Good standing position, with hands on hips and weight forward on toes. Walk on a straight line. Bring toe of rear foot against heel of forward foot. Toe in slightly and carry most of weight on outer border of foot (Fig. 130).

Exercise 9. Stand in good position, with back to wall, and with heels 4 inches from wall, hands on hips. Push away from wall with elbows. Walk across room, moving only at hip joints with short, stiff steps. Keep back flat and lower abdomen in. Carry most of weight on outer borders of foot.

Exercise 10. Good standing position. Feet in good alignment and toeing in slightly. Face wall with feet from 2 to 3 feet from wall. With hands placed against wall, sway slowly toward wall. Do not bend at knees and do not raise heels from floor. This exercise stretches a contracted Achilles tendon (Fig. 131).

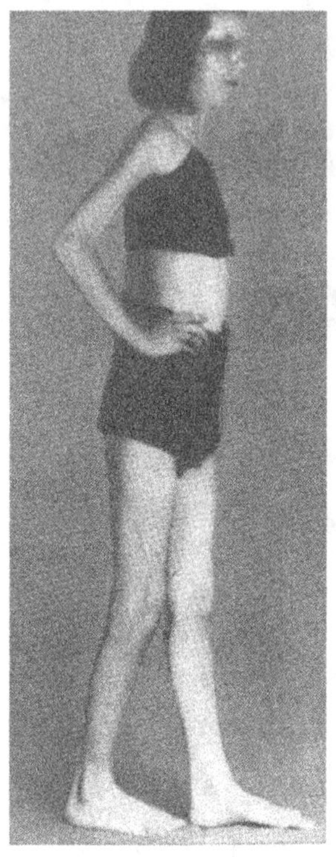

FIG.130. Exercise 8

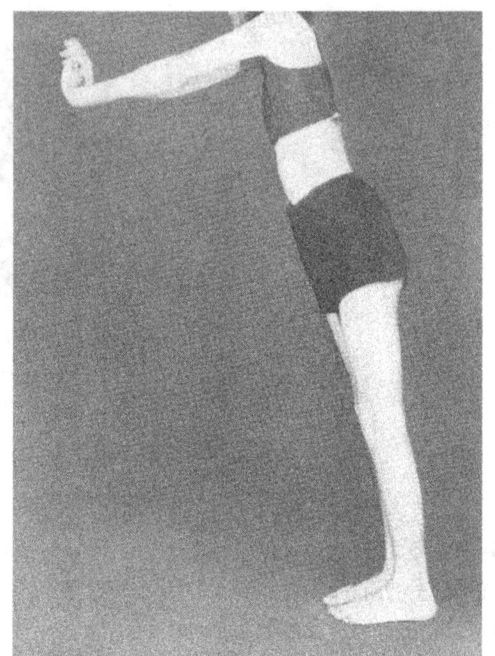

FIG.131. Exercise 10

These exercises can be modified and changed by the instructor to meet special needs or to put the emphasis upon the correction of various minor disabilities. In any changes the position of good body mechanics and proper alignment of the foot should be maintained. The exercises should be carried out from 5 to 10 times each and should be done 2 or 3 times each day. As the foot improves in position and function, the exercises are decreased and finally given up entirely after the patient has learned to use the foot in a normal manner.

SUPPORTS AND OPERATIVE TREATMENT

In childhood, unless there is fixed deformity, the only treatment required in most instances is proper shoes and correction of the faulty body mechanics. If there is much depression of the arches of the foot, a support often is fitted temporarily to hold the arches of the foot in good alignment until the foot can be held in better balance. Sometimes the foot is held rigidly in a valgus position by spasm in the peroneal muscles. Later, arthritic changes and adhesions develop in these feet held in valgus. This rigid valgus deformity is corrected by a manipulation of the foot while the patient is anesthetized. After the valgus is corrected, the foot usually is held in an over corrected position with a plaster cast. This cast is worn for about one week. Then a support is fitted to maintain better alignment of the foot, and exercises are given. Exercises are continued until the foot can be held in a good weight-bearing position by the supporting muscles. In addition, the mechanics of the body are corrected as much as possible. In the presence of severe congenital or acquired deformity of the foot, operations are occasionally necessary to regain satisfactory function in the foot and to permit good mechanical use of the body. Such operative procedures always should be simple, for a stiff foot in good alignment is better than a weak, unstable one. The operations most often required are correction of a hammer toe, correction of a hallux valgus, or an osteotomy, with reshaping of the posterior part of the foot. After operations, supports are used temporarily, and exercises are prescribed both for the feet and for the body mechanics. These are continued until good function and good alignment are obtained.

13

Public Health Aspects of Body Mechanics

It is a far greater achievement to prevent deformity and disease than to correct or to cure them after they have become evident. We believe that the same programs of education and training which have proved to be effective in preventing or minimizing the ravages of disease and improving health and well-being can be used in fostering good body mechanics. It is important for this purpose that physicians and public health officials have an understanding of their principles.

In the preceding chapters the effects of faulty body mechanics have been described, and methods for correction have been given. Treatment is concerned chiefly with the relief of symptoms and the correction of later deformities; but there are larger responsibilities which devolve upon physicians and others responsible for the physical education of the people. These include the prevention and the early correction of faulty body mechanics in order to avoid later ill-health and physical inefficiency.

Estimating Body Mechanics. In the past much confusion has resulted because of different methods for estimating body mechanics. They are many, varying from simple alignment of the body in a vertical line to complicated measurements of anteroposterior curvature of the spine and of displacement of the body masses from the center of gravity. Whatever method is used it should answer this question: How efficient mechanically is the body? There are four criteria that are helpful in determining this:

1. There should be no exaggeration of the antero-posterior curves of the spine. The body should be as tall as possible without strain.
2. The angle of the ribs at the xyphoid should be as near a right angle as possible.
3. The upper abdomen (just below the ribs) should be well developed and larger than the lower abdomen, which should be flat.
4. The natural chest girth at the lower end of the breastbone should be approximately halfway between that at full inspiration and that at full expiration.

Faulty body mechanics is an almost universal finding among children and untrained individuals. The chief reason advanced for this is that Man in the distant past had a plantigrade type of progression. In the evolution of the orthograde manner of walking no neuromuscular reflex mechanism has developed to maintain the upright carriage instinctively. The young of quadrupeds are usually able to stand and walk at birth, but for children from 1 to 2 years are required, since these are complex reflex acts which are learned only through long trial and error. If learning to stand and to walk is not guided properly, the result will be an imperfect one of resistance against the forces of gravity. With proper guidance, efficient use of the body can be learned in infancy.

Conditioned Reflexes. Good body mechanics, then, are not a part of the neuromuscular inheritance of the individual; they are the result of conditioned reflexes. Training in the acquisition of these can be begun at birth; in this way no bad habits and deformities will develop which must be corrected later. It is essential that the mother and the nurse give attention to the position in which the child sits or lies. While this may seem to be a trivial matter, mild deformities and bad habits in the use of supporting muscles are acquired readily. The child should be wholly recumbent until his muscles are strong enough to hold him in a sitting position. It has long been known that deformities can develop from too early assumption of sitting and standing positions. The healthy child, if unhindered, will sit and stand without urging when the musculature is strong enough.

Early Training. The clothing and the cribs and the chairs which the child uses can hinder the development of good body mechanics. Most of the baby's clothing is so made that it provides warmth without interfering with activity. Clothing should not hamper the normal movements of the extremities, nor should there be pressure on the upper abdominal and the thoracic muscles, which play so important a role in the maintenance of the upright position. Cribs should have firm mattresses so that marked sagging of the midportion of the body will be prevented (Fig. 132). The head should not be raised high with pillows, as this will cause increased flexion of the dorsal spine and flattening of the chest. When the child begins to sit up, and high chairs and baby carriages are used, an erect sitting position should be encouraged, with the head up, and with no undue flexion of the spine. A good sitting position can be aided by a small pillow placed to support the dorsolumbar spine.

During the first 6 months the baby is relatively passive and assumes the position of the surfaces on which he is placed. For this reason the child should be placed on a flat firm surface. When the child is held he should be held firmly against the adult's thorax with both hands. Holding the child loosely or with his spine markedly bent can produce a severe sprain in the muscles and the ligaments which can lead to chronic weakness in these structures. When the child begins to sit up for a half-hour or longer at a time, support should be provided both for the feet and the back. Most high-chairs and perambulators are not adjustable, but solid support for the back and for the feet can be provided by the use of firm pillows or books. In this way the child will sit in a good mechanical position. Sprain will be avoided, and the child will not develop faulty habits of balance. It is important during this first year that the child develop strength and co-ordination in the large muscular groups supporting the torso and the hips. Crawling should be encouraged for a long period before the child stands, and he should be permitted to climb on secure apparatus, such as a "jungle jim". If those in charge of the child are not too fearful, and permit the child to use his muscles in crawling, pulling and climbing, the child will have developed sufficient strength and control of his muscles to stand erect without fatigue and sag of his body.

As the child begins to stand, with, and later without, support, he can be taught to hold himself with the head up, the back almost flat, the abdomen retracted and the feet carrying the weight firmly without sagging. At first, assistance may be required, but the child will soon learn to hold his body in this position and use it without sagging. The pattern of carriage and gait which he assumes will in part be an imitation of those of the people around him. This training cannot be pushed but must follow the natural development of the child in strength and size; to succeed, there must also be adequate rest and good nutrition. After illness or during periods of rapid growth additional rest is often required.

Where no training in the proper use of the body has accompanied the early attempts in walking and standing, faulty habits of carriage and postural deformities soon become apparent. Every student of child psychology knows that the preschool age is one of the most important for the acquisition of many habits. The kindergarten and the nursery school have shown what can be accomplished in improving habits of health, in acquiring knowledge and in obeying moral codes. The teaching of good body mechanics is no more difficult. In a few progressive schools such efforts already have been made, with encouraging results. It is during the school years that the first organized effort is made to correct faulty body mechanics, when the child already is overburdened with things to be learned. If this were taught earlier, the task of maintaining correct posture in the school years would be simpler.

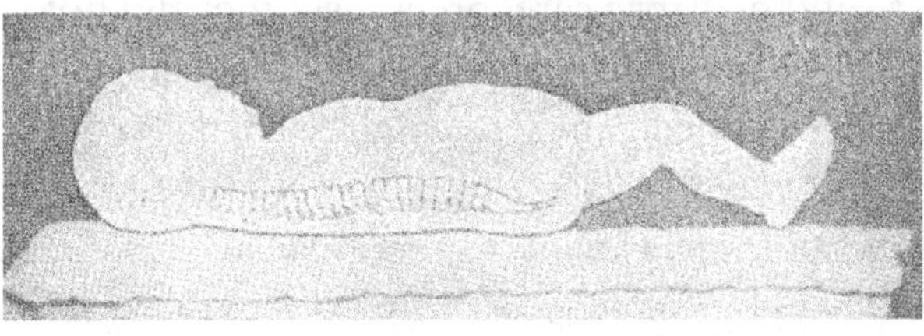

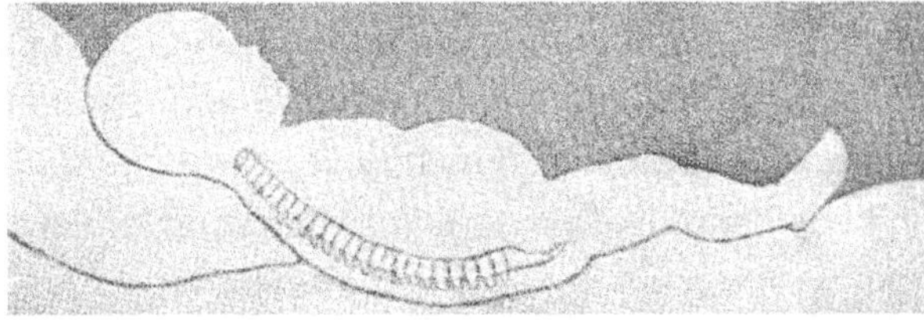

FIG. 132. (Top) Showing the child on a hard mattress, with good body mechanics. Note increased depth of the chest and the lessened prominence of the abdomen. In this position deformities of the chest occur less readily. (Bottom) Child in a soft bed, with pillows under the upper back and the head. Chest is flat, and abdomen is more prominent. Deformities of the shoulder girdle and the thoracic cage occur more readily in this position.

Training in Schools. The present system of correcting bad body mechanics in the schools is as follows: The worst cases are discovered by the school doctors in their periodic examinations of children, and treatment is recommended. It is given most frequently in special clinics or in hospitals. It commonly consists in the teaching of good mechanical use of the body in standing, and in exercises similar to those described in Chapter 10. Where the child's interest is aroused, and the co-operation of the parents is secured, rapid progress is observed. Often after from 3 to 6 months of training only occasional visits to the clinics or the hospitals are necessary. In schools which have competent instructors in physical education this training can be carried out as a part of the school program.

School furniture can be a help to the maintenance of good body mechanics, chiefly through lessening fatigue and preventing incorrect sitting posture. Attempts have been made to adjust school seats and desks to the sitting height of the child. In most school seats a support is provided for the dorsolumbar junction of the spine. Such adjustments are important when we consider that the child spends from 1/3; to 1/2 of his active daily life in the seats. However, no furniture will teach good body mechanics; it simply will make easier the assumption of good positions.

Rest Periods. In every school there are a fair percentage of children of lessened stamina who are absent frequently on account of minor illnesses. Often a medical examination shows no change from the normal except undernutrition and faulty body mechanics. Such children are usually slender and are growing rapidly. Their number has increased during the last few decades through improved hygiene and pediatric care; previously, they did not survive. Their condition, frequently called congenital visceroptosis, offers one of the most serious problems in body mechanics. Much more rest is needed for these children than is required by the ordinary child. They should have several rest periods, lying down, during the day, in addition to a long period in bed at night. In certain schools recumbent rest periods have resulted in marked improvement not only in physical well-being, but in progress in schoolwork as well.

Physical Education. In most schools the program of physical education is not concerned primarily with the acquiring of the ability to use the body correctly in the upright position. In the lower grades physical education is chiefly recreational and often is carried to the point of fatigue. A little later, elaborate drills are given which develop special skill in co-ordinating actions with spoken commands. These should follow, not precede or replace, training in good body mechanics. Much harm can follow too vigorous exercise, particularly in children who have not learned to use their bodies efficiently. The protective contraction of the muscles which holds the spine in balance and guards against the extremes of motion can be exhausted easily. This often results in strains, as well as in an increase in faulty body mechanics.

Recreational activities in the form of organized sports fill a large part of the program of physical education in schools but they fail to meet the needs of the majority of students. Those who are chosen for play and further training are usually those who need it least. They are commonly children who have well-co-ordinated neuro-muscular systems. They have learned, at least in sports, to use their bodies in a fairly efficient manner. This special training of the few with neglect of the great number who need it does not attain the aim of physical education. Nor do they secure later greater physical well-being and lessened physical disability for either the many or the few.

After preliminary training in good body mechanics, sports and recreational activities can be used for the large number of children who never will be athletes. Instruction in standing and running can be given so that it will add to the skill in playing the game while it teaches sound body mechanics. There are countless ways besides set exercises in which efficient use of the body can be learned and eventually made instinctive; unless this becomes habitual, it is valueless. The learning of a fixed position of the body which can be assumed momentarily and then forgotten does not add to the individual's co-ordination, stamina or physical well-being. Good body mechanics are not static, but dynamic-a way of using the whole body well all the time.

Probably much of the failure in teaching body mechanics in the past has been as much the fault of method as of aim. Commonly, the subject has been taught to groups and by group exercises. By such methods, considerable temporary improvement can be secured, as shown by Brown at Harvard and by Cook at Yale; but much of the benefit is lost as soon as instruction and supervision cease, since the students are not taught the application of proper carriage of the body to everyday activities. With continued instruction and with appreciation of the right use of the body all the time and in every activity, lasting improvement and continued good body mechanics can be expected.

Body Mechanics in Industry. In industry, an appreciation of body mechanics makes for efficiency and greater speed in work and less fatigue and strain in the worker. More consideration has been given to this problem in female workers, since the rate of absenteeism is greater in women. Here, studies have been. made of the factors which lead to fatigue and to periodic discomfort and lessened activity. Corporations which employ large numbers of women have found it to be profitable to study these problems. These studies have shown the effects of faulty body mechanics upon inefficient work and upon dysmenorrhea. Much sickness and absenteeism was prevented by correction of the body mechanics.

In both women and men, back sprains and shoulder sprains are common causes of disability. These can be prevented for the most part if the employees are taught how to sit and to stand properly and how to lift. Machines, with their levers, foot pedals and seats can be so placed that the body is not used for long periods in bad alignment.

The majority of young men and women who have left schools in the past have shown little conception of the right use of their bodies. They have gone into various vocations where poor body mechanics have resulted in many disabilities, with economic loss both to themselves and to their employers. The temporary loss of the services of skilled workmen has aroused the interest and the concern of industry and of insurance companies. Industry has found that it pays to foster better body mechanics in employees.

The first attempts in industry were directed to the obvious and tangible aspects of the problem. Physical examinations, with consideration of the body mechanics of the applicants were required, and those with defects or faults were rejected. Attention was a so directed to the seats and the workbenches. Seats were fitted to leg length, and workbenches were adjusted so that undue muscular strain or long-continued work in faulty attitudes was avoided. Even levers that had to be moved frequently or dials that required watching were placed advantageously so that frequent extension or flexion of the spine was avoided. Back rests were so placed that they gave support to the dorsolumbar junction and the lower dorsal region of the spine, the places where fatigue is usually felt. Seats often were tipped forward as much as 10°, and workbenches and desks were inclined as much as 20° to avoid unnecessary strain. The enlightened industries that made these changes found them to be profitable.

More recently, attention has been given to body mechanics in designing automobile seats and in making furniture and machines which are used in the home. The seats of automobiles can be so placed that undue sprain does not come on the neck and the upper back, and the low back is well supported. The brake and the clutch are so placed that the leg is held in slight flexion. In the home, chairs should support the lower back and permit the individual to sit on the gluteal muscles.

These simple measures, with their resulting lessened fatigue and strain from the assumption of better mechanical positions, naturally led to other methods of improving the physical efficiency of workmen. In certain industries employing large numbers of women, the teaching of good body mechanics has been found to be a helpful measure in lessening disability, particularly at the time of the catamenia. It has also lessened minor injuries, such as strains. In certain work requiring frequent stooping, an increased output has resulted from the giving of short rest periods during the day.

In the Army one has probably the best example of a concerted attempt to develop good body mechanics. The physical demands that are made in long marches, in maneuvers and in carrying heavy equipment have made it necessary to train the men to the greatest physical efficiency. In World War I it was shown by the number of rejections and by the necessity of prolonged training of a number of men after acceptance that good body mechanics had not been learned by the great mass of the population. In Massachusetts alone, 46 per cent of those called in the first selective draft were rejected, yet most of these men showed very little organic disease in their bodies. In the rest of the nation 33 per cent of the men examined were eliminated, the majority for minor physical defects. In France a number of the men who were sent first were found to be unfit for combat. Disabilities of the feet and the back were extremely common, and there was no stamina for continued effort. In special training battalions most of these men were able to do the work assigned to them after their body mechanics had been improved.

Prenatal and Postpartal Care. Symptoms and functional disturbances resulting from impairment of the body mechanics during or subsequent to pregnancy are common. The changes in the body during pregnancy often alter the alignment of the body. The upward extension and gradual enlargement of the uterus causes displacement of the small intestine, the transverse colon, and occasionally of the liver and the kidneys. The abdominal muscles become stretched. The diaphragm assumes a higher position, particularly during the last trimester of pregnancy. There is forward protrusion of the abdomen, with increased downward inclination of the pelvis. There is sprain upon the sacro-iliac joints. To balance the body in standing, the low back is held in greater extension. There is compensatory kyphosis of the dorsal spine, often with the head and the neck held forward.

In the latter part of pregnancy there is relaxation of the sacro-iliac joints and of the symphysis pubis leaves the pelvic joints much more vulnerable to sprains.

In addition to the changes in the spine and the pelvis, there may be pressure from the enlarged uterus upon the iliac veins which leads to interference with the return flow of blood. This may produce dilatation and varicosities in the superficial veins of the leg.

If the feet have been normal before pregnancy, and if normal footwear is worn, little disability of the feet should occur. However, foot disabilities are very common during pregnancy and occur from three main causes: an increase in weight, the forward inclination of the pelvis, with accompanying pronation of the feet and the faulty footwear that is worn. These usually lead to depression of the longitudinal and the transverse arches, with sprain and swelling about the ankles. During pregnancy many women take less and less exercise, stay indoors and wear loose, non-supporting slippers.

The common disabilities which arise from faulty body mechanics during pregnancy are backache, cramps in the muscles of the legs, varicosities and disabilities of the feet. The most common type of backache is a muscular and ligamentous sprain in the lumbar region. Occasionally sprain occurs in the cervical region and about the shoulder girdle. Sometimes an incapacitating backache occurs in the pelvis from relaxation of the sacro-iliac joints, with relaxation and weakness of the abdominal muscles. Muscular cramps can occur in the thigh or the calf muscles. They arise from overstretching of muscles and fascia and from circulatory interference in the veins from the muscles. Varicosities can develop during pregnancy and may become worse after delivery. They usually get worse with succeeding pregnancies. Foot disabilities can arise during pregnancy but are more commonly an aggravation of pre-existing disabilities.

Much can be done both to prevent and to correct these disabilities. Even if good body mechanics have not been secured before, they can be corrected during the first 6 months of pregnancy. This is done by the use of rest, support to the changing body and exercises. Breathing exercises, abdominal retraction, back flattening and pelvic-tilt exercises should be performed, with the patient lying down, three times a day. They tend to secure better co-ordination of the supporting musculature. During the last 3 months of pregnancy exercises for strengthening the abdominal muscles and exercises for relaxation seem to be most effective.

Since the musculature is stretched and often weakened, supports are usually necessary to hold better alignment at first, sometimes throughout the pregnancy. The best support to maintain better alignment is a firm corset that laces in the back. This is fitted to lift up the abdomen and to decrease the lumbar lordosis. As the uterus enlarges, eyes and laces are fitted to the side of the corset and are adjusted as necessary. In patients with very heavy breasts special brassieres with wide supporting straps fitted close to the base of the neck may be necessary. With marked relaxation of the sacro-iliac joints a firm canvas belt is used, buckled tightly around the pelvis.

More rest is required during pregnancy. Rest periods of ½ hour should be taken at least twice a day. At times it is more convenient to take a number of short rest periods throughout the day. This rest should be taken lying on a bed or a couch which does not sag. Only one small pillow or no pillow should be used. If there is backache, it is helpful to place a large cushion or pillow under the knees to flatten the lumbar spine. A folded towel under the lumbar spine in addition, lessens the sprain on the back.

If a little thought is taken, much can be done to avoid stooping and unusual sprains. Household furniture can be arranged to minimize fatigue and sprain. The pregnant woman should sit in a firm chair of usual height with a straight back. Tables should be at the height of the xyphoid bone. Long standing or sitting in one position should be avoided.

After delivery, with fatigue and stretched muscles, body mechanics may become worse. Backache is common, pelvic relaxation is frequent. Varicosities and phlebitis may appear only after delivery, and disabilities of the feet can become troublesome during this period. Usually there are four things related to body mechanics required for normal recovery. These are nutrition, rest periods, temporary support and exercises and activity. Fatigue and malnutrition must be eliminated. Support to the back and the abdomen is indicated if they cannot be held in good alignment. Support to the feet may be required also during the postpartal period. Venous disturbances can be helped by rest, elevation and occasion- ally by an elastic stocking or a pressure bandage. Exercises to improve the body mechanics can be started as soon as the involution of the uterus has occurred. Sometimes exercises are required also for the feet. In this way many disabilities which arise during or after pregnancy can be prevented.

Increase of General Well-being. A great mass of data has accumulated in regard to the value of good body mechanics. That they increase general well-being and that they are vital factors in the prevention of disease there can be no question. In the preceding chapters the physiologic disturbances which result have been explained, such as fatigue, strains, deformity, irritation of joints, and chronic arthritis and a host of disturbances in the thoracic and the abdominal viscera. The earlier in life that good body mechanics are taught, the easier becomes the teaching, and the less the deformity. They can be taught when the child first sits and stands. Whatever the method, the instruction must be continued until efficient use of the body all the time has become habitual.

When the teaching of good body mechanics becomes a more generally recognized public health measure, and when there is greater co-operation by the home and the school, with persistence and unity of aim, we shall see a great improvement in the physical well-being of the next generation. Training for adults is slow, tedious and costly. Industry and adult public health administration should not be required to solve this problem. The solution lies in the proper early training of the musculature which supports the body until this becomes not an occasional pose, but the habitual everyday use of the body at the maximum of efficiency and skill.

14

Geriatrics and Body Mechanics

INTRODUCTION

The number of individuals past 50 years of age in the general population is steadily increasing; today these people make up the major part of medical practice. The younger patients, except for acute infections and injuries, rarely require much medical treatment. As these younger patients become older, many definite disease processes appear which continue throughout life. Here, much disability and deformity can be prevented by training in good mechanics during childhood.

At the beginning of the nineteenth century the mean length of life was 35.5 years. At the beginning of the twentieth century it had risen to 50 years; today it is about 65 years. This increase in the average length of life is due almost entirely to better hygiene and the improved treatment of disease in childhood and early adult life. There has been very little change in the saving of life in individuals past 50. Life expectancy alter 50 has not been altered appreciably. The great increase in chronic disease is due largely to the fact that more people live longer, and chronic disease has a greater opportunity to make its appearance. Most of the diseases which we see in these older individuals fall into that group which we call degenerative diseases.

When we speak of old age it cannot be measured accurately in terms of years. Threescore and ten or even fourscore years of age are not necessarily synonymous with senility, nor do they connote serious chronic disease. While it is usual for various chronic ailments and disabilities to make their appearance with advancing age, this is not necessarily so. Aging is a normal physiologic process, part of the normal cycle of life; it is not, as is commonly believed, a terminal process, a final deterioration preceding death. While we cannot prevent aging, we can prevent or delay much of its accompanying discomfort and disability. The aging of the tissues and the organs of the body is dependent primarily upon these three factors: (1) Heredity, (2) the environment and (3) the internal condition of the body.

CHANGES IN THE AGING BODY

A number of structural changes are invariable accompaniments of aging. One of the most obvious is the change in carriage - the head is forward, with increased curve of the cervical spine, the back is bowed, with stiffness in the spinal and the costal joints; of the abdominal muscles and sagging and protrusion of the abdominal viscera appear; slight flexion of the knees an sagging of the arches of the feet are seen commonly. There is a slow progressive dehydration of the tissues, with a decrease in intracellular fluid. Connective tissue undergoes certain colloidal alterations, and collagen fibers decrease. With these changes, comes a greater tendency for these tissues to tear and to become less elastic. From these changes there is a gradual loss in weight and stature. The skin becomes thinner, and subcutaneous fat disappears. Wrinkles and pigmentation are common. The hair and the teeth tend to be lost. Changes take place in the special senses, so that they become less acute. There is gradual decalcification of the skeleton, but deposition of lime salts and of bone is common in cartilage and about the margins of joints. There is gradual degeneration of articular cartilage. Analogous to the changes externally discernible are changes in the internal organs. There is atrophy of the parenchyma and increase in the interstitial tissues. These lead to diminution in function. This function is frequently normal when the individual is under no physical strain, but a decreased functional capacity in the organ is evident as soon as unusual demands are made upon it. The reserves become gradually less and less. Later, from repeated strain, irreversible changes appear, and we have the clinical picture of chronic disease affecting various organs. Impairment of memory gradually becomes evident, but changes in personality are the result of frank disease or are the reaction of an unwanted and unemployed older individual to the community which makes no provision for him.

GENERAL MANAGEMENT

There is no simple plan to maintain usefulness and to prevent the progression of disease in the aged. Usually medical measures must be directed to improved individual hygiene, improved diet, the regulation of work and exercise, the prevention of lessening of disability, and the making of the environment as pleasant and wholesome as possible. For this, the usual periodic, stereotyped physical examination is wholly inadequate. A medical examination must survey the entire daily life and habits of the older individual. The aim is to preserve the aging person as a useful member of society as long as possible. Usually less food is required, but what is taken should contain adequate protein and vitamins. Treatment of disease in older persons usually comes late, since only disorders which hurt receive prompt attention. The common diseases which affect the older patient and lessen his activities are diseases of the cardiovascular system, various neoplasms, pneumonia and related pulmonary affections, diabetes, disturbances of digestion, chronic arthritis and the degenerative neurologic diseases.

CIRCULATORY DISTURBANCE5

In all of these conditions improvement in body mechanics frequently leads to a decrease in disability. In relation to the cardiovascular system the benefit of training in good body mechanics is discussed in Chapter 6. Treatment in these older individuals must often be less strenuous. Frequent assistive apparatus to help maintain good body mechanics must be worn permanently. By improving the action of the diaphragm, the return circulation is improved, greater vital capacity is maintained and functional capacity of circulatory system is maintained at its maximum efficiency. In older individuals also disturbances in the peripheral circulation are common. Varicose veins are observed frequently. Intermittent claudication and pains in the limbs at night, the result of arteriosclerosis with inadequate blood supply to the muscles of the extremities, make their appearance on exertion. In arteriosclerosis, the vessels to the kidneys, the heart and the brain are ones which most frequently cause serious symptoms. Function in all of these is helped by improvement in body mechanics.

TUMORS

The cause of tumors is unknown. Certain involutionary changes take place in the older people in certain organs and may precede the development of tumors. A number of the tumor formations are amenable to surgical treatment. In others, general measures to keep up the general condition of the individual and to maintain comfort are all that can be accomplished. In addition to the tumors, many functional disturbances which must be differentiated from tumors are found in various organs in older individuals.

GASTRO-INTESTINAL DISTURBANCES

There is usually a decreased secretion of the various digestive juices, particularly hydrochloric acid. The liver functions less well, and poorer drainage from the gall-bladder is seen. Gallstones are very common incidental findings in the aged. Flatulence, distention and faulty bowel elimination are common symptoms. Only when the functional disturbance becomes serious do the usual symptoms referable to various parts of the gastrointestinal system permit of an exact diagnosis. Symptoms referable to the gastro-intestinal system are probably the most common complaints which bring old people to their physicians. Many of these disturbances are helped by support and later by exercises which tend to keep the abdominal wall retracted and the viscera in their normal position.

DIABETES

Diabetes is found in steadily increasing frequency with advance in age. Most diabetic deaths occur during the seventh decade. In the older age group the development of diabetes is usually insidious, and a long time may pass before diagnosis is made Also, there usually are complications, and the manifestations of diabetes are frequently obscured by symptoms of other chronic diseases. Often diabetes can be controlled without insulin in the intelligent older person if it is not severe; but dietary regulation of aged individuals is difficult to maintain. Arteriosclerosis of severe grade is frequently present and leads to symptoms in the extremities. Usually, the older the individual when the diabetes was discovered, the more difficult is the management of the patient. In addition to supervision of the diet and the use of insulin to maintain the urine free of sugar, physical activity should be encouraged to the ability of the individual, as this increases the sugar tolerance of the individual. In addition to exercises graded to the patient's capacity, improvement in body mechanics will lead to improved circulation to the pancreas and other abdominal organs (Fig. 133). Where there is not too great damage to the islands of Langerhans, an improvement in the internal secretion of the pancreas may occur. Training in body mechanics also will improve the peripheral circulation when severe arteriosclerosis is present. Not infrequently, it will result in the disappearance of intermittent claudication and it has led often to the more rapid healing of ulcers after infection had been eliminated.

LUNG DISEASES

Chronic disease in the lungs is common in the aged. A certain amount of emphysema is considered to be the usual degenerative process in the lungs. Skeletal changes are probably an important cause. Calcification of the costal cartilages, limitation of motion at the costovertebral joints and degeneration of the intervertebral disks are usually found. Breathing is chiefly abdominal. There is a progressive decrease in respiratory function and in vital capacity. Accompanying this there are frequently cough and dyspnea. Recurring attacks of bronchitis are common. A sequel is often bronchopneumonia. Hernia in some weak part of the abdominal wall may occur.

While no treatment will restore the emphysematous lung to a normal condition, much can be done to arrest the progress of the disease and to relieve symptoms. A number of internists have noticed improvement in symptoms by the wearing of an abdominal belt. Breathing exercises have been stated to bring some symptomatic relief. When these are combined with improvement in body mechanics, often the patient can be kept at his usual vocation without the development of distressing symptoms (Fig. 134).

Tuberculosis. It has been stated that 25 per cent of all persons past the age of 50 have some evidence of tuberculous infection. There is a definite increase in deaths from tuberculosis after the age of 50. In most of these older individuals the infection is relatively quiescent; there is little fever, cough or sputum. Dyspnea and a rapid pulse are the most common symptoms. Overlooking the infection frequently does little harm to the elderly patient but it may result in the spread of the disease to other and younger members in the household. When it is discovered it is important that the patient does not become a menace to others. If proper personal hygiene is learned, often these patients can remain at home. Carefully supervised use of the principles of body mechanics frequently will improve symptoms greatly.

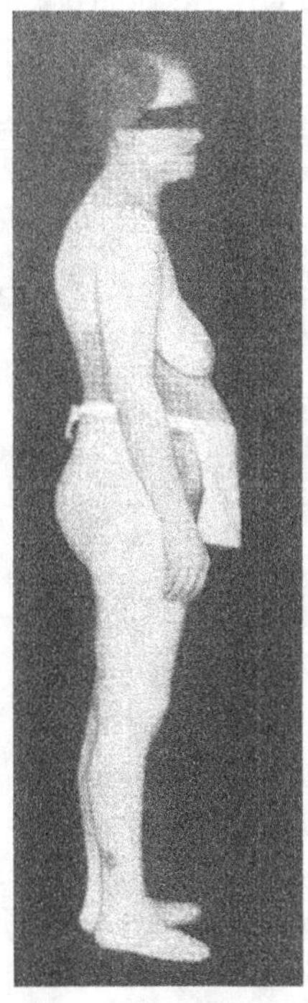

FIG. 133 (Left) Woman of 61 with severe diabetes. The chest is flat, and the upper abdomen has no great depth. The lower abdomen is very prominent.

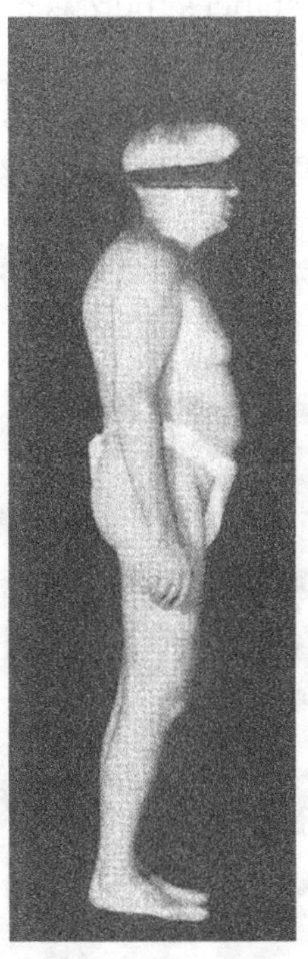

FIG. 134 (Right). Man of 62 with emphysema. There is bowing of the upper-dorsal spine. The chest is relatively fixed, and the abdomen is prominent.

NERVOUS DISEASES

Old age brings with it a slowing of function in the nervous system and evidence of degeneration in nervous tissue. A certain amount of involution takes place in the brain. Degeneration is dependent on a diminution of the circulation and arteriosclerosis. Tremors are common, and reflexes are diminished. One of the most common neurologic disorders in the aged is cerebral hemorrhage which is followed often by hemiplegia, a paralysis of varying degree on one side. This may lead to serious disability if not treated. The limbs should be protected by splints, preferably of plaster-of-paris, to prevent deformity. Later, exercises and correction of body mechanics are instituted to make the damaged limbs and the body work as efficiently as possible.

Paralysis agitans, sometimes called Parkinson's disease is another common disease of later life. It is probably a degenerative process affecting the midbrain and the basal ganglia. It is characterized by a certain amount of muscular rigidity and by tremor. Speech and gait become affected later. In all instances there is a forward progression of the head, with a great increase in curvature in the cervical spine. Medicines are of value in lessening the rigidity and the tremor. Occasionally apparatus is required for the neck, for the back and for the extremities. Lessening of the curvature in the neck and training to secure good body mechanics will prevent deformity in the thorax and will help to control disability in the arms and the legs. Balance and awkwardness improve when the lordosis of the cervical spine is decreased, and the back of the neck becomes relatively flat (Fig. 135).

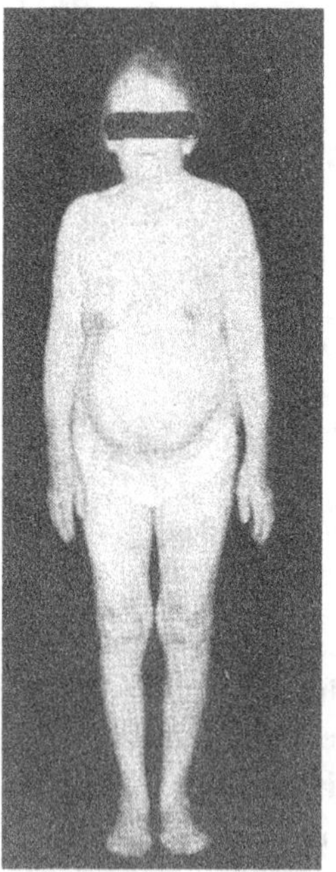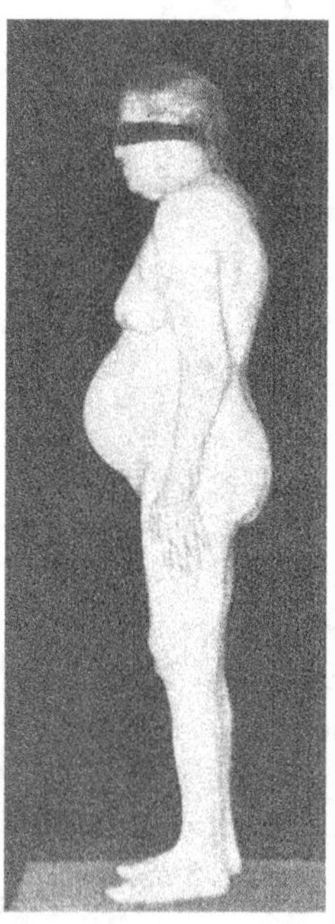

FIG. 135. Woman of 75 with paralysis agitans. The arms are rigid; the head is forward, with increased forward curvature of the cervical spine. There is also a senile kyphosis.

Multiple Sclerosis. The degenerative process in the spinal cord which commonly is called multiple sclerosis, as well as various neuromuscular dystrophies and atrophies, may be found in aging individuals. Here, in addition to general hygienic measures, an appraisal must be made of the patient's physical capabilities. Then, treatment must begin from here to prevent deformity and to improve function. Such treatment is begun most effectively by correction of the faulty body mechanics to as good a state as possible.

MENTAL DISEASE

Various mental deteriorations make their appearance in the aged. Thirty per cent of the patients admitted to institutions for mental disease are over 60 years of age. Senile dementia caused by advancing arteriosclerosis and failing blood supply to the brain is the most common mental disorder. It is slowly progressive. In the early stages much can be done by good hygiene and by improving the cerebral circulation with improvement in body mechanics. In the advanced stage the question of the mental competency of the individual may arise. Here, institutional care may be necessary to prevent the individual from being a hazard to the community. There is no sharp dividing line which permits us to say when the patient no longer can make decisions for himself.

ARTHRITIS

Chronic Arthritis. Among the most common symptoms in the aged are pain and stiffness in the back and the limbs. In most instances these are associated with arthritis, often hypertrophic arthritis, described in Chapter 9. Evidence of this disease is found in almost all persons past the age of 50. The joints which bear the greatest stress in man's upright posture are the ones which show the most evidence of hypertrophic arthritis. These joints are the knee, the hip, the spine and the pelvic joints. More rapid development of symptoms is encouraged by faulty body mechanics. In the spine, the usual locations of symptoms are in the neck and the lumbar spine. Since hypertrophic arthritis produces a decrease in the normal range of motion in the spine, sprains in the low back and the neck are common. In the hip, the name malum coxae senilis has been given to the condition. Thickening about the knees and pain in the knees on walking in elderly individuals are often found. Thickening about the terminal finger joints is found in most older individuals. Soreness in the fingers after prolonged use is common. In this type of arthritis there is little correlation between the symptoms and the changes shown in the roentgenograms.

While cure does not take place in this type of arthritis in older individuals, much can be done to make them more comfortable and less disabled. Dietary regulation, with lessening of obesity, is helpful. Simple medicines to relieve pain, to improve bowel function or to supplement an inadequate dietary intake have their place. But most benefit can be expected from increased rest, support to the inflamed joints, suitable apparatus and improvement in body mechanics. Any improvement will take place slowly in older persons. Support to maintain better alignment of the body usually must be worn for the remainder of the patient's life, but when he becomes accustomed to it he often can carry on with regular work without discomfort. Exercises to correct the body mechanics are given in small amounts. Often sufficient improvement in the alignment of joints occurs, so that symptoms disappear, and local support can be discarded.

Atrophic or rheumatoid arthritis is found quite often in aged individuals. It may be associated with a pre-existing hypertrophic arthritis and with the osteoporosis seen in the aged. Sometimes it is continuation or recurrence of an arthritis that began at a younger age. At times, a differentiation of types of arthritis and bony atrophy is difficult in these older persons. Fortunately, the treatment of all of them does not vary greatly at this age period. Treatment is that described in Chapter 10, but recovery is usually slow in the aged. Every effort should be made to prevent deformity and to maintain bodily vigor. Support to the inflamed joints helps greatly. Improvement in body mechanics is particularly beneficial in lessening sprains, in improving the circulation and in maintaining muscular strength and function.

MYOSITIS (FIBROSITIS)

Muscular soreness, often called myositis or fibrositis, is very common in the aged. Sometimes it represents only the reaction of the muscle to excessive use. At other times it seems to be the result of cold, injury or possibly some intoxication in the muscle. The symptoms are usually acute, with tenderness over the muscle and pain on motion. Treatment usually consists of proper elimination, heat and protection to the inflamed muscles until soreness subsides. Exercises are helpful after soreness abates and hasten convalescence. Improvement in body mechanics often prevents a recurrence of such muscular soreness.

BURSITIS

Bursitis, or a generalized stiffness about the shoulder, is another common disability of the aged. It results in very serious and often prolonged disability. The symptoms may be so severe as to interfere with sleep. Roentgenotherapy and heat to the shoulder are helpful. Manipulation is required sometimes to regain motion. Correction of body mechanics in order to bring the shoulder into a position of carriage which will be more stable hastens convalescence and often prevents recurrence.

SKELETAL DISTURBANCES

Osteoporosis of the Spine. There are a number of other conditions affecting the skeleton, peculiar to the aged, which sometimes result in a great deal of disability and increasing deformity. One that is almost universal is a gradually increasing osteoporosis of the spine. This also affects other parts of the skeleton and is the chief cause of the fractures, the brittle bones of the aged. In the spine, osteoporosis with lack of elasticity of the spinal ligaments and degeneration of the intervertebral disks often lead to a bowing of the spine, a senile kyphos.

This, with its associated disturbances in function in the heart and the lungs, can lead to serious disability. With proper diet and hygiene much of the osteoporosis can be prevented. If good body mechanics has been maintained in adult life, serious kyphos will occur rarely. Even when serious deformity has resulted the use of special positions and exercises to improve body mechanics will relieve the more serious symptoms.

Paget's disease (osteitis deformans) is one of the diseases affecting older people chiefly. There is usually thickening of the shaft of the bone, with bowing of the long bones. If there are symptoms they are usually a sense of pain and weakness, with a dull ache in the affected bone which may become severe at night. Support helps to prevent increase in deformity, and improvement in body mechanics relieves much of the discomfort (Fig. 97).

Fracture of the hip is a relatively common injury in the aged and often follows a mild fall. Healing is often slow, surgery is hazardous, and the end result not infrequently is a non union of the bone. Walking subsequently is painful and difficult. The hip joint then becomes unstable; the gluteal muscles become weak and atrophied. In the younger patient in good physical condition surgical procedures can be carried out sometimes to improve stability and to relieve pain. But in the aged patient, where this represents too great a risk, much can be done to make walking possible and less painful. A firm support about the pelvis relieves some discomfort and increases the stability of the hip. Exercises are given to improve the function of the gluteal muscles and to correct any flexion or adduction deformity. Correction of the body mechanics brings the weight-thrust upon the unstable femur most efficiently and helps greatly in improving the walking (Fig. 136).

Malignant Tumors of the Skeleton. One of the most distressing conditions found in older persons is the spread of malignant tumors to various parts of the skeleton. Here it may lead to severe pain, deformity, and fracture. Some relief of symptoms can be expected from roentgenotherapy . Protection of the involved portion of the skeleton may prevent fracture. Improvement in body mechanics relieves strain and helps in maintaining the best possible function in the involved limb.

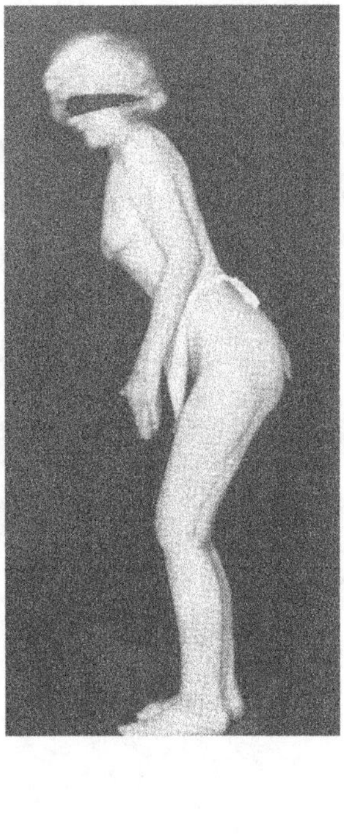

FIG. 136 Woman of 70 with ununited fracture of the left hip. Very faulty body mechanics is present. There is flexion and outward rotation of the left leg.

SUMMARY

The consequences of aging cannot be prevented but they can be delayed and modified. Therapy is chiefly palliative. An attempt is made to secure the best possible function in the aging body. Many of the symptoms resulting from senescence cannot be separated from those resulting from repeated illnesses and injuries. As one gets older repair tends to be slower and less complete. This results in an insidious decrease in functional capacity in various parts of the body. Nature has endowed the body with a tremendous reserve, estimated, for instance, to be over 400 per cent in the kidney, but with age this reserve is gradually broken down. Whatever treatment is given should be simple. Prolonged immobilization and rest are often hazardous in the aged. Exercise and physical exertion should be carried out in small amounts at frequent intervals. There should be little change in eating habits. No profound effect should be expected from medicines. The aim should be to maintain the reserves of the body at the maximum possible. When it is possible the cause of the symptoms should be corrected; the physiologic burden on organs and muscles should be reduced as much as possible. Nutrition should be kept as good as possible. In these aims correction of body mechanics should be an important part of the treatment in maintaining the aging body on as efficient a plane as one can.

Publishers Note:

The original text(s) had detailed references to many contemporary research studies, these references are available online at http://www.pranotherapy.com/bodymechanics

Index

Abdomen

cavity, effect of body mechanics, good or faulty, 109

shape, 53-55

organs, effects of pathologic conditions, in diaphragm, 50

pain, case history 118-1217

referred, from faulty body mechanics, 50-51

sag 14,90

upper, organs, effect of faulty body mechanics, 124

viscera, 53-55

arterial system, 55

effects of faulty body mechanics, 55

congestion, 55-57

diseases, 106-128

effects of faulty body mechanics, 53

position of organs and vessels, 106-108

affected by diaphragm, 108

venous system, 55-56

effects of faulty body mechanics, 55

Acetabulum, developmental deformities, 66

ACTH (adrenocorticotropliic hormone), for arthritis, 150

Adhesions, case history. 118

Adrenal cortex, and arthritis 150

Adrenocorticotrophic hormone- (ACTH), for arthritis, 150

Albuminuria, orthostatic, 55

Alignment of body, changes during pregnancy, 215

Anatomy, relation to disease, 13

Anemia, circulatory disturbances in slender body type. 115

Angina pectoris, 91,98,104

Ankle joint, anatomy, 198

developmental deformities, 66

Appendicitis, case history, 118

Arteries, 93

disease, from faulty body mechanics 93

Arteriosclerosis, in aged, 96-97,222

circulation disturbances, 93

treatment, exercises, 97

Arthritis, and adrenal cortex, 150

in aged 226-227

atrophic, 149,151-158,226

with bursitis, subcoracoid, case history, 164-166

case history, 159-162

causes, predisposing, 157-158

in childhood, case history, 162-163

clinical picture, 153-155

with psoriasis, case history, 163

spinal type, 155

treatment, 150,157

chronic, 148-170

causes, 148-149

treatment, 150

hypertrophic, 140,158-161

of spine, hips and knees, with visceroptosis, case history, 166-167

osteo-degenerative. See Arthritis, hypertrophic

proliferative. See Arthritis, atrophic

rheumatoid. See Arthritis, atrophic

Strumpell-Marie, 151,155

villous, of knee joint, 66

Arthrosclerosis, 96-97
"Athlete's foot" 201
Baby, clothing, 211
crawling, 211
cribs and mattresses, 211-212
early training in good body
mechanics, 211-214
high-chairs and perambulators 211
proper holding of child by
adult, 211-212
sitting position, 211
standing, 211
Backache, 68-74
basic mechanics, 68
case histories, 69-74,118-120
after delivery, 217
incidence, 68
in pregnancy, from faulty
body mechanics, 216
slender type of body, 70
symptoms, evaluation of, 69
treatment, 73-74
brace, 73
corset, 73
exercises, 74
operative, 79-82
fusion, 79-82
types, recognition of, 68-69
Beds and mattresses, relation to
good body mechanics, 212
Bladder, congestion, from
faulty body mechanics, 126
Blood pressure, 136
Body mechanics, criteria for
estimation of, 210
definition, 13, 32
general considerations, 32-35
good, from early training, 211-214
as result of conditioned reflexes 211
industry. See Industry, body
mechanics
public health aspects, 210-218
relation to disease, 13
training in schools. See
Schools
Body types. See Types of body
Bones, changes due to faulty
body mechanics, 35-39
diseases, from faulty body
mechanics, 58
Brace (s), 178-181
for back, 179
and abdomen, older men, 228
for backache, 73
corset, 181
jacket of leather or plaster, 181
shoulder strap, elastic, 180-181
spinal, intervertebral disk lesions 82
temporary use, 179-180
Breathing, impairment by obesity, 90-91
Buerger, disease of, circulation
disturbances, 93
Bunion, 200
Bursitis, in aged, 227
Calculi, urinary, with faulty
body mechanics, 126
Calluses, on foot, 202
Cecum, malposition from faulty
body mechanics, 125
slender type of body, 123
stocky type of body, 125
Cerebrum, circulation. 133
congestion, 131
Chest, 46-48
barrel, 90
developmental deformities, 60-62

drooped, 48
flat, 60
with other deformities,
funnel, 61
pigeon, 61
shape, in types of body, 46
See also Thorax
Child, training in good body
mechanics, physical education, 213-214
physical education, group
vs. individual instruction, 213-214
recreational activities, 213
in school, 213
furniture, 213
rest periods, 213
sports, 213
Circulation, control by solar
plexus, 55
disturbances, in aged, 221
in arteriosclerosis, 93
in Buerger's disease, 93
in extremities, 93
in Raynaud's disease, 93
rate, differences in type of
body, 28
return of blood, 85
interference by pressure
from enlarged uterus
during pregnancy, 216
of venous blood, impairment
by obesity, 90-91
Circulatory system, 84-97
Clavicle, developmental deformities, 60
Clubfoot, 199
Coccyx, bowing, 63
Colon, functional disturbances
from faulty body mechanics, 125
Compound E (cortisone), for

arthritis, 150
Constipation, 69
from faulty body mechanics, 57
Convulsions, from circulatory
congestion in cerebrum, 131
Correlation, mechanical, of body,
definition, 33-34,168
Corset, for backache, 73
for support during pregnancy, 218
as treatment brace, 180
Cortisone (Compound E)
for arthritis, 50
Coxa vara 66
Deformities, developmental, 58-67
extremities, lower, 66
upper, 66
head, 58-59
spine, 62-65
thorax, 62
Degeneration, Monckeberg's, 96
Dementia, senile, 226
Diabetes mellitus, in aged, 222-223
woman with gangrene of
foot, case history, 114-115
apparent, in a child, case history, 111-112
Diaphragm, 49-52
drag, 50
effects of body mechanics,
good or faulty, 49-52,84
functions, 50
nerves, effect of drag, 52
position, abnormal, from
faulty body mechanics, 108
with displacement of abdominal organs, 129
effect on abdominal organs, 109
respiratory excursion, 49
suspensory ligament, 18,50,51
Diplopia, with multiple sclerosis,

case history, 144-145

Disks, intervertebral, lesions, 82

herniation, 82

treatment, correction of

faulty body mechanics, 79

laminectomy and removal of disk

substance, 81,82

spinal brace, 79

Duodenum, malposition, from

faulty body mechanics, 107

Dysmenorrhea, from faulty

body mechanics, 126

Emphysema, 223

Epiphysitis, spinal, 62

Exercises as treatment,

abdominal muscles, 188

arm, neck and shoulder, 191

in arteriosclerosis, 96

backache, 74

after delivery, 216

habit of proper use of

muscles, 186

lying on back, 188

planned, 173

position, "face-prone" 175

horizontal, 174

hyperextension, 174

in pregnancy, 216

sitting, 192

standing, 192

trunk-muscle groups, 186

Extremities, circulation disturbances, 92

lower, developmental

deformities, 66

upper, developmental

deformities, 66

Eyestrain, from faulty body mechanics, 29

Face, asymmetry, 58

developmental deformities, 58

Factor-of-safety motion, 33

Femur, head, developmental

deformities, 66

neck, developmental deformities, 66

shaft, developmental deformities, 66

Fibrositis, in aged, 228

Flatfoot, acquired, 200

congenital, 200

Foot, anatomy, 197

'athlete's' 201

body mechanics, 196-203

circulation, disturbances, 201

deformities, 199

bunion, 200

calluses, 202

clubfoot, 199

depressed arches, correction, 207

developmental, 66

with faulty body mechanics, 203

flatfoot, acquired, 200

congenital, 200

hallux valgus, 203,204

operative treatment, 207

hammer toe, 200,204

operative treatment, 207

spread of forepart 200,204

tendo achillis, contracture, 199

development, 196-197

disabilities, during pregnancy, 216

sprains, muscular and ligamentous, 199

treatment, 204

symptoms and signs, 202

tests, 202

treatment, 204

types, 199

effects of constitutional diseases on, 201

exercises for correction of

faulty body mechanics, 205
function, disturbances in, 197
infections, 201
normal, 197,202
supports for depressed arches, 207
Forefoot, eversion, 66
Frame, Goldthwait, 182
Function, differences in body types, 30
Fusion as treatment, backache, 80
Gallbladder, disease, case history, 124
malposition, congestion from, 112
Gangrene, of foot, with diabetes mellitus
in elderly woman, case history, 114-115
Gastro-intestinal disturbances,
in aged, 222
Gastro-intestinal tract, slender
type of body, 28
stocky-type of body, 28
Geriatrics, arthritis, 226
and body mechanics, 220-229
changes in aging body, 220
bursitis, 227
circulatory disturbances, 221
diabetes, 222-223
gastro-intestinal disturbances, 222
general management of aged, 221
life expectancy, 220
lung diseases, 223
mental disease, 226
myositis (fibrositis), 227
nervous system diseases, 224
skeletal disturbances, 227
supports to maintain good
body mechanics, 229
tumors, 222
Glycosurias, from faulty body
mechanics, 110
Goldthwait frame, 182

Hallux valgus, 203,204
operative treatment, 207
Hammer toe, 200,204
operative treatment, 207
Harrison, groove of, 60
Harvard University chart for
grading body mechanics, 28
Head, developmental deformities, 58-59
tilt, 58
twist, 58
Heart, 84-97
change in shape from faulty
body mechanics, 86-87
disease, chronic, 89
displacement, 86
stretching of nerve fibers from, 136
dysfunction from obesity, 90-91
functional disturbances, 90
hypertrophy 88
in intermediate (normal)
type of body, 16
muscles, 88
referred pain, from faulty
body mechanics, 51
slender type of body, 13,18
stocky type of body, 13,18
strain, 88
valvular disease, chronic, 88
vertical or 'droplet, 87
Hemiplegia, after cerebral
hemorrhage in aged, 224
Hemorrhage, cerebral, in aged, 224
repeated, damage to cerebral
tissues from, 131
Hernia, femoral, from faulty
body mechanics, 51
inguinal, from faulty body mechanics 51
Hip joint, arthritis, from developmental

deformities of femur, 66
hypertrophic, with visceroptosis, case history, 166-167
fracture, in aged, 200
Hydronephrosis; from faulty body mechanics, 126
Hypertension, 92
Hypotension, 92
Ilia, crests, relation to sacrum, 38
Illness, chronic, problem of, 12-14
Indigestion, from congestion of abdominal organs, 55
Industry, body mechanics, 214
faulty, inefficiency from, 214
good, for prevention of disabilities, 214
design of products for good body mechanics, 215
equipment, adjustment and design for good body mechanics, 215
physical examinations. 215
problems with women workers, 215
rest periods, 215
Infantile paralysis. 140
Intestine, large, congestion, 55
in intermediate (normal) type of body, 16
slender type of body, 21-23
stocky type of body, 23-24
small, malposition from faulty body mechanics, 123
slender type of body. 18,54,123,126
stocky type of body. 25,28,125
Jacket for treatment, 147
Joints. See individual joints
Kidney congestion, 57
from faulty body mechanics, 126
diseases, effects of faulty body mechanics, 126

Kidneys, floating, case history, 118-120
with faulty posture, 126
in intermediate (normal) type of body, 16
Knee, flexed or hyperextended, 66
joint, arthritis, hypertrophic, with visceroptosis, case history, 166-167
villous, 66
developmental deformities, 66
epiphyses, distortion in growth, 66
knock, 66
Kyphosis, adolescent juvenile, 62
Legs, bowing, 66
Life expectancy, 220
Ligament(s), of foot, sprains, 199
limitation of motion in joint by, 33-35
suspensory, of diaphragm, 50
Liver. malposition, congestion from, 109
Lordosis, cervical, 90
lumbar, 62
effect on sacrum, 36-38
Lungs, diseases, of aged, 223
tuberculosis, 223
in intermediate (normal) type of body, 16
Malnutrition, 116
Menorrhagia, from faulty body mechanics, 126
Menstruation, irregular, from faulty body mechanics, 126
Mental disease, in aged, 226
Metabolism, basal, test, 177
Military service, aspects of body mechanics, good or faulty, 215
Monckeberg, degeneration of, 96
Muscles, atrophy, 141

case history, 147
control, development, 176
disease, from faulty body mechanics, 58
dystrophy, 142
of foot,sprains, 200
functions, 35
heart, 88
of legs, cramps during pregnancy
from faulty body mechanics, 215
re-education as treatment, 181-183
abdominal group, 187
exercises, 188
balance, 184
exercises, lying on back, 188-190
sitting, 192
standing, 192-194
habit of proper use, 186
exercises, 186
requirements, 182
sitting position, 184
standing position, 183
trunk alignment, 185
re-education as treatment
trunk group, 186
exercises, 186
Myositis, in aged, 227
Nerves, phrenic, effects of drag
of diaphragm, 50
Nervous system, diseases, 130-147
of aged, 224-225
hemiplegia, 224
hemorrhage, cerebral, 224
multiple sclerosis, 225
paralysis agitans, 225
circulatory disturbances, 131
from anemia, 131
from congestion, cerebral, 131
from hemorrhages, 131

mechanical irritation, 139
multiple sclerosis, 141,143
with diplopia, case history, 144
with extreme disability,
case history, 143
with slowly increasing
disability from faulty
body mechanics, case history, 146
muscles, atrophy, case history, 147
progressive involvement, 139
response to sensory stimuli, 139
root pains, 139
structural changes in nerve tissue, 130
divisions, 134
infantile paralysis, 140
injuries, 131
mental states, association
with faulty body mechanics, 142
muscles, atrophy, 141
dystrophy, 142
paralysis agitans, 141
vegetative, 134-135
diagrammatic sketch, 138
body mechanics, 134
disturbances by faulty body
mechanics, 134-135
cervical portion, 135
parasympathetic, 135
sympathetic (autonomic), 135-137
disturbances, by faulty
body mechanics, 137
in ganglia, 136
venous drainage impairment
by faulty body mechanics, 132
Obesity, breathing impaired by, 90
cardiac dysfunction from, 90
circulation of venous blood
impaired by, 91

Os calcis, valgus,66
Osteitis deformans, 167
in aged, 228
case history, 169-170
Osteoporosis of spine in aged, 227
Osteotomy for correction of
foot deformities, 208
Paget, disease of, 167
in aged, 228
case history, 169-170
Pancreas, diseases of, from
faulty body mechanics, 110
treatment, 110
pressure on, from faulty body
mechanics, 110
Paralysis agitans, 141,225
Parkinson, disease of. See
Paralysis agitans
Pelvis, developmental deformities, 66
female, slender type of body, 36
stocky type of body, 36
organs, effects, of body mechanics, good or
faulty, 126
of pathologic conditions
of diaphragm, 51
female, congestion, 57
malignancy, 57
functional disturbances from
faulty body mechanics, 126
male, congestion, 57
malignancy, 57
Pericardium, shape, 85
Phlebitis, 94
after delivery, 217
Physical examinations, in
industry, 215
Physiologic processes, slender
type of body, 29

stocky type of body, 29
Plexus (es), solar (celiac), 105,138
control of circulation, 55-56
sympathetic, about aorta and
heart, 136
Poise, imperfect, 116
Posture, types of body, intermediate
(normal), 27
slender, 27
stocky, 27
Pregnancy, gynecologic disability and
weakness after, from faulty
body mechanics, 57
varicosities in legs during
and after ,95
Prostate gland, congestion, 57
from faulty body mechanics, 126
malignancy, 57
Pseudo-angina, 91
Psoriasis, with atrophic arthritis,
case history, 164
Psychological characteristics,
slender type of body, 29
stocky type of body, 29
Psychoses, with faulty body mechanics, 142
Public health aspects of body
mechanics, 210-218
increase of general wellbeing, 217
teaching and training, 217-218
Pylorus, malposition, from
faulty body mechanics, 115-116
Raynaud, disease of, circulation
disturbances, 94
Recovery from disease, relation
to treatment, 12-14
Reflexes, conditioned, good
body mechanics as result of, 212
Rest, during pregnancy, 217

Ribs, 46
floating, 79
joints, 77
costotransverse, 76
costovertebral, 76
range of motion, 77
referred pain, 78
sprains and strains, 78
treatment, 79
mechanical supports, 79
structure, 76
transverse processes, 76
Sacrum, bowing, 63
concave, in lumbar lordosis, 36
flat, 36
position, relation to ilia crests, 37-38
slender type of body, 38
stocky type of body, 39
types, 25
Sag, body, 14
Scapula, developmental deformities, 61
Sciatica, 71,77
Schools, furniture, proper, for
maintenance of good body mechanics, 213
physical education, 213
physical education-
group vs. individual instruction
in body mechanics, 214
recreational activities, 213
rest periods, 213
sports, 214
training in good body mechanics, 213
Sclerosis, multiple, 142,226
with diplopia, case history, 144
with extreme disability,
case history, 143
with slowly increasing disability from faulty
body mechanics, case history, 146

Scoliosis, 64
Shoes, correct type for good
body mechanics, 204
high-heeled, faulty body mechanics
from, 200
pads or plates, for correction
of disabilities of foot, 205
Skeleton, disturbances, in aged, 227
slender type of body, 48
stocky type of body, 48
tumors, malignant, in aged, 222
Spine, 39-46
arthritis, atrophic, 149,151-158
hypertrophic. with visceroptosis.
case history. 166-167
cervical, 44
referred pain from, 74
sprains and strains, 75
curvature, lateral, 62
developmental deformities, 58-67
dorsal, 42
dorsolumbar, 44
epiphysitis, 62
in intermediate (normal) body, 16
lumbosacral, effects of body
mechanics, good or faulty, 40
osteoporosis, in aged, 227
processes, 39
articular, 39
impingement, 62
transverse, 39
scoliosis, 64
slender type of body, 20
spondylolisthesis, 65
sprains, 74-79
stocky type of body, 20,24-26
thoracic, referred pain from, 76
sprains and strains, 74-79

See also Vertebrae
Spleen, displacement, by faulty
body mechanics, 115
Spondylitis, ankylosing, 154-155
Spondylolisthesis, 63
Standards and tests, in body
mechanics, 32-34
Stasis, urinary, from faulty
body mechanics, 126
Sternum, 46-47
developmental deformities, 60
Harrison's groove, 60
slender type of body, 47
stocky type of body, 47
Still, disease of, case history, 162
Stomach, congestion, 57
'cow's horn' (transverse), 116
diseases, from faulty body
mechanics, 115-116
fishhook type, 22,53,115
in intermediate (normal)
type of body, 16
]. See Stomach, fishhook type
slender type of body, 19,23,115
stocky type of body, 24,115
transverse ('cow's horn'), 115
Strumpell-Marie arthritis, 151,155
Supports, for aged, for maintenance
of good, body mechanics, 228
for depressed arches, 206
for foot after operative treatment, 207
in pregnancy, brassiere, corset, 217
Susceptibility to disease,
slender type of body, 30
stocky type of body, 30
Symphysis pubis, slender type
of body, 38
stocky type of body, 38

Teeth, malocclusion, from distortion
of mandible, 59
Tendo achillis, contracture, 203,205
Test, basal metabolism, 177
Thorax, cavity, change in size
from faulty body mechanics, 85-86
effects of body mechanics,
good or faulty, 54
structure, 52
suspensory ligament, 84
developmental deformities, 60
See also Chest
Thrombophlebitis, 94
Treatment, braces. See Braces
co-operation of patient, 172
development of muscle control, 176
of disease, relation to recovery, 12-14
education of patient, 173
exercises. See Exercises
general considerations, 172-178
Goldthwait frame, 181
muscles, re-education, 181
abdominal group, 187
balance, 184
habit of proper use, 186
requirements, 182
sitting position, 184
standing position, 185
trunk, alignment, 185
muscle group, 186
pads, 175-176
plaster-of-paris shell, 175
supports. See Braces and
Supports
work, active, resumption of, 176
See also individual diseases
Tuberculosis, in aged, 223
Tumors, in aged, 222

malignant, in skeleton of aged, 228
Types of body, 16-31
differentiation, 26
intermediate (normal) 16-18
normal. See Types of body,
intermediate
slender, 19-22
comparison with intermediate, 18
synonyms, 18
stocky, 24-26
comparison with slender, 24
synonyms, 18
Ulcer, duodenal, 124
from congestion in abdominal
organs, 56
gastric, case history. 124
from congestion in abdominal
organs 56
Ureter, kinked, from faulty
body mechanics, 126
Valgus of os calcis, 66
Vascular system, 91-97
angina pectoris, 98,104
arteries, 93
disease, from faulty bod)
mechanics, 93
arteriosclerosis, senile. 96
blood pressure, 92
disturbances in circulation in
extremities, 93
hypertension, 92
hypotension, 92
peripheral circulatory disturbances, 93
case history, 93
pseudo-angina, 91
veins. See Veins
Veins, 94
phlebitis, 94

thrombophlebitis, 94
varicose, 95
in aged, 222
after delivery, 95,217
from faulty body mechanics, 127
during pregnancy, 95,217
Vertebrae, cervical, 44
effects of faulty body mechanics, 37
thoracic, 43
wedging, anteroposterior, 62
Viscera, damage by faulty
mechanics, 14
Visceroptosis, case history 121
congenital, 116
case history, 118
from faulty body mechanics 125
Vomiting, cyclic, 116
case history, 116
Women, in industry, special
problems, 215
prenatal care, 215
alignment of body, alteration
during pregnancy, 216
common disabilities from
faulty body mechanics, 216
exercises, 216
foot disabilities, 216
interference with return flow of
blood by pressure of enlarged
uterus, 216
rest, 217
supports, 217
varicose veins of legs, 95,217
postpartal care, 215
Wrist, extension, 33

PIONEERS OF MANUAL THERAPY SERIES

VOLUME 1

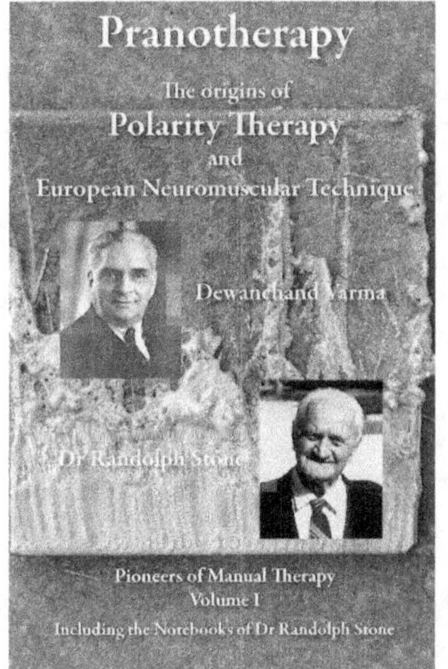

In this volume, which includes a faithful reproduction of Dewanchand Varma's original book on Pranotherapy, the reader can trace one of the early developmental branches of modern manual therapy and learn something of the eccentric life of one its early pioneers in the West. Phil Young has drawn the threads of this development together with the inclusion of the previously unpublished notebooks of another such pioneer, Dr Randolph Stone, a contemporary of Varma who, like Stanley Lief the founder of modern European Neuromuscular Technique, was influenced by Varma's work. Stone was the founder of his own system of manual therapy, which he called Polarity Therapy, and although it is similar to Varma's work, it has maintained to this day more of the original vitalistic, energy approach.
ISBN:78-0-9565803-3-7

VOLUME 11

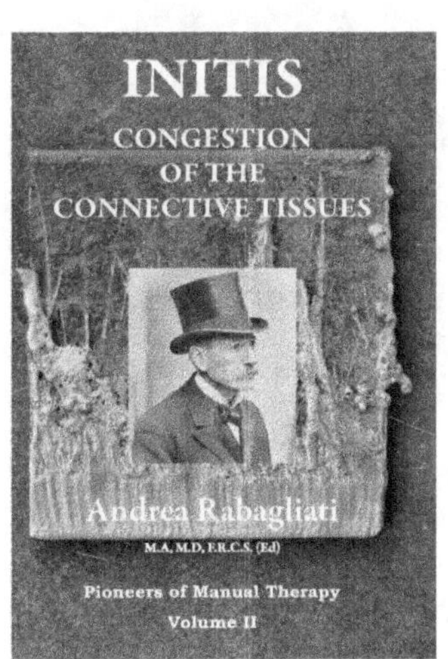

Dr Rabagliati's book "INITIS - Nutrition and Exercises" first published in 1916, is faithfully reproduced with the original photographs of his self-help exercises. The book is a delightful mix of the scientific and the esoteric, containing his unique viewpoints on the body and its ailments. His work is as valuable today as it was at the beginning of the 1900s.
ISBN: 978-0-9565803-4-4

To learn more about Varma, Stone and Rabagliati visit:
http://www.pranotherapy.com

Available at all good bookstores or online

www.ingramcontent.com/pod-product-compliance
Lightning Source LLC
Chambersburg PA
CBHW082247060726
47592CB00021B/2938